The
**Pandemic
Divide**

The Pandemic Divide

HOW COVID INCREASED INEQUALITY IN AMERICA

EDITED BY

**Gwendolyn L. Wright,
Lucas Hubbard, and
William A. Darity Jr.**

DUKE UNIVERSITY PRESS
Durham and London   2022

Typeset in Whitman and Scala Sans Pro
by Westchester Publishing Services.

Cover art: Face mask.
Courtesy dorisj/Getty
Images.

Library of Congress Cataloging-in-Publication Data
Names: Wright, Gwendolyn L., [date] editor. | Hubbard,
Lucas (Freelance writer), editor. | Darity, William A., Jr.,
[date] editor.
Title: The pandemic divide : how COVID increased inequality
in America / edited by Gwendolyn L. Wright, Lucas Hubbard,
William A. Darity Jr.
Description: Durham : Duke University Press, 2022. |
Includes bibliographical references and index.
Identifiers: LCCN 2021970057 (print)
LCCN 2021970058 (ebook)
ISBN 9781478015888 (hardcover)
ISBN 9781478018537 (paperback)
ISBN 9781478023135 (ebook)
Subjects: LCSH: COVID-19 Pandemic, 2020-—Social aspects—
United States. | COVID-19 Pandemic, 2020-—Economic
aspects—United States. | Racism—Health aspects—United
States. | Health and race—United States. | BISAC: MEDICAL /
Public Health | SOCIAL SCIENCE / Sociology / General
Classification: LCC RA644.C67 P364 2022 (print) | LCC
RA644.C67 (ebook) | DDC 362.1962/414—dc23/eng/20220322
LC record available at https:// lccn.loc.gov/2021970057
LC ebook record available at https:// lccn.loc.gov/2021970058

This book is dedicated to the memory of our beloved colleague and friend Dr. Marta Sánchez—a scholar, advocate, and tireless warrior for truth and justice.

Contents

Given that the time frame of analysis contained in this book predates the arrival in America of notable variant strains, including the Delta strain of SARS-CoV-2, we will refer to the initial strain of the disease caused by SARS-CoV-2 as COVID-19 and the era in which it became widespread as the COVID-19 pandemic. Newer (or alternate) strains of SARS-CoV-2 will be identified as such.

Furthermore, given this collection's focus on racial disparities as related to the COVID-19 pandemic, we use a variety of terms to refer to different races and ethnicities. While we recognize each term has strengths and shortcomings, we are inclined primarily to use *black* and *white*—both lowercase—to reflect that race, despite having deleterious and disparate effects, is a construct rather than a biological classification—to denote individuals, families, and communities of those skin tones.

Moreover, when discussing individuals of the Latino community, we will typically employ the term *Latinos* or *Latinx*, a decision that is further explained in the chapter by Sánchez and colleagues. When the term *Hispanic* is used in the data sets that are utilized throughout the book, we use that term in the text for clarity and consistency.

Foreword

MARY T. BASSETT

In 2020, COVID-19 swept the world. By the time 2021 came to an end, the US death toll had surpassed 825,000, a figure that is officially acknowledged as an undercount. The United States continues to experience a disproportionate share of the global COVID-19 burden, a distinction that is especially true when comparing the United States to other wealthy nations. In *The Pandemic Divide: How COVID Increased Inequality in America*, the Samuel DuBois Cook Center on Social Equity at Duke University brings together essays that help us to understand why the pandemic's lethal toll in the United States could and should have been anticipated—despite the fact that the United States can boast many world-renowned scientists and outstanding healthcare institutions, and despite the astonishing speed of development of an effective vaccine.

COVID-19 pulled back the curtain on the extent of racialized inequality in the United States. In this experience lies a lesson: today's dizzying levels of income and wealth inequality and the continued impact of racial hierarchy, driven by the ideology of white supremacy, make these contemporary economic arrangements dangerous for lives and livelihoods. These essays detail the destructive effects of such arrangements, revealing their impact on national well-being. Importantly, the authors make major policy recommendations for change.

There are at least three important messages in this book. First, the policy impact of white supremacy virtually made inevitable an excess *exposure* to COVID-19 among communities of color. Who continued to go to work? Who worked under unsafe conditions? Who lived in crowded, often multigenerational housing? The answers to these key questions are the same, always disproportionately featuring black and brown populations. Second, the *susceptibility* to severe or fatal COVID-19 was enhanced by the already higher rates of many common conditions among communities of color, a pattern itself attributable to bad policies that keep a decent life out of reach. Barriers range from the high cost of housing to a lack of access to healthy food, the difficulties in rapid initiation of personal medical care, the lack of paid sick leave, and the high cost of care.

Third, and most significant, the scholarship collected in this volume by the Samuel DuBois Cook Center on Social Equity builds on decades of scholarship about the racial partitioning of American life: in employment, wealth acquisition, educational attainment, housing, and more. An intriguing chapter describes how black church attendance, a mainstay of community resilience and defiance, might have been more beneficial than the risk posed by in-person worship. A similar calculus also took people of all races/ethnicities to the streets to protest the murder of George Floyd.

Much of this expanding intellectual enterprise has been pioneered by black scholars and other scholars of color. Their work has not received the attention it deserves, and this must change if we are to understand, fully, how COVID-19 has affected our lives. An effective vaccine will not alter the vulnerabilities that this virus revealed. Only concerted policy action will produce the change we need.

Looking back, we recall that the first person in the United States with COVID-19 was diagnosed in January 2020. The first death was reported in February, and almost immediately, in March, local jurisdictions began to report an overrepresentation of African Americans among the dead. Careful inspection reveals another fact: not only have black, Latinx and indigenous people died at higher rates, but they also have died at younger ages.

A preventable death is always a tragedy. The terrible toll among elders carries a high social cost. For example, indigenous communities lost treasured native speakers of their languages. But deaths among younger people leave families without wage earners, leave children without parents. These have consequences for families and communities.

Then came the murder of George Floyd: a man's life casually snuffed out over the allegation of a counterfeit $20 bill as he and bystanders pled for his life. The combination of these phenomena—a pandemic roaring through the country and the graphic display of racial terror—led to a historic display of public outrage at the enduring impact of white supremacy across both the nation and the globe.

This racial reckoning has made the phrase *structural racism* into common parlance. *Structural racism* and its sister concept *systemic racism* are now frequently referenced by leaders in both public and private sectors, in academia, and in philanthropy.

This book details the broad reach of structural racism—how it is embedded in this nation's history, its economy, across its institutions and our culture and beliefs. I hope this volume, among the other work carefully referenced throughout, will move to the center of our national discourse. There is much bad news here, but above all the message is that structural racism is not in our genes. Concerted action, drawing upon the work of these and other scholars, can dismantle it.

Introduction. Six Feet and Miles Apart: Structural Racism in the United States and Racially Disparate Outcomes during the COVID-19 Pandemic

LUCAS HUBBARD, GWENDOLYN L. WRIGHT,
AND WILLIAM A. DARITY JR.

The effects of the COVID-19 pandemic in America have been staggering: at the end of 2021, more than fifty-four million confirmed cases have been reported, with the Centers for Disease Control and Prevention (CDC) estimating that less than one-quarter of all cases have been diagnosed (CDC 2021a). The pandemic has resulted in more US deaths than any military engagement in the country's history. With the US death toll north of 825,000 at the start of 2022, higher than that of any other country, the COVID-19 pandemic is the most fatal in recent US history, having long surpassed the 1918 flu pandemic's toll of 675,000 deaths (CDC 2018). By the time this book arrives on shelves, it seems likely that the number of deaths in America will have surpassed one million people, an unconscionable total.

The importance of any undertaking like *The Pandemic Divide: How COVID Increased Inequality in America*, which attempts to comprehend this terrible disease and its effects, is self-evident. However, the inequities this pandemic has exposed and exacerbated mean that any thorough examination of this period must take the approach pursued here. The investigation must apply a critical lens to the spheres most affected by COVID-19, assessing how these sectors had previously established disparities while examining how these disparities heightened from March 2020 onward. In addition, the study must emphasize that "returning to normal" after the pandemic is woefully insufficient. Moreover, as it is becoming increasingly likely (in early 2022) that this pandemic will never be fully eradicated—that there may never be a prospect of a "return to normal"—the analysis must propose policies and practices that promote equity in both the near and long term, policies that will reduce disparities both in the presence of COVID-19 and in its absence.

The COVID-19 pandemic has become a rich source for research, both because of its extensive impact and because of how it intersects and reflects social disparities in many aspects of American life. It underscores and amplifies inequities in health outcomes experienced by different social groups in the United

States. And it has managed to take such a toll—in terms of mortality, morbidity, financial instability, and general fragility—because of developments across the rest of society.

Foremost of these developments is an economy that, in combination with a ravaged social safety net, has forced wage earners to make the impossible choice between the risk of catching a deadly virus at their workplace and not feeding their families. For example, as of July 2021 in the editors' home state of North Carolina, black persons constituted 22 percent and Latinos constituted 9.5 percent of the state's population, but they amounted to 36 percent and 17 percent of the state's COVID-19 deaths, respectively (Off, Alexander, and Sánchez-Guerra 2021). Black and Latino workers disproportionately held "essential" jobs, often with low pay, that put them at greater risk of contracting the virus. North Carolina's death records indicate that black and Latino workers were 87 percent of food-production workers, 67 percent of food-service workers, 58 percent of construction workers, and 44 percent of healthcare workers who died during the course of the pandemic. Nationally, only 20 percent of black workers and 16 percent of Latino workers had employment where they could work remotely, unlike 30 percent of white workers (Off, Alexander, and Sánchez-Guerra 2021).

The pandemic also has exposed an entrepreneurial environment in which access to public and private capital is dictated largely by race. Nationwide, between February and April 2020, 40 percent of black-owned businesses went out of operation. The shock of the coronavirus predictably had a more devastating effect on black entrepreneurs. Prior to the pandemic, a Federal Reserve Bank of New York study reported that "about 58 percent of black-owned businesses were at risk of financial distress . . . compared with about 27 percent of white-owned businesses" (Washington 2021).

Underlying this black entrepreneurial disadvantage is the enormous racial gulf in wealth. In 2019, the Federal Reserve's 2019 Survey of Consumer Finances revealed that the average black household had a net worth $840,900 less than the average white household, and the average Hispanic household had a net worth $817,900 less than the average white household (Bhutta et al. 2020).

Moreover, a racially tiered educational system and a depleted infrastructure have been highly visible. Predominantly black and Latino students in poorly funded schools, with teachers frequently assigned classes outside of their fields of specialization, were already falling behind. But insufficient home resources (personal computers, dedicated workspaces) for these groups to foster a sound remote-learning environment during the pandemic, not to mention barriers to high-speed internet for both rural and poor Americans, have resulted in their amplified learning losses.

The pandemic also has exploited inequities in living conditions. Not only has mass incarceration dehumanized disproportionately black and brown individuals and destabilized their families, but during the course of the COVID-19 pandemic outbreaks in these institutionalized settings have caused inmate mortality to increase sharply (ACLU West Virginia 2020). Housing shortages—stemming from decades of racially discriminatory actions on the part of banks, sellers, realtors, and the government coupled with hostile whites and their violent protests against neighborhood desegregation—have left black families behind. Bereft of wealth, many black families have been forced into areas without access to adequate healthcare, grocery stores, or green space: vital amenities in a health crisis (Smith et al. 2019). Furthermore, the pandemic has exacerbated racial disparities in homelessness across the country, and an evolving eviction crisis threatens to worsen the disparity (National Law Center on Homelessness and Poverty 2020, 1). Corresponding health consequences have been palpable, with surges in COVID-19 infections occurring in shelters in San Francisco, Boston, Los Angeles, and Dallas (National Law Center on Homelessness and Poverty 2020, 2).

These inequalities, without fail, favor the white population and disadvantage blacks and Latinos. White Americans were less likely to find themselves laid off; they were less likely to find themselves in environments conducive to coronavirus outbreaks—most notably, factories full of essential workers and prisons—and they were more equipped, via access to better technological infrastructure and amenities, to make a seamless transition to remote work and remote education. Conversely, black and brown Americans bore the brunt of the country's response, or lack thereof, to the unfolding crisis.

It didn't have to be this way. In Australia, for example, the government has met the health needs of its long-subjugated indigenous population: giving priority to more at-risk indigenous groups in the vaccination process and granting community health workers the contact-tracing tools of state health authorities (Pannett 2021). By April 2021, these communities were six times less likely than the general population to contract COVID-19.

Australia's action—and success—shows how America chose instead to ignore and sacrifice its most vulnerable and marginalized. These people could have been prioritized and protected during this period of extreme crisis, but they weren't. This book asks, and answers, a simple question: Why did these groups, particularly blacks and Latinos, suffer so much in America during the COVID-19 pandemic?

It is crucial to state clearly what we are not arguing. We are starting with the recognition that race is a social construct, and ethno-racial social groups are neither inherently nor innately different. Moreover, this is not a book that harps on personal responsibility or cultural values as explanations for these disparate outcomes.

Instead, we recognize that, while race and racial differences have no basis in biology, the categorization of individuals by their skin color and their ethnicity has been an essential element in structuring American social hierarchy—dictating which groups are privileged and which groups are denigrated, and which groups are given opportunities to survive and succeed and which groups are treated as expendable. Race matters because it has been made to matter: race is not biogenetic, but it is powerfully politically salient.

Contributors to this volume examine the systems that have failed or, at least, have been disrupted by the COVID-19 pandemic. The chapters here explore how inequities have evolved since March 2020, repeatedly demonstrating how the inequities of the pandemic aggravate prepandemic disparities. Those prior disparities were not caused by an unforeseen outbreak like COVID-19 but were caused, instead, by policy design. By understanding these two processes in tandem—how certain systems developed to marginalize certain groups, and how COVID-19's spread magnified the effects of those systems—we can answer our initial question, and we can begin to answer the logical follow-up: How can we prevent suffering and inequity in the next outbreak?

So, before we look to the future, we must study the past. Specifically, we must examine the progression of the COVID-19 pandemic in America and the creation and structure of the social environments in which it spread to disparate effect.

The Path to Now: The COVID-19 Pandemic

In January 2020, America was on edge. The Democratic presidential primary was lurching toward its first contest in Iowa. A debate on January 14 between the six top candidates featured discussions of a potential war with Iran and an impending impeachment trial against the president. In the transcript of the debate, the words *virus*, *COVID-19*, and related variations are nowhere to be found (*Des Moines Register* 2020). It was, quite simply, a different era.

The national unemployment rate was 3.6 percent, down from 4 percent a year prior; average life expectancy had held steady from 2010 to 2018 at just north of 78.5 years (US Bureau of Labor Statistics 2020a; Woolf, Masters, and Aron 2021). The numbers for both metrics, when broken out by race, were less favorable for black Americans, and things were about to get seismically worse.

The *New York Times* first mentioned COVID-19 ("the new virus, a coronavirus") on January 8, 2020, noting an initial outbreak in Wuhan, China, that had infected dozens of individuals in late December (Wee and McNeil 2020). On January 21, after returning from Wuhan, a Washington resident became the first confirmed case in the United States. By late January, the State Department and the Centers for Disease Control and Prevention (CDC) were recommending that nonessential travel to China be placed on deferral. By the first week of February, global air traffic began undergoing restrictions, and the United States had declared a national public-health emergency.

By the second week of March, the United States—and the rest of the world—was in full-blown panic as the World Health Organization officially recognized the growing global crisis as a pandemic. The stock markets, which had been trending downward on the winds of increasingly ominous news, finally crashed on March 9, with the Dow Jones Industrial Average having its largest-ever single-day fall in points (a drop soon surpassed on March 12 and March 16). The unemployment rate creeped up slightly in March, from 3.5 percent to 4.4 percent, before skyrocketing in April to 14.7 percent, with the black unemployment rate 2.5 percentage points above the white unemployment rate (US Bureau of Labor Statistics 2020b). This development actually represented a momentary reduction in the black-white unemployment disparity, but during the recovery in months to come, the traditional two-to-one ratio—with the black unemployment rate doubling that of whites—would reemerge.

In early April, as New York City was in the midst of its first outbreak, early data suggested that black and Latino people were dying at twice the rate of white people (NYC Health 2020). Myriad explanations were advanced for the disparity. Black workers who retained their jobs were more likely to be working in essential front-line jobs—typically lower-paying positions in service industries—and were thus less able to physically distance or work remotely to protect themselves and their families from COVID-19. They were more likely to live in the poorer neighborhoods where outbreaks were pronounced (more outbreaks occurred in these neighborhoods, in part because residents in richer neighborhoods lived under less crowded conditions and often could decamp from the city to second homes with minimal fuss). They were more likely to be in jobs with fewer benefits, in particular those with fewer paid sick days and less flexible work arrangements. And, given existing income and poverty disparities, they could least afford to stop working.

With unemployment rising nationally, financial stimulus arrived—at least, in theory. The Coronavirus Aid, Relief, and Economic Security (CARES) Act passed on March 27, 2020, the largest economic stimulus package—$2.2 trillion—in US history. Providing billions in one-time cash payments (rather than recurring monthly payments as some had proposed), business relief, extended unemployment benefits, corporate loans, and more, it quickly became clear that it would not level the playing field but heighten the tilt.

While some individuals received their direct deposit checks starting in mid-April, the process—only expedited for those whose bank information (from recent tax filings) had been stored with the Internal Revenue Service—led to delays for many. A Brookings analysis showed that renters, low-income, low-asset, and unbanked individuals were significantly more likely to experience delays in receiving payments. In total, black households were 8 percent more likely to experience this delay, and Latino households were 11 percent more likely (Roll and Grinstein-Weiss 2020). Moreover, as millions found themselves applying for unemployment benefits in spring 2020, black potential recipients were pushed, again, to the back of the line. A study from Howard University researchers found that from April to June, only 13 percent of unemployed black workers received unemployment checks, whereas in the same timeframe, 24 percent of white workers and 22 percent of Hispanic workers received checks. This disparity was partially a function of (disproportionately black) southern states being slow to expand these benefits (Menton 2020).

Similar patterns appeared in the business world. With the CARES Act came the formation of the federal Paycheck Protection Program (or PPP), which allowed businesses to apply for low-interest loans to continue paying their employees and meet other business costs. Despite its sizable sticker price ($953 billion), the PPP failed to deliver funds equitably or deliver funds to many who needed it.

Census tract-level analyses revealed that in many metro areas, majority-white tracts received loans at substantially higher rates than majority-black and majority-Latino areas (Morel, Al Elew, and Harris 2021). Most of the money also went to larger firms, with the top five percent of businesses sopping up more than half of the PPP loans—including six hundred companies that claimed the maximum $10 million in relief (Van Dam and O'Connell 2020). With banks receiving more in fees through these big loans, this distribution—in combination with the billions offered in tax breaks through the CARES Act—helped ensure that the spring 2020 stimulus package, rather than help the poor, delivered most of its benefits to the already wealthy (Hall, Wieder, and Nehamas 2020). The already wealthy, of course, were predominantly white.

Summer brought misguided hope, with daily case tallies in early June—while still in the thousands—nearly half those of two months prior. However, case counts would not be this low again until May 2021. Many states began loosening stay-at-home restrictions after just seven disciplined weeks; cases would subsequently skyrocket in the South and West, in both rural and urban areas.

Outrage over the videotaped murder of George Floyd by policeman Derek Chauvin sparked mass worldwide protests (largely outdoor and masked), while mass incarceration and the pandemic became overtly intertwined as major disease outbreaks occurred in prisons across the country. Counties with the largest proportion of persons incarcerated had significantly more, new COVID-19 cases from May to August 2020 (Hooks and Sawyer 2020). The *New York Times* reported that the overall rate of infection in US prisons, a disproportionately black and brown population, was more than three times the rate in the general population (ACLU 2020; Burkhalter et al. 2021; Hooks and Sawyer 2020).

In the fall, it was the education system's turn to assist COVID-19's spread. College campuses reopened well before any vaccines were available, welcoming students back to dormitories and/or in-person classes, leading to sizable jumps in cases in the surrounding communities. K-12 school districts that returned to in-person instruction also contributed to the surge. A review of school reopenings in Texas found that, in the two months following reopenings, this had contributed to 43,000 additional COVID-19 cases and 800 additional fatalities (Courtemanche et al. 2021). But remote schooling, with its attendant learning loss, only amplified demands for in-person instruction. A McKinsey analysis anticipated that, in part because of the digital divide and the increased reliance on remote instruction, black and Latino students might experience a learning loss 50 percent greater than their white counterparts (Dorn et al. 2021).

By early November, US daily case counts had risen past the unthinkable threshold of 100,000; on January 8, 2021, they would peak just above 300,000.[1] For a nearly three-month period, the seven-day average death toll from COVID-19 never fell below 2,000. The racial disparities first identified in the spring, while somewhat mitigated as the disease spread to more rural areas, persisted, with black, Latino, and Asian populations more likely to be hospitalized with COVID-19 across all regions of the United States.[2]

By this time, the economy had recovered nominally, at least for the most well-off. The stock market, after its collapse in March, reached new heights by November, resulting in the rich—at least those who had survived the initial downturn—recouping all of their losses and in fact getting wealthier in just nine months. The job market demonstrated a "K-shaped recovery": a bifurcated response that saw the number of high-wage jobs actually increase since January 2020 and 20 percent of low-wage jobs get eliminated, largely in the hospitality and service sectors—jobs occupied by many black and Latino workers (Gould and Kassa 2021).

In late December, nearly nine months into the pandemic, a second COVID-19 relief package, the Consolidated Appropriations Act, was passed, providing recipients an additional $600—an amount that even the Republican president called "ridiculously low" (Calia 2020). Delays in payment arose again, as they had with the CARES Act payments in spring 2020.

Hope arrived via the rapid development of multiple high-efficacy vaccines. In December, the Food and Drug Administration approved the use of two vaccines—from Pfizer-BioNTech and Moderna—for widespread use. Vaccination rollout began slowly. By year's end, the country had only delivered shots to 2.8 million individuals, well short of the declared goal of 20 million; logistical problems and mismanagement slowed the rollout.

Even as the Biden administration took office in January and accelerated the rate of vaccination, disparities began to reappear. Notably, black vaccination rates lagged behind their higher rates of infection and death from COVID-19. While initially attributed to vaccine hesitancy because of centuries of medical mistreatment (a hesitancy that disappeared throughout the rollout), the more accurate structural explanation was that vaccine sites were disproportionately located in white neighborhoods and, hence, less accessible to black and Latino populations (Hamel, Sparks, and Brodie 2021; McMinn et al. 2021). From December to May, a period in which more than half of the US population received at least one shot, the proportionate decline in deaths for black and Latino populations remained lower than for the white population (Hamel, Sparks, and Brodie 2021; McMinn et al. 2021).

Through November 2021, adjusting for population age differences, the CDC estimated that Native Americans, Latinos, and blacks are 120 percent, 90 percent, and 70 percent, respectively, more likely than non-Hispanic whites to die from the virus (CDC 2021b).[3] But the pandemic's impact also can be seen through the lens of life expectancy: COVID-19's arrival led, in 2020, to the greatest drop in life expectancy in the United States since 1943, in the midst of World War II (Santhanam 2021). The unprecedented outcome grows starker when considering race. While the non-Hispanic white population saw its average life expectancy fall by 1.36 years between 2018 and 2020, the non-Hispanic black population saw its average life expectancy fall by 3.25 years; for the Hispanic population, the decline was 3.88 years (Woolf, Masters, and Aron 2021). These varying drops in life expectancy can be tied to working and living conditions: fewer black and Latino workers were able to telecommute during the pandemic. Given the acute financial pressures these groups face, it makes sense that they, nevertheless, might take the calculated risk to continue to work.

With the overall unemployment rate in December 2021 now almost returned to its prepandemic level (3.9 percent vs. 3.5 percent), the racial disparities in these rates have expanded, with the black unemployment rate more than twice that of the white unemployment rate (7.1 vs. 3.2 percent) (Vinopal 2022). Just as the

Great Recession ballooned both general economic inequality and racial economic inequality—a reality that was not fully observable until years after the crisis had abated—the COVID-19 pandemic appears to be doing the same.

The Path to Now: Racial Disparities

A complete summary of how America achieved such rampant, robust racial disparities prior to the COVID-19 pandemic would require a project orders of magnitude larger than this entire volume, let alone a section of its introduction. Suffice it to say, condensing this history into a few pages will elide some crucial details.

While readers will learn more of this history in subsequent chapters of *The Pandemic Divide*, particularly the first two, we encourage readers to seek out additional pre-COVID-19 analyses, including, but not limited to, Ira Katznelson's *When Affirmative Action Was White: An Untold History of Racial Inequality in the Twentieth-Century America*; Keeanga-Yamahtta Taylor's *Race for Profit: How Banks and the Real Estate Industry Undermined Black Homeownership*; Isabel Wilkerson's *Caste: The Origins of Our Discontents*; Richard Rothstein's *The Color of Law: A Forgotten History of How Our Government Segregated America*; Mehrsa Baradaran's *The Color of Money: Black Banks and the Racial Wealth Gap*; and William A. Darity Jr. and A. Kirsten Mullen's *From Here to Equality: Reparations for Black Americans in the Twenty-First Century*.

Since its inception in 1776, the United States of America has upheld a racial hierarchy. The settler colonialists, after forming a new nation, waged war against and otherwise subjugated and denied rights to the indigenous peoples. They fostered and benefitted from eighty-nine years of black enslavement. They sanctioned a century of legal segregation and white violence directed against the black population. They instituted nativist immigration policies that, in conjunction with the country's bellicose actions and general meddling in Latin America, created a situation in which the United States has been seen as the preferred but often unattainable landing spot for unmoored populations.

The effects of these past and present actions are tangible, intertwined, and widespread. In terms of medical care, black and Latino populations are less likely to have health insurance—in part because of America's reliance on employers to provide health coverage—and are more likely to avoid seeking care because of cost barriers (Buchmueller and Levy 2020). When these populations do receive treatment, their experiences are marred by negligence and bias, and their outcomes are worse. For example, pregnant black women have a maternal mortality rate more than triple that of white women as well as an infant mortality rate twice as high—a rate that is highest for the most highly educated black women (Smith et al. 2018; National WIC Association 2019).

Inequities also have arisen from housing policies that have long kept certain populations from the necessary amenities for a healthy life. In addition to individual bigotry displayed by landlords, bankers, and citizens who have refused to rent to, loan to, or live alongside black and Latino families, government actions are to blame. From the Reconstruction era, when the formerly enslaved were denied land allocations promised in General William T. Sherman's "forty acres" field order and in the first Freedmen's Bureau Act; to the New Deal, notably, the systematic redlining of "risky" all-black neighborhoods; to the racially disparate application of the GI Bill in granting mortgage support to soldiers returning from World War II; to the mid- to-late-twentieth century urban renewal projects that cleaved black neighborhoods in two; the US government has created policies that have fostered residential disparities and, in turn, extreme levels of wealth inequality.

Today, black and racially mixed neighborhoods are more likely to be both food deserts (with a lack of access to fresh fruit and vegetables) and food swamps (with a surplus of fast food and other unhealthy food options). These neighborhoods are also more likely to feature a dearth of safe spaces for recreation, and they are more likely to be exposed to air pollution and other environmental hazards (Smith et al. 2019). Given these conditions, it follows that both black and Latino populations have higher rates of obesity and diabetes—blacks also have higher rates of hypertension—notable risk factors for worse outcomes after contracting COVID-19.

Perhaps the most comprehensive explanation of these racial disparities arises via the triple lens of employment, education, and wealth. For generations, blacks in America, initially brought here enslaved to exploit their labor, were denied wealth-building opportunities. Once freed and denied the promised initial asset of forty-acre land grants, persistent discrimination and white violence ensured they had little opportunity for advancement.

While not all Latinos have arrived in the United States in poverty (Cuban immigrants following the installation of the Castro regime and phenotypically white immigrants from southern cone countries are two notable exceptions), many arrivals have started from behind and then faced headwinds in American labor markets. Unemployment rates for Latinos and blacks have long outstripped the white unemployment rate—with the black unemployment rate the highest of all three (US Bureau of Labor Statistics 2011; Stone 2020). Moreover, the jobs that these groups can find typically offer worse pay and fewer benefits: prepandemic data shows that blacks and Latinos are more likely than whites to work jobs with no form of paid time off and no health insurance (Mason and Acosta 2021).

Attempts to overcome discrimination have met continued resistance. After the judicial mandate of public-school desegregation following *Brown v. Board of Education* in 1954, school desegregation met with defiant opposition and protests from whites. In Prince Edward County, Virginia, an all-white school board chose to close all of the public schools rather than allow black and white children to attend school together.

The growth of private schools, in conjunction with continued residential segregation, has helped manifest a pattern of school resegregation (Clotfelter 2006). The implementation of affirmative action policies in the 1960s briefly promised an improvement in the relative economic position of these groups through reduced exclusion from better employment opportunities, but the half-century since has proven otherwise. Affirmative action has been critiqued, attacked, and weakened to the point of being largely ineffective.

This cycle of little-to-no initial wealth for these groups, combined with narrow or blocked avenues to accrue wealth, means marginalized groups fall further behind their white peers with no avenue to catch up. Initial wealth disparities lead to heightened gaps for future generations, as many (white) individuals whose ancestors possessed wealth can inherit a foundational sum with years of interest gained in addition to benefitting from the security and safety net that familial wealth provides.

Today, the average black family has $840,900 less net worth than the average white family; Latino families have $817,900 less on average (Bhutta et al. 2020). Moreover, even if any of the oft-declared routes to economic success— greater employment, greater educational attainment, greater entrepreneurship, greater family stability—are realized, likely they will not have a significant effect in reducing the racial wealth chasm (Darity et al. 2018). These initial wealth disparities and their enduring effects mean that many mechanisms that could have alleviated worse outcomes from the COVID-19 pandemic for black and Latino populations will remain unattainable—at least without a substantial and deliberate transfer of wealth to these groups.

At the start of the COVID-19 pandemic, the popular refrain that rang out claimed "we're all in this together," as if stressors lessen disparities rather than accentuate them. But the history of America, and how it has fostered inequities in its past and present, means that the statement cannot be true. The COVID-19 pandemic cannot affect all groups equally because all groups in America have not been treated as equals. In other words, the virus has been mimicking the behavior of its host population.

The Pandemic Divide, in Brief

It is with this understanding of the events of the COVID-19 pandemic and of this country's history that we have compiled *The Pandemic Divide*. The following eleven chapters and postscript focus on a particular area of American life affected by the pandemic. Each chapter includes answers to the following questions:

- How have past (and ongoing) inequities in this field made certain populations especially vulnerable to the COVID-19 pandemic?
- How does viewing the COVID-19 pandemic through this lens reflect both the frustrations felt by these populations and the shortcomings elsewhere in society that are contributing to their marginalization?
- What remedies are needed in this area to alleviate inequities—both during pandemic and nonpandemic times?

The opening section lays the historical groundwork for much of the rest of the volume, exploring the development of racial disparities in health and labor outcomes and the confluence of factors contributing to both. The first chapter, by Keisha L. Bentley-Edwards, Melissa J. Scott, and Paul A. Robbins, analyzes how the prevalence of preexisting health conditions among black Americans—including hypertension, diabetes, asthma, obesity, kidney disease, and cardiovascular disease—contributed to their worse outcomes from COVID-19. Further, the authors consider the environmental and neighborhood factors that paved the way for such preconditions to develop: a lack of social resources (such as green spaces and supermarkets) provided in black neighborhoods and a greater exposure to environmental hazards. These racial disparities are better understood, the authors explain, when viewed in conjunction with black America's lack of access to the healthcare system and overrepresentation in jobs that do not provide health insurance or related benefits.

In the volume's second chapter, Joe William Trotter Jr. assesses the relationship between epidemics and pandemics and African American labor history. As black Americans travelled north during the Great Migration in search of new opportunities, however, they landed "at the bottom of the occupational hierarchy in the most hazardous and unhealthy jobs in the industrial economy," Trotter writes.

Their situation in their domestic lives was no better; they were shunted into overpriced, segregated residential neighborhoods and forced to live in crowded and unsanitary conditions. However, despite these circumstances, and in part because of civic institutions in urban settings, African Americans were able to generate activism and resistance to pressure health services and other government entities to recognize and improve their treatment.

The next section considers two institutions—the church and the prison system—that have long affected America's black population and have continued doing so since March 2020.

Sandra L. Barnes's chapter, "'God Is in Control': Race, Religion, Family, and Community during the COVID-19 Pandemic," explores the interplay between religious practices and pandemic behaviors and attitudes. Through interviews with a multigenerational black Christian family living in various COVID-19 hotspots, Barnes teases out the relationship between race and religion in 2020 and situates these dynamics alongside larger spiritual and religious racial trends. She notes the affirmation of black Christians' faith in the wake of the pandemic and concludes by saying, given the long-standing significant role of the church in the black community, "for some blacks today, closed churches may be just as damaging as open ones."

Arvind Krishnamurthy's chapter, "COVID-19, Race, and Mass Incarceration," looks at the effects of American mass incarceration on the spread of and disparate infection and mortality rates from COVID-19. The country's predilection for imprisonment as a means of "justice" (America accounts for more than one-fifth of all prisoners worldwide, a disproportionate number of whom are black and Latino) is damaging in nonpandemic times—and catastrophic in the presence of a deadly airborne virus. With thousands of individuals held in indoor facilities with insufficient spacing for distancing, the impact of the coronavirus has been devastating.

In light of these circumstances, Krishnamurthy explains, some (albeit too few) states implemented a variety of policy changes to reduce the prison population—with varying degrees of effectiveness. Larger scale policy adjustments and mitigation strategies—early releases of the incarcerated and forgoing prison sentences for low-level offenses—could have saved significant numbers of lives. Given the racialized nature of the prison population that Krishnamurthy notes, these practices further exacerbated the racially disparate effects of COVID-19.

Section III, the largest section of the book, explores the financial effects of the COVID-19 pandemic. Fenaba R. Addo and Adam Hollowell's chapter studies the effects of the pandemic on housing, schooling, and employment for black families. In particular, the authors note how housing precarity (and the comparative lack of homeownership) among black families constructs a barrier to wealth accumulation for this population.

Addo and Hollowell detail how housing inequality also has contributed to uneven learning environments in the pandemic, as students in low-income areas often lack access to a computer and/or high-speed internet. Crucially, they connect disparities in schooling to labor market bias to show that the cost of pursuing higher education is ultimately higher for blacks relative to their economic resources.

For black students, pursuing higher education entails taking on copious amounts of student debt to earn a degree before landing in a job that, typically, provides lower compensation than that of their white counterparts with similar levels of educational attainment. Addo and Hollowell enumerate a range of policies to combat these interlocking structures of inequality, which include student debt cancellation, reinvestment in black-owned businesses, and a further amplification and reinforcement of the Fair Housing Act.

Henry Clay McKoy Jr., in his chapter "Race, Entrepreneurship, and COVID-19," considers the impact of the pandemic on the landscape of black entrepreneurship. Prior to the pandemic, black-owned businesses were drastically smaller and far less sustainable than their white counterparts. As McKoy states, their ecosystem has been in "perpetual crisis" as a consequence of more than two centuries of "fiscal exclusions and economic discriminations." Unfortunately, this pattern has continued with the CARES Act and the one-sided allocation of PPP loans.

McKoy argues that in order to put black businesses on a more equitable footing, direct aid and deliberate action must occur. In this fashion, he outlines a permanently funded US Black Business Development Block Grant Program, which would provide short-term cash infusions to businesses in need and distribute funds to local governments and other civic institutions to support programs "creating more equitable local entrepreneurial, business, and economic ecosystems."

In their chapter titled "COVID-19 Effects on Black Business-Owner Households," Chris Wheat, Fiona Greig, and Damon Jones expand the analysis of black business ownership during the pandemic. Utilizing a novel administrative data set drawn from bank data on households and small businesses as well as publicly available voter registration information, the authors examine household and small-business finances, cash flows, and liquidity.

In particular, they study the initial effects of the pandemic's onset and the subsequent attempts to alleviate financial distress in the wake of the CARES Act. They find that a key constraint for these households is their lack of liquidity, with black business owners possessing smaller reserves of cash than their non-black peers. Accordingly, they demonstrate that stimulus payouts and other income supports led to greater consumer spending among lower-income groups, and they posit that targeting these programs and policies toward black business owners will lead to greater survival rates for these enterprises.

In the last chapter of section III, Jane Dokko and Jung Sakong contemplate and compare a number of possible policy interventions in the wake of widening economic racial disparities. Separating these policies between those applied to "high-return" and "low-return" groups, the authors advocate a range of actions that operate upstream and target the next generation. They recommend bolstering children's health and education, supporting parents of children, and preventing youth from entering the prison pipeline.

Furthermore, they consider meaningful proposals regarding homeownership, wealth accrual, entrepreneurship, and geographic investment programs. Their analysis points toward questions lingering in each of these areas, noting that some form of these types of interventions—beyond those that emphasize boosting human capital—will likely be necessary to promote higher returns in the future.

The final section of the book shines a light on educational inequities in three different arenas: the struggles of Latino/Latina American families navigating remote learning for their school-aged children, rising disparities in higher education under COVID-19, and amplified achievement gaps and slumps in K-12 education exacerbated by the move to virtual classrooms.

In their chapter, "Latinx Immigrant Parents and Their Children in Times of COVID-19," Marta Sánchez, Melania DiPietro, Leslie Babinski, Steven J. Amendum, and Steven Knotek review a novel survey of fifty-one Latino parents of kindergarten and first grade (K-1) students in a southern school district. The researchers asked respondents a number of questions about their experience during the pandemic, with particular weight given to their responses about remote schooling.

Through their inquiry, the authors are able to identify the difficulties these families face, ranging from obstacles using the technology or accessing the virtual classroom to frustration encountered by parents lacking the training to support their child in this learning environment. Grounding their analysis in the historical circumstances Latino families have faced in American schools and the conditions many Latino workers face in their essential (and dangerous) occupations, the researchers provide a holistic look at stressors confronting these families and delineate the vital support structures lost during the pandemic.

In "COVID-19, Higher Education, and Social Inequality," Adam Hollowell and N. Joyce Payne explore how an already tilted scale of higher education became more unbalanced in 2020. The authors, in contrast to the popular emphasis on billion-dollar endowments at America's prestigious universities, detail the vulnerability of many higher education institutions in the United States, including a vast majority of Historically Black Colleges and Universities (HBCUS).

With the expected reduction in endowments (as philanthropic giving has declined in recent economic recessions) and enrollments (the latter in part due to colleges' constrained ability to award adequate financial aid), prospects for many colleges and universities are bleak. These pressures are intensified at historically black institutions; generally, they have significantly smaller endowments and are more reliant on tuition dollars to stay in operation. With enrollment numbers already declining since 2011, any acceleration of this descent, like that brought on by the COVID-19 pandemic, has ominous implications for HBCUs.

The authors argue that this is the moment for bold policy implementation, in the form of student debt relief and a renewed commitment to improving and valuing the experiences of black students, staff, and faculty as well as for greater investment in HBCUs. It is paramount, Hollowell and Payne state, for higher education to, generally, become more accessible, rather than less; only if the academy "promotes and expands social mobility" can it truly empower the populace.

In the chapter that follows this, Kristen R. Stephens, Kisha N. Daniels, and Erica R. Phillips explore the difficult conditions that emerged in US elementary, middle, and high schools throughout most of 2020 and the first half of 2021. They begin their discussion with a profile of the current realities associated with K-12 public education in America—school systems that are underresourced, understaffed, and long plagued by racial and income-based achievement gaps. Their chapter summarizes how, across the board, the COVID-19 pandemic has amplified these disparities and insufficiencies.

Stephens, Daniels, and Phillips call for a "critical and systematic deep dive into [the] fissures" of the American public education system. In their plan for re-envisioning and rejuvenating this critical institution, the authors emphasize their sense of optimism for the nation's emergence from this moment of intense crisis.

Finally, Eugene T. Richardson's postscript, "COVID-19 and the Path Forward," provides a succinct capstone to the arguments advanced in the volume. Richardson directs his ire at the guiding, consistent ideology at the heart of all these disparities: white supremacy. As the connective tissue that draws together the country's history and the concomitant failure to urgently respond to the COVID-19 pandemic, white supremacy is the dragon Richardson identifies that must be slayed in order to change the future of American life.

Further (and Future) Considerations

The chapters in this volume summarize key issues concerning racial inequality and the COVID-19 pandemic. Before concluding this introduction, we consider a range of other topics that also warrant discussion, with hopes that future editions of *The Pandemic Divide* may undertake additional treatment of these topics and that readers will bear in mind these issues as they proceed through the volume.

First, this volume does not address the experiences of Asian Americans during the COVID-19 pandemic. With the origins of COVID-19 traced to Wuhan, China, and the racist if not outright xenophobic attitudes that America has long displayed, it is unsurprising that Asian Americans have been on the receiving end of heightened vitriol, hatred, and violence during this period. Attitudes toward Asian Americans soured as COVID-19 spread, and they persisted even as the pandemic's worst effects abated. Stop AAPI Hate, a group tracking and responding to racist incidents targeting Asian Americans and Pacific Islanders in the United States, documented more than 6,600 attacks from March 2020 to March 2021, with police data showing that attacks on these groups rose 164 percent in the first quarter of 2021 (Healy 2021; Farivar 2021). Asian American youths were slower to return to in-person schools in light of these threats, and Asian American small businesses saw the biggest decline during the pandemic, with the number of working businesses falling by 20 percent (Rogers 2021).

We do not ignore these atrocities. Rather, we are exploring how initial, preexisting racial disparities contributed to further inequities in the wake of the COVID-19 pandemic. While Asian Americans have been victims of discrimination and bigotry in America, they have not experienced disparities in their health and economic outcomes on par with the groups highlighted here (notably, in terms of familial wealth and life expectancy). However, given the hatred that we have seen in the wake of the COVID-19 pandemic and the economic ill effects that it has had on the Asian American population, the group's relatively strong position may prove to be precarious. Moving forward, Asian American well-being warrants close attention. As with other groups, and perhaps even more so, the full burden of the COVID-19 pandemic on the Asian American population may only become visible years after it has passed.

Similarly, a number of analyses have shown the varying effects of the pandemic on different genders and age cohorts of individuals (Heggeness 2021; Chatters, Taylor, and Taylor 2020). A prime example occurred in December 2020, when women accounted for all of the jobs lost in the economy: the economic sector lost 140,000 jobs, but men actually gained 16,000 jobs, meaning that women alone lost 156,000 jobs (Rasta 2021). Addo and Hollowell explore gender-differentiated outcomes from the pandemic in their chapter, but readers should note how the disparities described in this book have not been confined to the nonwhite population, writ large, but also have had an aggravated impact across the intersectional lines of race and gender.

Nor does this book examine in depth the shortcomings of the provision of healthcare in America. Not all health treatment is equal here: community and safety-net hospitals—those that accepted patients without insurance or with insurance that did not cover treatment at more prestigious medical centers—were often overwhelmed with COVID-19 patients (Fink and Kosoksky 2021; Dwyer 2020). America's web of public and private hospitals, combined with its patchwork health insurance system, led to numerous logistical crises across major cities, misallocations of resources, and, ultimately, unnecessary death. Responses that have been more just—the rollout of free-of-charge COVID-19 vaccines to US residents and, eventually, of at-home tests to all US households—suggest that there exist other, less punitive possibilities.

We embrace the notion that structural changes in the financing of public health should be considered in hopes of greater equity and effectiveness. However, national health insurance alone cannot mitigate racial disparities. In the UK, for example, the COVID-19 mortality risk for ethnic minority groups is twice that of white British patients; one early analysis found that 63 percent of health and social care workers who died were of black or Asian descent—a group that comprised 21 percent of NHS workers (Razai et al. 2021).

Finally, this project coincided with two seismic events in America: the reactivation of Black Lives Matter protests during the 2020 summer in the wake of numerous high-profile police and extrajudicial killings of black individuals and the 2020 presidential primary and general elections. Both attending these protests and voting in these elections became causes for anxiety as gathering in the streets or at voting precincts put participants at greater risk for catching the airborne virus.

To suggest how either the protests or elections would have turned out sans COVID-19 is conjectural; however, it is worth stating these elements were intertwined (NAACP 2020) While the pandemic provided an excuse for mayors and other officials to enact municipality-wide curfews to quell protests, much of the outrage and racial reckoning over the summer of 2020 has been attributed to the stasis, financial uncertainty, and racial inequities of the pandemic (Arora 2020; Michener 2020). Racial disparities that contributed to black morbidity and mortality under COVID-19 stem partly from the overpolicing of black individuals and their subsequent incarceration (as Krishnamurthy describes in his chapter). Overpolicing and excessive use of force by the police historically has limited black individuals' capacity to accrue wealth to weather this sort of disaster; for the incarcerated, it placed them in the virus' path as the virus made its way through the unsanitary, socially undistanced prison system.

Voting similarly underwent changes in response to the pandemic, as an unprecedented number of citizens opted to vote early (during less crowded times) or absentee (through the postal service). Nevertheless, in the 2020 November election, much like in past elections, nonwhite neighborhoods were more likely to experience greater wait times when voting (Quealy and Parlapiano 2021). While the danger that the pandemic would provide an opportunity to suppress black votes and steal the presidential election failed to manifest, the tightly bracketed Senate and the Republican gains in the House in 2020 arose in no small part because of various forms of voter suppression. With restricted access to the ballot under consideration in states across the country in 2021 and beyond, an exploration of these potential dangers might still be valuable for similar scenarios in the future—given that black voters were the most likely demographic to vote in person during the 2020 presidential election (Lopez and Noe-Bustamante 2021).

Tangentially, the COVID-19 pandemic became increasingly intertwined with the partisan responses in public-health policies (mask mandates, curfews, indoor occupation restrictions) enacted by state governors and governments. As COVID-19 made inroads, a political divide emerged, with Republican-led states more likely to preemptively reopen, leading to their having higher case counts from summer 2020 onward (VanDusky-Allen and Shvetsova 2021). When Republican leaders urged their state citizens to stay home, they received a more positive response from Democratic-leaning counties than from Republican-leaning counties, indication of a "backlash" effect for Republican leaders who dared to contradict their national party figureheads (Grossman et al. 2020).

But these states also made decisions in the past—including refusing to expand Medicaid—that have hurt their constituents in the COVID-19 era. Moreover, Republican states continue to lag behind in vaccination rates, largely failing to persuade their citizens of the vaccine's utility and delaying the nation from reaching its goal of herd immunity. As countries like Australia have highlighted the success of centralized policy and public health mandates, America is perhaps the prime demonstrator of the drawbacks of piecemeal epidemiology. Clear and consistent national policy will be necessary to manage the COVID-19 pandemic and navigate future crises of this nature.

Reducing the Distance

This book aims to help promote an understanding of these disparate realities so that necessary improvements can be made to abate them. To achieve this, the discussion must translate into action and policy. Many of the chapters here propose policy changes to improve the plight of black Americans—and all marginalized groups—in future pandemics. We endorse these suggestions and wish to highlight two of our own that will improve the position of these groups and enhance their capacity to respond in similar future disasters.

The first such policy, also discussed in the chapter by Addo and Hollowell, is a federal job guarantee (FJG) of the type outlined by Paul, Darity, and Hamilton (2018). The COVID-19 pandemic has reflected, horrifically, the volatility and precarity of America's overreliance on private sector employment. The implementation of an FJG, though no small task, would ensure millions of Americans would not starve in the face of lengthy if not indefinite unemployment; moreover, because the FJG would include health insurance for all its full-time workers, individuals and families would no longer risk having to experience the two-fold setback of losing their job and their health insurance. Notably, this policy, while universal, would disproportionately help black and Latino Americans mitigate risk during pandemics, given their greater degree of unemployment and—when employed—their lower likelihood of working jobs that provide health benefits.

Similarly, we propose reparations for black Americans, both as a matter of justice and as a preventative tool to minimize the disparities highlighted here. The restitutive and compensatory case for reparations has been covered in depth elsewhere (see Mullen and Darity 2020). But reparations can also function as a public-health tool. A 2021 article from Eugene T. Richardson and colleagues explores how areas with greater social equity (South Korea) demonstrate lower transmission rates than those with less equity (Louisiana). The authors' analysis suggests that a successful reparations program would have reduced the initial transmission curve of the relevant population by 31–68 percent, which, in turn, would have helped to slow the transmission of the disease in the overall population.

This analysis suggests that greater equity can beget greater equity and promote better outcomes for all. However, the converse is also true. As much as COVID-19 is presented as unprecedented, its effects—heightening inequities, particularly racial inequities—are not. This collection of essays argues that understanding the disparate societal conditions that preceded COVID-19, as well as the racial inequality that pervades all walks of American life, is essential to determining the necessary steps forward.

NOTES

1. This moment would represent the height of the pandemic until the rise of the highly transmissible Omicron variant in winter 2021–2022, during which cases peaked at more than 800,000 per day.

2. The disparity for the latter group is surprising and still somewhat unexplained, given that the Asian population typically has the best health outcomes of all other Americans. However, they are more likely to work in jobs in vulnerable sectors that don't allow for telecommuting, and they are more likely to live in multigenerational housing with greater risk of COVID-19 transmission. Moreover, it is feasible that the hatred directed toward Asian Americans in the wake of the COVID-19 pandemic has heightened barriers to testing and healthcare, as they are more hesitant to leave their homes (Yee 2021).

3. Indeed, evidence suggests that Native Americans may have the worst COVID-19 outcomes in terms of deaths and hospitalizations of any racial/ethnic group (Artiga, Hill, and Haldar 2021). Given their well-established history in America as the victims of genocide, subjugation, and wealth-stripping, their situation would make sense to highlight in this volume. Unfortunately, the data on this group is more limited: a function of their smaller population (they constitute about 2 percent of Americans), an indication of the difficulty of applying traditional unemployment measures to this population (see Kleinfeld and Kruse 1982), and a reflection of a larger pattern of their exclusion from the public consciousness. Notably, Native Americans are not included in the US Bureau of Labor Statistics monthly jobs reports, which are crucial for analyzing granular economic changes in response to the ever-evolving COVID-19 pandemic, nor are they given their own category in the Survey of Consumer Finances data set that summarizes the modern racial wealth gap (Sanchez, Maxim, and Foxworth 2021; Bhutta et al. 2020).

This lack of data is a hindrance, and it must not become permanent. "Oil and Blood: The Color of Wealth in Tulsa, Oklahoma," co-authored by an editor of this volume, shows it is possible to collect detailed financial and wealth data not just for all Native Americans but for specific tribal affiliations (Lee et al. 2021). Detailed, deliberate research must be conducted regarding these populations so that the small sample size excuse does not become a crutch, enabling ignorance and blindness to these long-standing injustices.

REFERENCES

ACLU (American Civil Liberties Union) West Virginia. 2020. "Racial Disparities in Jails and Prisons: COVID-19's Impact on the Black Community." June 12. https://www.acluwv.org/en/news/racial-disparities-jails-and-prisons-covid-19s-impact-black-community.

Artiga, Samantha, Latoya Hill, and Sweta Haldar. 2021. "COVID-19 Cases and Deaths by Race/Ethnicity: Current Data and Changes over Time." KFF (Kaiser Family Foundation). October 8. https://www.kff.org/racial-equity-and-health-policy/issue-brief/covid-19-cases-and-deaths-by-race-ethnicity-current-data-and-changes-over-time/.

Arora, Maneesh. 2020. "How the Coronavirus Pandemic Helped the Floyd Protests Become the Biggest in U.S. History." *Washington Post*, August 4. https://www.washingtonpost.com/politics/2020/08/05/how-coronavirus-pandemic-helped-floyd-protests-become-biggest-us-history/.

Bhutta, Neil, Andrew C. Chang, Lisa J. Dettling, and Joanna W. Hsu. 2020. "Disparities in Wealth by Race and Ethnicity in the 2019 Survey of Consumer Finances." Board of Governors of the Federal Reserve System. FEDS Notes. September 28. https://

www.federalreserve.gov/econres/notes/feds-notes/disparities-in-wealth-by-race-and
-ethnicity-in-the-2019-survey-of-consumer-finances-20200928.htm.

Buchmueller, Thomas C., and Helen G. Levy. 2020. "The ACA's Impact on Racial and
Ethnic Disparities in Health Insurance Coverage and Access to Care." *Health Affairs* 39
(3): 395–402. https://doi.org/10.1377/hlthaff.2019.01394.

Burkhalter, Eddie, Izzy Colón, Brendon Derr, Lazaro Gamio, Rebecca Griesbach, Ann
Hinga Klein, and Danya Issawi. 2021. "Incarcerated and Infected: How the Virus Tore
through the US Prison System." *New York Times*, April 10. https://www.nytimes.com
/interactive/2021/04/10/us/covid-prison-outbreak.html.

Calia, Mike. 2020. "Trump Calls COVID Relief Bill Unsuitable and Demands Congress
Add Bigger Stimulus Payments." CNBC. December 22. https://www.cnbc.com/2020
/12/22/trump-calls-covid-relief-bill-unsuitable-and-demands-congress-add-higher
-stimulus-payments.html.

CDC (Centers for Disease Control and Prevention). 2018. "History of 1918 Flu Pandemic." March 21. https://www.cdc.gov/flu/pandemic-resources/1918-commemoration
/1918-pandemic-history.htm.

CDC (Centers for Disease Control and Prevention). 2021a. "Estimated COVID-19 Burden." May 19. https://www.cdc.gov/coronavirus/2019-ncov/cases-updates/burden.html.

CDC (Centers for Disease Control and Prevention). 2021b. "Risk for COVID-19 Infection,
Hospitalization, and Death by Race/Ethnicity." November 22. https://www.cdc.gov
/coronavirus/2019-ncov/covid-data/investigations-discovery/hospitalization-death-by
-race-ethnicity.html.

Chatters, Linda M., Harry Owen Taylor, and Robert Joseph Taylor. 2020. "Older Black
Americans During COVID-19: Race and Age Double Jeopardy." *Health Education and
Behavior* 47 (6): 855–60. https://doi.org/10.1177/1090198120965513.

Clotfelter, Charles T. 2006. *After Brown: The Rise and Retreat of School Desegregation.*
Princeton, NJ: Princeton University Press.

Courtemanche, Charles, Anh Le, Aaron Yelowitz, and Ron Zimmer. 2021. "School
Reopenings, Mobility, and COVID-19 Spread: Evidence from Texas." Working Paper
w28753, National Bureau of Economic Research, Cambridge, MA. https://doi.org/10
.3386/w28753.

Darity, William, Darrick Hamilton, Mark Paul, Alan Aja, Anne Price, Antonio Moore,
and Caterina Chiopris. 2018. "What We Get Wrong about Closing the Racial Wealth
Gap." Durham, NC: Samuel DuBois Cook Center on Social Equity at Duke University. April. https://socialequity.duke.edu/wp-content/uploads/2020/01/what-we-get
-wrong.pdf.

Des Moines Register. 2020. "Read the Full Transcript of Tuesday Night's CNN/*Des
Moines Register* Debate." January 14. https://www.desmoinesregister.com/story/news
/elections/presidential/caucus/2020/01/14/democratic-debate-transcript-what-the
-candidates-said-quotes/4460789002/.

Dorn, Emma, Bryan Hancock, Jimmy Sarakatsannis, and Ellen Viruleg. 2021. "COVID-19
and Learning Loss—Disparities Grow and Students Need Help." McKinsey and Company. March 1. https://www.mckinsey.com/industries/public-and-social-sector/our
-insights/covid-19-and-learning-loss-disparities-grow-and-students-need-help#.

Dwyer, Jim. 2020. "One Hospital Was Besieged by the Virus. Nearby Was 'Plenty of Space.'" *New York Times*. May 14. https://www.nytimes.com/2020/05/14/nyregion/coronavirus-ny-hospitals.html.

Farivar, Masood. 2021. "Attacks on Asian Americans Spiked by 164 Percent in First Quarter of 2021." Voice of America. April 30. https://www.voanews.com/usa/attacks-asian-americans-spiked-164-first-quarter-2021.

Fink, Sheri, and Isadora Kosofsky. 2021. "Dying of COVID in a 'Separate and Unequal' LA Hospital." *New York Times*. February 8. https://www.nytimes.com/2021/02/08/us/covid-los-angeles.html.

Gould, Elise, and Melat Kassa. 2021. "Low-Wage, Low-Hours Workers Were Hit Hardest in the COVID-19 Recession." Economic Policy Institute. May 20. https://www.epi.org/publication/swa-2020-employment-report/.

Grossman, Guy, Soojong Kim, Jonah M. Rexer, and Harsha Thirumurthy. 2020. "Political Partisanship Influences Behavioral Responses to Governors' Recommendations for COVID-19 Prevention in the United States." PNAS (National Academy of Sciences). September 29. https://www.pnas.org/content/117/39/24144.

Hall, Kevin G., Ben Wieder, and Nicholas Nehamas. 2020. "Big Banks Generated Billions in Fees from Paycheck Protection Program." *Miami Herald*. December 3. https://www.miamiherald.com/news/coronavirus/article247562870.html.

Hamel, Liz, Grace Sparks, and Mollyann Brodie. 2021. "KFF COVID-19 Vaccine Monitor: February 2021." KFF (Kaiser Family Foundation). February 26. https://www.kff.org/coronavirus-covid-19/poll-finding/kff-covid-19-vaccine-monitor-february-2021/.

Healy, Jack. 2021. "For Asian Americans Wary of Attacks, Reopening Is Not an Option." *New York Times*, June 8. https://www.nytimes.com/2021/06/08/us/asian-american-attacks.html.

Heggeness, Misty L. 2020. "Estimating the Immediate Impact of the COVID-19 Shock on Parental Attachment to the Labor Market and the Double Bind of Mothers." *Review of Economics of the Household* 18, no. 4: 1053–78. https://doi.org/10.1007/s11150-020-09514-x.

Hooks, Gregory, and Wendy Sawyer. 2020. "Mass Incarceration, COVID-19, and Community Spread." Prison Policy Initiative. December. https://www.prisonpolicy.org/reports/covidspread.html.

Kleinfeld, Judith, and John A. Kruse. 1982. "Native Americans in the Labor Force: Hunting for an Accurate Measure." *Monthly Labor Review* 105, no. 7 (July): 47–51. http://www.jstor.org/stable/41841850.

Lee, C. Aujean, Randall Akee, Raffi E. García, Lauren Russell, Jorge Zumaeta, and William A. Darity Jr. 2021. "Oil and Blood: The Color of Wealth in Tulsa, Oklahoma." Durham, NC: Samuel DuBois Cook Center on Social Equity at Duke University. https://socialequity.duke.edu/wp-content/uploads/2021/11/50088_Tulsa-Report_111321_print.pdf.

Lopez, Mark Hugo, and Luis Noe-Bustamante. 2021. "Black Voters Were Most Likely to Say November Election Was Run Very Well." Pew Research Center. January 12. https://www.pewresearch.org/fact-tank/2021/01/12/black-voters-were-most-likely-to-say-november-election-was-run-very-well/.

Mason, Jessica, and Paula Molina Acosta. 2021. "Called to Care: A Racially Just Recovery Demands Paid Family and Medical Leave." National Partnership for Women and Families. March. https://www.nationalpartnership.org/our-work/resources/economic -justice/paid-leave/called-to-care-a-racially-just-recovery-demands-paid-family-and -medical-leave.pdf.

McMinn, Sean, Shalina Chatlani, Ashley Lopez, Sam Whitehead, Ruth Talbot, and Austin Fast. 2021. "Across the South, COVID-19 Vaccine Sites Missing from Black and Hispanic Neighborhoods." NPR. February 5. https://www.npr.org/2021/02/05/962946721 /across-the-south-covid-19-vaccine-sites-missing-from-black-and-hispanic-neighbor.

Menton, Jessica. 2020. "Unemployment Benefits: Racial Disparity in Jobless Aid Grows as Congress Stalls on COVID-19 Stimulus." USA Today. October 27. https://www .usatoday.com/story/money/2020/10/22/stimulus-check-black-unemployment-rate -racial-disparity-coronavirus-trump-biden/3650844001/.

Michener, Jamila. 2020. "George Floyd's Killing Was Just the Spark. Here's What Really Made the Protests Explode." Washington Post. June 11. https://www.washingtonpost .com/politics/2020/06/11/george-floyds-killing-was-just-spark-heres-what-really-made -protests-explode/.

Morel, Laura C., Mohamed Al Elew, and Emily Harris. 2021. "Hundreds of Billions of Dollars in PPP Loans Marred by Racial Inequity." Reveal. June 30. https://revealnews .org/article/rampant-racial-disparities-plagued-how-billions-of-dollars-in-ppp-loans -were-distributed-in-the-u-s/.

Mullen, A. Kirsten, and William A. Darity. 2020. From Here to Equality: Reparations for Black Americans in the Twenty-First Century. Chapel Hill: The University of North Carolina Press.

NAACP (National Association for the Advancement of Colored People). 2020. "2020 American Election Eve Poll Finds Coronavirus Pandemic and Racial Justice among Most Important Issues for African American Voters." November 10. https://naacp .org/latest/2020-american-election-eve-poll-finds-coronavirus-pandemic-and-racial -justice-among-most-important-issues-for-african-american-voters/.

National Law Center on Homelessness and Poverty. 2020. "Racism, Homelessness, and Poverty." May. https://nlchp.org/wp-content/uploads/2020/05/Racism-Homelessness -and-COVID-19-Fact-Sheet-_Final_2.pdf.

National WIC Association. 2019. "Maternal Mortality in the US: The Role of WIC in Addressing the Crisis." https://s3.amazonaws.com/aws.upl/nwica.org/2019-wic-maternal -mortality.pdf.

NYC Health. 2020. "Age Adjusted Rate of Fatal Lab Confirmed Cases per 100,000 by racial/ethnic group." April 6. https://www1.nyc.gov/assets/doh/downloads/pdf/imm /covid-19-deaths-race-ethnicity-04242020-1.pdf.

Off, Gavin, Ames Alexander, and Aaron Sánchez-Guerra. 2021. "Black, Latino NC Workers Had to Play 'Russian Roulette' during COVID. The Toll Was Steep." Charlotte Observer. June 9. https://www.charlotteobserver.com/news/state/north-carolina /article251871898.html.

Pannett, Rachel. 2021. "Australia Made a Plan to Protect Indigenous Elders from COVID-19. It Worked." Washington Post. April 14. https://www.washingtonpost.com/world/asia

_pacific/australia-coronavirus-aboriginal-indigenous/2021/04/09/7acd4d56-96a4-11eb -8f0a-3384cf4fb399_story.html.

Paul, Mark, William A. Darity, and Darrick Hamilton. 2018. "The Federal Job Guarantee—A Policy to Achieve Permanent Full Employment." *Center on Budget and Policy Priorities*. March 9. https://www.cbpp.org/research/full-employment/the-federal-job -guarantee-a-policy-to-achieve-permanent-full-employment.

Quealy, Kevin, and Alicia Parlapiano. 2021. "Election Day Voting in 2020 Took Longer in America's Poorest Neighborhoods." *New York Times*. January 4. https://www.nytimes .com/interactive/2021/01/04/upshot/voting-wait-times.html.

Rasta, Anoushah. 2021. "Women Account for 100 percent of Job Losses in December: Report." NBC Bay Area. January 14. https://www.nbcbayarea.com/news/local/women -account-for-100-of-job-losses-in-december-report/2445853/.

Razai, Mohamed S., Hayden K.N. Kankam, Azeem Majeed, Aneez Esmail, and David R. William. 2021. "Mitigating Ethnic Disparities in COVID-19 and Beyond." BMJ. https:// www.bmj.com/content/372/bmj.m4921.

Richardson, Eugene T., Momin M. Malik, William A. Darity, A. Kirsten Mullen, Michelle E. Morse, Maya Malik, Aletha Maybank, Mary T. Bassett, Paul E. Farmer, Lee Worden, and James Holland Jones. 2021. "Reparations for Black American Descendants of Persons Enslaved in the US and Their Potential Impact on SARS CoV-2 Transmission." *Social Science and Medicine* 276 (May): 113741. https://doi.org/10.1016/j .socscimed.2021.113741.

Rogers, Kate. 2021. "Asian-Owned Small Businesses Saw an Outsized Pandemic Impact Last Year." CNBC. March 3. https://www.cnbc.com/2021/03/03/asian-owned-small -businesses-saw-an-outsized-pandemic-impact-last-year-.html.

Roll, Stephen, and Michal Grinstein-Weiss. 2020. "Did CARES Act Benefits Reach Vulnerable Americans? Evidence from a National Survey." Brookings. August 25. https:// www.brookings.edu/research/did-cares-act-benefits-reach-vulnerable-americans -evidence-from-a-national-survey/.

Sanchez, Gabriel R., Robert Maxim, and Raymond Foxworth. 2021. "The Monthly Jobs Report Ignores Native Americans. How Are They Faring Economically?" Brookings. November 10. https://www.brookings.edu/blog/the-avenue/2021 /11/10/the-monthly-jobs-report-ignores-native-americans-how-are-they-faring -economically/.

Santhanam, Laura. 2021. "Covid Helped Cause the Biggest Drop in U.S. Life Expectancy since WWII. " PBS NewsHour. December 22. https://www.pbs.org/newshour/health /covid-helped-cause-the-biggest-drop-in-u-s-life-expectancy-since-wwii.

Smith, Imari Z. Loneke T. Blackman Carr, Salimah El-Amin, Keisha L. Bentley-Edwards, and William A. Darity Jr. 2019. "Inequity in Place: Obesity Disparities and the Legacy of Racial Residential Segregation and Social Immobility." Durham, NC: Samuel DuBois Cook Center on Social Equity at Duke University. https://socialequity.duke .edu/wp-content/uploads/2019/10/Inequity-In-Place.pdf.

Smith, Imari Z., Salimah El-Amin, Keisha L. Bentley-Edwards, and William A. Darity Jr. 2018. "Fighting at Birth: Eradicating the Black-White Infant Mortality Gap." Durham, NC: Samuel DuBois Cook Center on Social Equity at Duke University.

https://socialequity.duke.edu/wp-content/uploads/2019/12/Eradicating-Black-Infant
-Mortality-March-2018.pdf.

Stone, Chad. 2020. "Robust Unemployment Insurance, Other Relief Needed to Mitigate
Racial and Ethnic Unemployment Disparities." Center on Budget and Policy Priorities.
August 5. https://www.cbpp.org/research/economy/robust-unemployment-insurance
-other-relief-needed-to-mitigate-racial-and-ethnic.

US Bureau of Labor Statistics. 2011. "Unemployment Rates by Race and Ethnicity,
2010." TED: The Economics Daily. October 5. https://www.bls.gov/opub/ted/2011/ted
_20111005.htm.

US Bureau of Labor Statistics. 2020a. "Unemployment Rate 2.0 Percent for College
Grads, 3.8 Percent for High School Grads in January 2020." TED: The Economics Daily.
February 12. https://www.bls.gov/opub/ted/2020/unemployment-rate-2-percent-for
-college-grads-3-8-percent-for-high-school-grads-in-january-2020.htm.

US Bureau of Labor Statistics. 2020b. "Unemployment Rate Rises to Record
High 14.7 Percent in April 2020." May 13. https://www.bls.gov/opub/ted/2020
/unemployment-rate-rises-to-record-high-14-point-7-percent-in-april-2020.htm.

Van Dam, Andrew, and Jonathan O'Connell. 2020. "More Than Half of Emergency
Small-Business Funds Went to Larger Businesses, New Data Shows." Washington Post.
December 9. https://www.washingtonpost.com/business/2020/12/01/ppp-sba-data/.

VanDusky-Allen, Julie, and Olga Shvetsova. 2021. "How America's Partisan Divide over
Pandemic Responses Played Out in the States." The Conversation. May 12. https://
theconversation.com/how-americas-partisan-divide-over-pandemic-responses-played
-out-in-the-states-157565.

Vinopal, Courtney. 2022. "Black Americans Were the Only US Group to See Unemployment Tick up in December." Quartz. January 7. https://qz.com/2110476/unemployment
-among-black-workers-ticked-up-in-december-2021/.

Washington, Kemberley. 2021. "COVID-19 Has Had a Disproportionate Financial Impact
on Black Small Businesses." Forbes. July 7. https://www.forbes.com/advisor/personal
-finance/covid19-financial-impact-on-black-businesses/.

Wee, Sui-Lee, and Donald G. McNeil Jr. 2020. "From Jan. 2020: China Identifies New
Virus Causing Pneumonialike Illness." New York Times. January 9. https://www
.nytimes.com/2020/01/08/health/china-pneumonia-outbreak-virus.html.

Woolf, Steven H., Ryan K. Masters, and Laudan Y. Aron. 2021. "Effect of the COVID-19
Pandemic in 2020 on Life Expectancy across Populations in the USA and Other High
Income Countries: Simulations of Provisional Mortality Data." BMJ. https://doi.org/10
.1136/bmj.n1343.

Yee, Amy. 2021. "COVID's Outsize Impact on Asian Americans Is Being Ignored." Scientific American. May 6. https://www.scientificamerican.com/article/covids-outsize
-impact-on-asian-americans-is-being-ignored/.

COVID-19 in Context

1. How Systemic Racism and Preexisting Conditions Contributed to COVID-19 Disparities for Black Americans

KEISHA L. BENTLEY-EDWARDS, MELISSA J. SCOTT,
AND PAUL A. ROBBINS

The initial reporting of COVID-19 presented two dominant narratives. The first painted a picture in which all people in the United States faced a similar public-health threat. Popular media narratives and public-health campaigns asserted that COVID-19 was an invisible enemy that would strike indiscriminately. The second narrative was that black people were immune to COVID-19 because of both the low prevalence of the virus in Africa and too few known cases for black people prior to April 2020. These myths were quickly dispelled once researchers and public-health officials began disaggregating and analyzing data along racial lines. The data revealed precisely what anyone with a rudimentary understanding of racial health disparities would expect: this illness could be added to an extensive list of preventable diseases that disproportionately impact black Americans.

Race, the social construction that supports racial hierarchies, is not based on genetic differences (Yudell et al. 2016), and black people are neither immune nor susceptible to COVID-19 because of race-based genetics (Carter and Sandford III 2020). Data analyzed by the Centers for Disease Control and Prevention (CDC) indicate that from March to mid-November 2020, African Americans were 3.7 times more likely to be hospitalized and 2.1 times more likely to die because of COVID-19 compared to white Americans (Centers for Disease Control and Prevention 2020). With minimal scrutiny, this health disparity could simply be attributed to the large portions of black people who live in the major cities and densely populated neighborhoods that were greatly affected early on, such as New York and Detroit. However, white people who were living in adjacent densely populated neighborhoods had lower odds of contracting and dying from COVID-19. Thus, rationales for the observed racial group differences in COVID-19 outcomes plausibly extend beyond genetics, geographic location, and urbanicity; disparities are likely attributable to other social factors. This chapter argues that this virus is a unique threat to the health of black Americans because of ongoing systemic health disparities in preexisting conditions, access to quality healthcare, and differences in lived experiences, all of which have been major catalysts for dissimilar COVID-19 outcomes.

Social Determinants of Preexisting Conditions

To understand why this disease and many others are particularly perilous for black Americans, it is important to consider how daily engagement with the racial biases that are embedded in the socioecological structures of the United States generate and exacerbate racial health gaps (Williams and Mohammed 2013a). These systems consistently endanger black people by exposing them to uneven risk without providing equitable support structures to mitigate the burden on black health. As a result, black Americans—especially those who were born in the United States rather than those who immigrated here—are more likely to have adverse health conditions such as hypertension, diabetes, asthma, obesity, kidney disease, and cardiovascular disease (Benjamin et al. 2019; Mazurek and Syamlal 2018). Typically, these comorbidities are more debilitating and often are deadlier among US-born black people. Each of these preexisting conditions has also been associated with suffering moderate to severe symptoms and greater mortality from COVID-19.[1]

Prior to the pandemic, black Americans had higher rates of the comorbid illnesses that make COVID-19 more dangerous, and they tended to develop many of these diseases at earlier ages than non-Hispanic, white Americans. For example, although the prevalence and mortality rates of cardiovascular disease are similar for black and white adults over the age of 65, young and middle-aged black adults have higher prevalence rates than their white counterparts that cannot be wholly explained by clinical and socioeconomic indicators (Jolly et al. 2010). The existence of such health disparities means that the population of black people who are vulnerable to the pandemic includes a wider age range than epidemiologists might predict for Americans in general. Relatedly, reports claimed that people who were 65 years or older were at substantially greater risk for COVID-19 complications than younger adults, often without acknowledging that these data were not disaggregated by race *and* age. Conducting a deeper analysis of the data for which race was available, people who are over 65 years comprised the majority of COVID-19 hospitalizations among whites—but the same age group comprised less than 40 percent among blacks in the United States (Centers for Disease Control and Prevention 2021a). For black Americans, the majority of hospitalizations occurred in those who were thought to be at lower risk: adults younger than 65 years old. Black Americans began the pandemic with higher rates of medical conditions that exacerbate COVID-19, so their distinct susceptibility to COVID-19 should have been anticipated.

Still, a singular focus on the higher likelihood of having underlying health conditions overlooks the larger social systems that contribute to black overrepresentation among the less healthy in the United States. Specifically, this emphasis on individual health trivializes how racially biased social, medical, and environmental systems reliably produce worse outcomes for black Americans compared to their white peers. Recognizing systemic failures does not take away from an individual's personal agency around health behaviors; to the contrary, it recognizes that people's health behaviors, conditions, *and* outcomes are informed by the society and structures in which they live, play, and work. The interplay between systemic racism and individual outcomes and behaviors complicates the relentless focus of poor outcomes resulting from a combination of poor individual choices. Instead, a recursive approach clarifies how disparities in preexisting conditions are produced by black people being sorted into contexts of social and health immobility (Colen et al. 2018; Yancy 2020). These social determinants of health make it more likely that, collectively, black people will become and remain in poorer health regardless of their financial and social capital (Williams, Priest, and Anderson 2016; Smith et al. 2018).

Many of the racial gaps in the health conditions that have been linked to worse COVID-19 outcomes can be partially attributed to differences in access to the US healthcare system. Not only are black people overrepresented among the uninsured and underinsured, but a sizable portion reside in areas that lack quality medical facilities. As is outlined in other chapters of this book, black Americans have lower incomes and less wealth than white Americans, which limits their access to private insurance and their ability to pay for medical care if they are uninsured. Furthermore, the majority of black Americans live in southern states, many of which have rejected federal funding for Medicaid expansion without providing adequate alternatives.

Also contributing to black Americans' lack of access to the healthcare system is their overrepresentation in jobs that do not subsidize or provide sufficient insurance benefits and paid sick leave (Brundage Jr. 2020). The drastic rise in unemployment due to COVID-19-related restrictions and expiring pandemic-related safety nets have expanded disparities in the labor force, which, in turn, have negatively impacted black Americans' access to health insurance (Groeger 2020; Garfield and Tolbert 2020). People without health insurance are often dissuaded from scheduling doctor visits for nonemergencies because of the out-of-pocket costs of covering preventative healthcare. At times, they avoid going to the doctor if they believe that they could be diagnosed with a serious illness or one that would require significant time and money for proper treatment. Those without or with only minimal paid sick leave sometimes are made to choose between missing shifts to receive a professional assessment of their symptoms or working while ill. For workers who are paid by the hour, missing work to see a physician means they will lose some of the money they would have earned as well as the opportunity to make additional money. The combined lack of financial resources and public or private protections decreases black Americans' inclination and agency to seek routine wellness screenings and medical treatment, adding to their likelihood of having undiagnosed and untreated preexisting conditions that leave them susceptible to COVID-19.

Essential Workers and Health Risk

Aside from the lack of wages and insurance coverage provided to black employees, many of their jobs directly contributed to their risk of exposure to COVID-19. Black Americans are overrepresented within service occupations, such as public service, food service, manufacturing, food processing, postal service, package delivery, custodial, healthcare support, and gig economy (e.g., ride-share and grocery delivery) jobs (US Bureau of Labor Statistics 2018). Many of these jobs cannot be performed remotely and require close, direct contact with clients, customers, or coworkers and left black workers disproportionately vulnerable to COVID-19 exposure, which likely increased their risk of contracting and dying from the disease (Rogers et al. 2020). As states implemented stay-at-home orders and business restrictions, many service occupations were deemed essential and did not suspend operations; some even increased their business. Many traveled to and from these jobs as either a passenger on or an employee of public transportation systems, which added another potential point of exposure (Dwyer 2020).

During widespread uncertainty about the prevalence of this respiratory pathogen or effective mitigation strategies, these employees were expected to risk their own health to not only ensure societal stability in some instances but also support the comfort and consumerist conveniences of their fellow citizens. For many, taking this risk was not a choice. Workers who were unwilling to make this sacrifice during a time when so many others had either permanently or temporarily lost their jobs learned that essential workers were, in fact, disposable. The volatility of employment in this sector likely disincentivized employees who were symptomatic from reporting COVID-19 symptoms or potential exposure. Moreover, many of these workers risked spreading the virus to others and caused outbreaks because they could not afford to get precautionary testing or engage in extended quarantines and risk being replaced, especially if they were asymptomatic. Having to work in these circumstances placed many black workers, especially those who had other health conditions, at risk of being disproportionately impacted by COVID-19.

As businesses and restaurants continue to reopen, many states have assumed that essential workers are not returning to the workforce because of pandemic-related enhanced unemployment benefits rather than because of health concerns and trauma. Essential workers, particularly black essential workers, personally witnessed the dire repercussions of COVID-19. A study found that in California, black retail workers experienced a 36 percent increase of mortality in 2020 (from March to October) that can be attributed to the COVID-19 pandemic (Chen et al. 2021).

Neighborhood and Environmental Factors

The health risks for black Americans do not end at work, as many went back to homes and neighborhoods, shaped by racialized contexts, that bolstered the threat of contact with COVID-19 and amplified the illnesses that exacerbate COVID-19's effects. Since many of the early pandemic mitigation strategies were based on the assumption that people would be safer at home, it is important to reflect on how and why black Americans live in homes and neighborhoods that do not necessarily decrease their susceptibility to COVID-19 or the comorbid illnesses that worsen its effects. To begin, inequitable social and economic systems make black people more likely to live in multigenerational, multifamily, and overcrowded congregate living situations or public housing, irrespective of income and urbanicity (Marquez-Velarde 2020). Living in these circumstances during a highly communicable, respiratory pandemic obviously can facilitate widespread contagion among older people and those with preexisting conditions.

Once outside of their homes, black Americans face disparately unhealthy outcomes in their neighborhood contexts through at least two primary methods. First, many black people who live in racially and economically segregated areas have insufficient access to mechanisms that support overall health and well-being (White and Borrell 2011). Second, they often live in settings with higher exposure to hazardous pollutants that have also been linked to many of the wide-ranging health problems that predispose people to poor COVID-19 outcomes (Bullard 2007; Winkler and Flowers 2017; Bullard 1994). Explicitly, neighborhood design and environment contribute to disparate rates of preexisting conditions and, subsequently, disparities in COVID-19 outcomes.

Neighborhood-level variation in supports and barriers affects the health of residents. For instance, those who live in safe areas with features that promote physical activity—such as sidewalks, bike lanes, and green spaces—have more opportunities to walk to their destinations (Casagrande et al. 2011). Additionally, having access to businesses that carry nutritious and affordable food is an important part of ensuring healthy neighborhoods (Cooksey Stowers et al. 2020). Regularly participating in active transportation or exercise and having access to healthy food can decrease the likelihood of developing cardiovascular disease, hypertension, diabetes, obesity, and neurological conditions. However, structural systems that determine resource allocations and business locations have constrained black proximity to activity spaces and inexpensive grocery stores. Instead, black neighborhoods contain more fast food and convenience stores and fewer supermarkets than white neighborhoods of similar socioeconomic status (Singleton, Affuso, and Sen 2016; Powell et al. 2007). Those who live in these areas experience the corresponding health burden (Kelli et al. 2017).

Even when black people live in adequately resourced neighborhoods, they are disproportionately exposed to environmental hazards that are beyond their control. For instance, black people tend to live in areas with greater air pollution than whites, even though white consumerism and travel cause more of this contamination (Tessum et al. 2019; Mikati et al. 2018). Black people in urban communities encounter compounded pollutants from cars, bus stations, and airports as well as from factories and toxic waste disposal plants. Those living in rural areas might avoid toxins from massive transportation corridors, but they may live close to or work at heavy polluters such as large farms, meat producers, manufacturers, and chemical and solid waste disposal sites. Notably, this is not simply a matter of public infrastructure and businesses arbitrarily depositing their waste in neighborhoods that lack resources (Winkler and Flowers 2017). Entities that contribute to large-scale environmental pollution are more likely to be located in areas that expose black people and other minority populations, even after controlling for neighborhood socioeconomic factors (Mohai et al. 2009).

There is substantial evidence that, even at low levels, exposure to ambient air pollution and other toxins contributes to higher rates of cardiovascular disease, cancer, diabetes, hypertension, asthma, and respiratory disease (Papadogeorgou et al. 2019; Brender, Maantay, and Chakraborty 2011; Ruiz et al. 2018). Thus, many of the same illnesses that are linked to environmental hazards have been identified as preexisting conditions that predict worse COVID-19 outcomes. Predictably, there is evidence that people who live near higher levels of air pollution have an increased risk of COVID-19 mortality. Specifically, small increases in the amount of exposure to long-term air pollution predicted increased county-level COVID-19 death rates in parts of the United States, even after adjusting for factors on various socioecological levels (Wu et al. 2020). Black Americans' inordinate exposure to contaminants likely puts them at risk of developing the diseases that worsen COVID-19, while also making them more susceptible to COVID-19 morbidity and mortality even if they do not suffer from an underlying medical condition.

Disparities in Vaccine Rollout

In December 2020, the Food and Drug Administration provided emergency use authorization for two vaccines, commonly known as the Moderna and Pfizer COVID-19 vaccines (US Food and Drug Administration 2020). Like at the onset of COVID-19 earlier in the year, the vaccine rollout bore the weight of overarching narratives that specifically affected black Americans. The first narrative, was that black people would not get the COVID-19 vaccine because of *vaccine hesitancy*, which refers to "delay in acceptance or refusal of vaccination despite availability of vaccination services" (MacDonald 2015, 4163). The second narrative was that everyone had an equal likelihood of accessing the COVID-19 vaccines. The realities of these narratives are much more complex.

When vaccines became available in December 2020, polls revealed that if available, 39 percent of black adults wanted to delay vaccination, while 9 percent said that they would refuse the vaccine if available (Kaiser Family Foundation 2021). In comparison to other groups, black adults had the highest vaccine hesitancy. These findings of black people's vaccine hesitancy were met with equal parts urgency to understand black people's mistrust of the government and health systems and dismissal of their concerns. Some of the most common concerns of black Americans included the perception that the vaccine was experimental and not sufficiently tested, discomfort with large-scale vaccination sites (as opposed to a doctor's office), prior discrimination in healthcare settings, and a mistrust of government health initiatives based upon a history of medical experimentation and mistreatment (Shah et al. 2021). Interestingly, upon closer inspection, those same polls revealed that, were a dose available, 36 percent of white adults wanted to delay vaccination, while 15 percent said that they would refuse the vaccine if available (Kaiser Family Foundation 2021). Despite the similarly low enthusiasm for the COVID-19 vaccine in December across races, the public-health activities at that time were focused on *educating* black people about the vaccine while *vaccinating* white people.

This leads to the second narrative around vaccines: access. The initial rollout was determined by each state. Most states loosely followed the CDC's vaccine priority tiers and phases (Dooling et al. 2020). With this structure, healthcare personnel and long-term care facility residents were given first access to the vaccine across most states. Some states quickly realized that an age priority for residents who were 75 and over, as recommended by the CDC, created a racial equity issue and reduced the age requirement in the second tier to 65 years. People of color in the United States skew younger than white people; moreover, black life expectancy in 2019 was 74.7 years in comparison to white life expectancy of 78.8 years (Arias, Tejada-Vera, and Ahmad 2021). The priority age group recommended by the CDC extended beyond the life expectancy of black Americans, further delaying this population access to the vaccine.

As demand for the vaccine grew beyond the supply, priority status to the vaccine became politicized. Essential workers who were initially included in the second tier were pushed further and further down the priority list for vaccines, while occupations that typically have low black representation (such as teachers) were moved higher on the list (Watson 2021). As executed, the vaccine rollout prioritized people who *interacted* with people at greatest risk for COVID-19 infection rather than those who were actually at greatest risk themselves.

As supply increased and could theoretically meet demand, President Biden approved the vaccine to all residents sixteen years and older in mid-April 2021. After a quick surge from those who were high in vaccine enthusiasm, once again, the issues of hesitancy and access came to the forefront. Disaggregated data on vaccine enthusiasm collected in May 2021 revealed that refusal sentiments were highest among white adults (15 percent), Republicans (27 percent), and those living in rural communities (24 percent). Whereas vaccine refusal remained consistent for these populations, vaccine refusal sentiments fell from 10 percent in December 2020 to 6 percent in May 2021. Although the desire to delay vaccination remained highest for black Americans, the percentage polled fell to 22 percent (Kaiser Family Foundation 2021).

As of June 2021, black Americans had the lowest vaccination rates of any racial or ethnic group (Centers for Disease Control and Prevention 2021b).

Rather than focusing on why black people who are unvaccinated have not been vaccinated, some polls asked why they will eventually get vaccinated (Shah et al. 2021). For the most part, the reasons were family focused: protecting family members or keeping children from losing a parent to COVID-19, as well as wanting to safely return to family celebrations. The COVID-19 pandemic as a whole—and specifically the vaccine rollout—has crystallized the need for racial equity in health implementation strategies and health communications.

Health Communication

While health communications about the risks of COVID-19 have been effective among older adult Americans, there are multiple issues with communication and messaging among other age groups. There has been communication about who is at greatest risk of COVID-19-related hospitalizations and death—specifically in consideration of age (people of 65 years and above). As noted earlier, for black Americans, risk for adverse outcomes related to COVID-19 is rather high across adulthood. Additionally, the heavy communication about high-risk age groups has implied that young adults and children have no or negligible risk for COVID-19-related morbidity and mortality. The consequences of being told throughout the pandemic that young adults are not at risk can be seen in the low vaccine uptake among young adults as well as in the reluctance of black parents (30 percent refusal, 22 percent unsure) to vaccinate their children (Shah et al. 2021).

Health communication strategies must remain nimble to manage evolving recommendations. The confusion around sometimes contradictory COVID-19 health guidelines provides opportunities for misinformation to thrive. For example, some social media misinformation campaigns will distort contemporary and historical racial health disparities, social justice initiatives, and medical experimentation to dissuade black people from getting the COVID-19 vaccine (Stone 2021). Often by deceiving respected scholars into providing interviews and statements, these antivaccine strategies specifically target black Americans by acknowledging structural racism while also discouraging black people from seeking healthcare. Improving health communication that specifically addresses the concerns of black Americans is among our recommendations.

Recommendations and Conclusions

Respect Black Patient Advocacy. The prevalence and death disparities related to COVID-19 closely mimic the outcomes of most racial health disparities in America—that is, they strongly evidence systemic racism. For example, early in the pandemic, black people in Detroit and Chicago reported that their family members were denied testing or sent home from hospitals prematurely—and died shortly thereafter (Eligon and Burch 2020). These narratives echoed the stories of black women whose perinatal concerns were ignored, resulting in infant and maternal deaths or severe morbidity (Cottom 2018; Martin and Montagne 2017; Scott, Britton, and McLemore 2019). Black patient advocacy is often ignored or seen as threatening because black patients and their family's composure can take precedence over the urgency of their health needs.

Disaggregate the Data. It is necessary to emphasize the importance of disaggregating data in order to better understand the prevalence, treatment, and consequences of COVID-19. Broad generalizations do not capture the severity of risk and the depth of protection for black Americans overall, nor do they do so for intersectional identities. As discussed in this chapter, age was seen as a key indicator for complications and deaths related to COVID-19, yet disaggregated data revealed increased hospitalization rates for black Americans in young and middle adulthood (Centers for Disease Control and Prevention 2021a).

At the beginning of the pandemic, the Centers for Disease Control and Prevention found that the COVID-19 hospitalization rates for black people were higher across the lifespan than for white people (Centers for Disease Control and Prevention 2020). Black children, adults 18–49 years old, and adults 50–64 years old had hospitalization rates that were 5.1, 5.4, and 4.7 times higher, respectively, than for similarly aged white people. As of June 2021, age adjusted hospitalization rates for black Americans were 2.9 times higher than for white Americans (Centers for Disease Control and Prevention 2021a). In the 2020–2021 winter, a major surge point of the pandemic, black adults over 65 years had the greatest hospitalization rate ratio of any group of 1,168.2 per 100,000, which was 3.4 times higher than for older white adults. In sum, without disaggregated data, prevention efforts and treatment of COVID-19 would ignore the vulnerabilities of younger black people and make the concerns of older black adults invisible, even though they still face an outsized health burden.

Children, Native Americans, and the Latinx Community. Although African Americans had the highest COVID-19 mortality rates at the beginning of the outbreak in the United States, the prevalence of the disease and hospitalization rates among Latinx people rose at an alarming rate (Centers for Disease Control and Prevention 2020; APM Research Lab 2020, 2021). As of March 2, 2021, the cumulative age adjusted mortality rates for Latinos and Native Americans were 2.4 and 3.3 times higher, respectively, than for white Americans. Prior to March 2, 2021, the cumulative age adjusted mortality rates for Latinos and Native Americans were 3.2 and 3.1 times higher, respectively, than for white Americans (APM Research Lab 2020, 2021). Thus, the age adjusted mortality rates for Latinos went down compared to that of white Americans, whereas the age adjusted mortality rates for Native Americans increased compared to that of white Americans. Native Americans have the highest COVID-19 mortality rate among all racial or ethnic groups (APM Research Lab 2021).

For reasons that are not clearly understood, children are generally spared from the most severe illness associated with COVID-19. This has been the overarching reason why many schools reopened in fall 2020. In September 2020, the CDC revealed that although children under twenty-one years old accounted for less than 1 percent of all COVID-19 deaths, 45 percent were Latinx, and 29 percent were black (Bixler et al. 2020). The fact that one-quarter of these children had no underlying health condition, and that roughly half had either obesity or asthma, should raise alarms about the vulnerability of black and Latinx children to COVID-19. As noted above, obesity and asthma are noted for their association with environmental racism in adults, and children are not immune to their effects. As of June 2021, white children aged 0–4 years old have had the highest percentage of COVID-19 deaths (50 percent), whereas Hispanic and black children aged 0–4 years old have experienced the second and third most COVID-19 deaths at 24 percent and 18 percent, respectively. This trend remains the same for ages 5–17 years old. Black children are overrepresented in their share of COVID-19-related deaths in comparison to their population.

It should be noted that the onset of the Omicron variant in winter 2021–2022 saw a surge of COVID-19-related pediatric hospitalizations, with a particularly large increase among children who were four years old and younger and who were ineligible for COVID-19 vaccination at the time. Early data that are not disaggregated by race show that COVID-19 hospitalizations for children four years old and younger went from a low case count of four in mid-June 2021 to a case count of 239 in early January 2022 (Centers for Disease Control and Prevention, 2022).

Community Partnerships. Evidence shows that community partnerships with universities in the vaccine rollout have been effective at getting black Americans and Latinos vaccinated. Trusted community health and faith organizations as well as state and local governments joined forces with universities to provide free COVID-19 testing, resources for care, free ride shares to services, space, and COVID-19 vaccinations regardless of immigration or insurance status. A breakthrough in vaccination efforts in Philadelphia occurred through the Black Doctors Consortium at the University of Pennsylvania, led by Dr. Ala Stanford. Expanding on their successful COVID-19 testing strategies, the Consortium brought the COVID-19 vaccine to black and other underserved communities by having round-the-clock availability; engaging with neighborhood block captains, churches, and community organizations; and utilizing mobile testing and vaccination sites (Jaklevic 2021; Marrett 2021). Moving forward, the question is how do university and government health systems maintain these community partnerships so that they are mutually beneficial, shared collaborations and so they can spark innovation in eliminating health disparities and their underlying causes?

Eliminate Systemic Racism. A 2017 report, "Discrimination in America: Experiences and Views of African Americans," found that 32 percent of the African Americans in the study stated that they had been discriminated in healthcare settings, and 22 percent avoided medical care out of fear of discrimination (National Public Radio, Robert Wood Johnson Foundation, and Harvard T. H. Chan School of Public Health 2017). The healthcare system has a discrimination problem that extends beyond interpersonal dynamics. If these problems were truly about an individual provider or healthcare worker that treats black patients poorly, then eliminating or retraining these individuals would end these disparities in care. Yet, these individuals persist within healthcare systems because their perceived talent or status is seen as having greater value than the health of the black people they serve. We must address systems where accountability and blame for outcomes are not balanced between institutions and patients.

Ultimately, we must decide that the health disparities that allow COVID-19 to proliferate among black Americans is both unacceptable and actionable. Public-health initiatives must balance campaigns that address individual behavior with those that eliminate institutionalized racism. The more than 825,000 lives lost in the United States at 2021's end because of COVID-19 is truly unconscionable. But we must also recognize that in the first year and a half of the pandemic, if black Americans died of COVID-19 at the same rate as white Americans, more than forty-four thousand black people would still be alive (APM Research Lab 2020; Centers for Disease Control and Prevention 2021c).

NOTE

1. For a well-developed framework on the impact of racism on health outcomes, see the work of Williams and Mohammed (2013b, 2013a).

REFERENCES

APM Research Lab. 2020. *The Color of Coronavirus: COVID-19 Deaths by Race and Ethnicity in the US.* October 15. https://www.apmresearchlab.org/covid/deaths-by-race.

APM Research Lab. 2021. *The Color of Coronavirus: COVID-19 Deaths by Race and Ethnicity in the US.* March 5. https://www.apmresearchlab.org/covid/deaths-by-race.

Arias, Elizabeth, Betzaida Tejada-Vera, and Farida Ahmad. 2021. *Provisional Life Expectancy Estimates for January through June, 2020.* National Center for Health Statistics, Centers for Disease Control and Prevention. February. https://dx.doi.org/10.15620/cdc:100392.

Benjamin, Emelia J., Paul Muntner, Alvaro Alonso, Marcio S. Bittencourt, Clifton W. Callaway, April P. Carson, Alanna M. Chamberlain et al. 2019. "Heart Disease and Stroke Statistics—2019 Update: A Report from the American Heart Association." *Circulation* 139, no. 10: e56–e528. https://doi.org/doi:10.1161/CIR.0000000000000659.

Bixler, Danae, Allison D. Miller, Claire P. Mattison, Burnestine Taylor, Kenneth Komatsu, Xandy Peterson Pompa, Steve Moon et al. 2020. "SARS-CoV-2–Associated Deaths Among Persons Aged <21 Years—United States, February 12–July 31, 2020." *Morbidity and Mortality Weekly Report (MMWR)* 69, no. 37 (September 18): 1324–29. https://doi.org/10.15585/mmwr.mm6937e4.

Brender, Jean D., Juliana A. Maantay, and Jayajit Chakraborty. 2011. "Residential Proximity to Environmental Hazards and Adverse Health Outcomes." *American Journal of Public Health* 101, no. S1 (December): S37–S52. https://doi.org/10.2105/AJPH.2011.300183.

Brundage, Vernon, Jr. 2020. *Labor Market Activity of Blacks in the United States.* Division of Labor Force Statistics, US Bureau of Labor Statistics. https://www.bls.gov/spotlight/2020/african-american-history-month/home.htm.

Bullard, Robert D. 1994. *Unequal Protection: Environmental Justice and Communities of Color.* San Francisco: Sierra Club Books.

Bullard, Robert D. 2007. *The Black Metropolis in the Twenty-First Century: Race, Power, and Politics of Place.* Lanham: Rowman and Littlefield.

Carter, Chelsea, and Ezelle Sandford III. 2020. "The Myth of Black Immunity: Racialized Disease during the COVID-19 Pandemic." *Black Perspectives* (blog), African American Intellectual History Society. April 3. https://www.aaihs.org/racializeddiseaseandpandemic/.

Casagrande, Sarah Stark, Joel Gittelsohn, Alan B. Zonderman, Michele K. Evans, and Tiffany L. Gary-Webb. 2011. "Association of Walkability with Obesity in Baltimore City, Maryland." *American Journal of Public Health* 101, no. S1 (December): S318–S324. https://doi.org/10.2105/ajph.2009.187492.

Centers for Disease Control and Prevention (CDC). 2020. *COVID View: A Weekly Surveillance Summary of US COVID-19 Activity.* https://www.cdc.gov/coronavirus/2019-ncov/cases-updates/cases-in-us.html.

Centers for Disease Control and Prevention (CDC). 2021a. *COVID-NET: COVID-19-Associated Hospitalization Surveillance Network.* June 25. https://gis.cdc.gov/grasp/COVIDNet/COVID19_5.html.

Centers for Disease Control and Prevention (CDC). 2021b. *Demographic Characteristics of People Receiving COVID-19 Vaccinations in the United States.* COVID Data Tracker. https://covid.cdc.gov/covid-data-tracker/#vaccination-demographic.

Centers for Disease Control and Prevention (CDC). 2021c. *Health Disparities: Provisional Death Counts for Coronavirus Disease 2019 (COVID-19).* https://www.cdc.gov/nchs/nvss /vsrr/covid19/health_disparities.htm.

Centers for Disease Control and Prevention (CDC). 2022. *COVID-NET: Covid-19-Associated Hospitalization Surveillance Network.* February 3. https://gis.cdc.gov/grasp/COVIDNet /COVID19_5.html.

Chen, Yea-Hung, Maria Glymour, Alicia Riley, John Balmes, Kate Duchowny, Robert Harrison, Ellicott Matthay, and Kirsten Bibbins-Domingo. 2021. "Excess Mortality Associated with the COVID-19 Pandemic among Californians 18–65 Years of Age, by Occupational Sector and Occupation: March through November 2020." *PLOS ONE* 16, no. 6 (June): e0252454. https://doi.org/10.1371/journal.pone.0252454.

Colen, Cynthia G., David M. Ramey, Elizabeth C. Cooksey, and David R. Williams. 2018. "Racial Disparities in Health among Nonpoor African Americans and Hispanics: The Role of Acute and Chronic Discrimination." *Social Science and Medicine* 199: 167–80.

Cooksey Stowers, Kristen, Qianxia Jiang, Abiodun T. Atoloye, Sean Lucan, and Kim Gans. 2020. "Racial Differences in Perceived Food Swamp and Food Desert Exposure and Disparities in Self-Reported Dietary Habits." *International Journal of Environmental Research and Public Health* 17, no. 19: 7143. https://doi.org/10.3390/ijerph17197143.

Cottom, Tressie McMillan. 2018. *Thick and Other Essays.* New York: New Press.

Dooling, Kathleen, Mona Marin, Megan Wallace, Nancy McClung, Mary Chamberland, Grace Lee, Keipp Talbot, José Romero, Beth Bell, and Sara Oliver. 2020. *The Advisory Committee on Immunization Practices' Updated Interim Recommendation for Allocation of COVID-19 Vaccine—United States, December 2020.* Centers for Disease Control and Prevention, Atlanta, GA. https://doi.org/10.15585/mmwr.mm695152e2.

Dwyer, Colin. 2020. "'Take This Serious': Bus Driver Dies of COVID-19 after Calling Out Coughing Rider." National Public Radio. April 3. https://www.npr.org/sections /coronavirus-live-updates/2020/04/03/826817866/take-this-serious-bus-driver-dies-of -covid-19-after-calling-out-coughing-rider.

Eligon, John, and Audra D. S. Burch. 2020. "Questions of Bias in COVID-19 Treatment Add to the Mourning for Black Families." *New York Times*, May 11. https://nyti.ms /2xPIo4Z.

Garfield, Rachel, and Jennifer Tolbert. 2020. *What We Do and Don't Know about Recent Trends in Health Insurance Coverage in the US.* KFF (Kaiser Family Foundation). https:// www.kff.org/policy-watch/what-we-do-and-dont-know-about-recent-trends-in-health -insurance-coverage-in-the-us/.

Groeger, Lena V. 2020. "What Coronavirus Job Losses Reveal about Racism in America." ProPublica. July 20. https://projects.propublica.org/coronavirus-unemployment/.

Jaklevic, Mary Chris. 2021. "Surgeon Fills COVID-19 Testing Gap in Philadelphia's Black Neighborhoods." *JAMA* 325, no. 1: 14–16. https://doi.org/10.1001/jama.2020.22796.

Jolly, Stacey, Eric Vittinghoff, Arpita Chattopadhyay, and Kirsten Bibbins-Domingo. 2010. "Higher Cardiovascular Disease Prevalence and Mortality among Younger

Blacks Compared to Whites." *American Journal of Medicine* 123, no. 9: 811–18. https://doi.org/10.1016/j.amjmed.2010.04.020.

Kaiser Family Foundation. 2021. KFF COVID-19 Vaccine Monitor. https://www.kff.org/coronavirus-covid-19/dashboard/kff-covid-19-vaccine-monitor-dashboard/.

Kelli, Heval M., Muhammad Hammadah, Hina Ahmed, Yi-An Ko, Matthew Topel, Ayman Samman-Tahhan, Mossab Awad, Keyur Patel, Kareem Mohammed, and Laurence S Sperling. 2017. "Association between Living in Food Deserts and Cardiovascular Risk." *Circulation: Cardiovascular Quality and Outcomes* 10, no. 9: e003532.

MacDonald, Noni E. 2015. "Vaccine Hesitancy: Definition, Scope and Determinants." *Vaccine* 33, no. 34: 4161–64. https://doi.org/10.1016/j.vaccine.2015.04.036.

Marquez-Velarde, Guadalupe. 2020. "Multigenerational Households: A Descriptive Approach to Distinctive Definitions." In *International Handbook on the Demography of Marriage and the Family*, edited by D. Nicole Farris and A. J. H. Borque, 215–25. New York: Springer.

Marrett, Cora B. 2021. "Racial Disparities and COVID-19: the Social Context." *Journal of Racial and Ethnic Health Disparities* 8, no. 3: 794–97. https://doi.org/10.1007/s40615-021-00988-8.

Martin, Nina, and Renee Montagne. 2017. "The Last Person You'd Expect to Die in Childbirth." ProPublica. May 12. https://www.propublica.org/article/die-in-childbirth-maternal-death-rate-health-care-system.

Mazurek, Jacek M., and Girija Syamlal. 2018. "Prevalence of Asthma, Asthma Attacks, and Emergency Department Visits for Asthma among Working Adults—National Health Interview Survey, 2011–2016." *Morbidity and Mortality Weekly Report* 67, no. 13: 377–86. https://doi.org/10.15585/mmwr.mm6713a1.

Mikati, Ihab, Adam F. Benson, Thomas J. Luben, Jason D. Sacks, and Jennifer Richmond-Bryant. 2018. "Disparities in Distribution of Particulate Matter Emission Sources by Race and Poverty Status." *American Journal of Public Health* 108, no. 4: 480–85.

Mohai, Paul, Paula M. Lantz, Jeffrey Morenoff, James S. House, and Richard P. Mero. 2009. "Racial and Socioeconomic Disparities in Residential Proximity to Polluting Industrial Facilities: Evidence from the Americans' Changing Lives Study." *American Journal of Public Health* 99, no. S3: S649–S656.

National Public Radio, Robert Wood Johnson Foundation, and Harvard T. H. Chan School of Public Health. 2017. *Discrimination in America: Experiences and Views of African Americans.* https://www.rwjf.org/en/library/research/2017/10/discrimination-in-america—experiences-and-views.html.

Papadogeorgou, Georgia, Marianthi-Anna Kioumourtzoglou, Danielle Braun, and Antonella Zanobetti. 2019. "Low Levels of Air Pollution and Health: Effect Estimates, Methodological Challenges, and Future Directions." *Current Environmental Health Reports* 6, no. 3: 105–15.

Powell, Lisa M., Sandy Slater, Donka Mirtcheva, Yanjun Bao, and Frank J. Chaloupka. 2007. "Food Store Availability and Neighborhood Characteristics in the United States." *Preventive Medicine* 44, no. 3: 189–95.

Rogers, Tiana N., Charles R. Rogers, Elizabeth VanSant-Webb, Lily Y. Gu, Bin Yan, and Fares Qeadan. 2020. "Racial Disparities in COVID-19 Mortality among Essential Work-

ers in the United States." *World Medical and Health Policy* 12, no. 3: 311–27. https://doi
.org/10.1002/wmh3.358.

Ruiz, Daniel, Marisol Becerra, Jyotsna S. Jagai, Kerry Ard, and Robert M. Sargis. 2018.
"Disparities in Environmental Exposures to Endocrine-Disrupting Chemicals and
Diabetes Risk in Vulnerable Populations." *Diabetes Care* 41, no. 1: 193–205.

Scott, Karen A., Laura Britton, and Monica R. McLemore. 2019. "The Ethics of Perinatal
Care for Black Women: Dismantling the Structural Racism in 'Mother Blame' Narratives." *Journal of Perinatal and Neonatal Nursing* 33, no. 2: 108–15. https://doi.org/10
.1097/jpn.0000000000000394.

Shah, Arnav, Eric C. Schneider, Laurie Zephyrin, Ray Block Barreto, Gabriel R. Sanchez,
and Henry Fernandez. 2021. *What Do Americans Think about Getting Vaccinated against
COVID-19?* African American Research Collaborative, Commonwealth Fund. June 16.
https://www.commonwealthfund.org/publications/2021/jun/what-do-americans-think
-about-getting-vaccinated-against-covid-19.

Singleton, Chelsea R., Olivia Affuso, and Bisakha Sen. 2016. "Decomposing Racial
Disparities in Obesity Prevalence: Variations in Retail Food Environment." *American
Journal of Preventive Medicine* 50, no. 3: 365–72.

Smith, Imari Z., Keisha L. Bentley-Edwards, Salimah El-Amin, and William Darity Jr.
2018. "Fighting at Birth: Eradicating the Black-White Infant Mortality Gap." Durham,
NC: Samuel DuBois Cook Center on Social Equity and Insight Center on Community
Economic Development. http://socialequity.duke.edu/sites/socialequity.duke.edu/files
/site-images/EradicatingBlackInfantMortality-March2018-DRAFT4.pdf.

Stone, Will. 2021. "Untangling Disinformation: An Anti-vaccine Film Targeted to Black
Americans Spreads False Information." *All Things Considered*. National Public Radio.
June 8. https://www.npr.org/sections/health-shots/2021/06/08/1004214189/anti
-vaccine-film-targeted-to-black-americans-spreads-false-information.

Tessum, Christopher W., Joshua S. Apte, Andrew L. Goodkind, Nicholas Z. Muller,
Kimberley A. Mullins, David A. Paolella, Stephen Polasky, Nathaniel P. Springer,
Sumil K. Thakrar, and Julian D. Marshall. 2019. "Inequity in Consumption of Goods
and Services Adds to Racial–Ethnic Disparities in Air Pollution Exposure." *Proceedings of the National Academy of Sciences* 116, no. 13: 6001–6.

US Bureau of Labor Statistics. 2018. *Employed Persons by Detailed Industry, Sex, Race, and
Hispanic or Latino Ethnicity.* https://www.bls.gov/cps/cpsaat18.htm.

US Food and Drug Administration. 2020. "Coronavirus (COVID-19) Update: December 17, 2020." https://www.fda.gov/news-events/press-announcements/coronavirus
-covid-19-update-december-17-2020.

Watson, Kathryn. 2021. "Biden Says Teachers and Support Staff Should Move Up on
Vaccine Priority List." *CBS News*. February 17. https://www.cbsnews.com/news/biden
-covid-vaccine-teachers-schools/.

White, Kellee, and Luisa N. Borrell. 2011. "Racial/Ethnic Residential Segregation:
Framing the Context of Health Risk and Health Disparities." *Health and Place* 17, no. 2:
438–48. https://doi.org/10.1016/j.healthplace.2010.12.002. https://www.ncbi.nlm.nih
.gov/pmc/articles/PMC3056936.

Williams, David R., and Selina A. Mohammed. 2013a. "Racism and Health I: Pathways and Scientific Evidence." *American Behavioral Scientist* 57, no. 8: 10.1177/0002764213487340. https://doi.org/10.1177/0002764213487340. http://www.ncbi.nlm.nih.gov/pmc/articles/PMC3863357/.

Williams, David R., and Selina A. Mohammed. 2013b. "Racism and Health II: A Needed Research Agenda for Effective Interventions." *American Behavioral Scientist* 57, no. 8: 1200–26. https://doi.org/10.1177/0002764213487341.

Williams, David R., Naomi Priest, and Norman B Anderson. 2016. "Understanding Associations among Race, Socioeconomic Status, and Health: Patterns and Prospects." *Health Psychology* 35, no. 4: 407–11.

Winkler, Inga T., and Catherine Coleman Flowers. 2017. "America's Dirty Secret: The Human Right to Sanitation in Alabama's Black Belt." *Columbia Human Rights Law Review* 49, no. 1: 181–228.

Wu, Xiao, Rachel C. Nethery, Benjamin M. Sabath, Danielle Braun, and Francesca Dominici. 2020. "Exposure to Air Pollution and COVID-19 Mortality in the United States." *medRxiv* (April). https://www.medrxiv.org/content/medrxiv/early/2020/04/27/2020.04.05.20054502.full.pdf.

Yancy, Clyde W. 2020. "COVID-19 and African Americans." *JAMA* 323, no. 19: 1891–92. https://doi.org/10.1001/jama.2020.6548.

Yudell, Michael, Dorothy Roberts, Rob Desalle, and Sarah Tishkoff. 2016. "Taking Race out of Human Genetics." *Science* 351, no. 6273: 564–65. https://doi.org/10.1126/science.aac4951.

2. Labor History and Pandemic Response: The Overlapping Experiences of Work, Housing, and Neighborhood Conditions

JOE WILLIAM TROTTER JR.

The initial onset of the COVID-19 pandemic produced disturbing comments that black Americans were not being severely affected by the disease or that they were less likely to be infected; however, evidence of alarming racial disparities swiftly demolished the foundation of such notions (Charles 2020; Walsh 2020). The emerging racial profile of the pandemic also called attention to the need for more knowledge of health inequality in historical perspective—one that not only uncovers the roots of contemporary health disparities in the past but also reveals how poor and working-class black people forged paths toward their own recovery and survival. Accordingly, this chapter provides a historical backdrop for understanding the unequal class and racial impact of COVID-19 and responses by black Americans.

Focusing on the overlapping experiences of work, housing, and living conditions, this chapter examines the life and labor experiences of poor and working-class blacks in America from the advent of the transatlantic slave trade to the early twenty-first century. Beginning with the preindustrial world of southern agriculture, it charts certain continuities and changes in the African American experience during the industrial era and its subsequent demise as the new digital age got underway. While this chapter emphasizes how debilitating work and living conditions repeatedly exposed black Americans to disproportionately high rates of disease and deaths, it also discusses the strategies that black people devised to address the challenges of their own lives under shifting historical conditions.

Enslavement

Some fifteen million African people arrived in the Americas during the transatlantic slave trade. An estimated half million of the enslaved Africans disembarked in North America. After surviving the horrors of the Middle Passage, they confronted dreadful work routines and health and living conditions on American soil. In colonial North America, Europeans quickly turned to enslaved African labor to produce a variety of staple crops for international markets. The labor requirements of staple production varied from crop to crop, but the work regimen in sugar, rice, tobacco, and cotton took a huge toll on the health and lives of African people (Berlin 2010, 14–15; Smallwood 2007; Byrd 2008; Rediker 2007).

In the Chesapeake region, enslaved workers cultivated the delicate tobacco crop, which required both strenuous labor and meticulous care. The planter John Carter described tobacco as "a very tender plant" that acquired a much-deserved reputation as "a plant of perpetual trouble and difficulty." A wide range of circumstances and conditions could destroy the crop—including late planting, the tobacco fly, "worms, disease, [and] weeds, excessive moisture left in the leaves, and too much pressure applied during packing" (Morgan 1998, 169). In early Virginia and Maryland, enslaved Africans worked side by side with white indentured servants. However, as the colonies defined African people as "slaves for life" during the late seventeenth and early eighteenth centuries, the rise of large tobacco plantations tied the Chesapeake region to enslaved African labor, especially in Virginia (Morgan 1998, 1–23, 165–66; Berlin 1998, 29–46, 109–17; Jones 1998, 26–31; Clark et al. 2008, 68–74; Berlin and Morgan 1993, 170–99).

Rising numbers of enslaved African people fueled the Chesapeake's tobacco economy. Production involved a long cultivation cycle that stretched from January through late fall. The new season commenced in January and February, when gangs of enslaved workers, under strict supervision of overseers cleared "new lands or old beds" for planting the tobacco seeds. By early March, workers sowed the seed in the "newly cleared beds of fine mulch." Tobacco plants were "too delicate" for sowing in "unprotected open fields," and as the seedlings made their appearance by April, the work of enslaved people intensified. Thereafter, they tended the small plants until they were ready to be transplanted to the tobacco fields. When a spring or early summer rain occurred, the plants were carefully removed from their beds and transplanted. Blacks worked feverishly to complete the job before the ground dried and destroyed the small seedlings (Walsh and Morgan 1993).

Tobacco entered its peak growing season between June and August. Most new Africans arrived to the Chesapeake region during this period, when the crop demanded consistent hoeing, weeding, and plowing. They faced the difficult chore of harvesting and preparing the plants for market. After cutting stalks to the ground, they transported bundles to well-ventilated tobacco houses, where they hung plants for curing. Once cured, Africans carefully sorted the stalks by quality and then removed the tobacco leaves. Finally, they bound, pressed, and prepared the crop for shipping (Morgan 1998, 166–68). Some planters required that they work at night, often by firelight, but they "rarely received equivalent food, shelter, and medical attention" (Berlin 1998, 116–17).

Cultivating tobacco frequently strained "every nerve" of the bondsmen and bondswomen's bodies, but life and labor was even more difficult in the lower South, where rice production predominated during the colonial era. During the early to mid-eighteenth century, South Carolina moved from a mixed economy of small farming and cattle raising for the West Indian market to an increased dependence on rice production and international trade. Rice produced by en-slaved Africans emerged at the center of the South Carolina Lowcountry econ-omy. One late eighteenth century observer, James Glen, remarked that, "The only Commodity of Consequence produced in *South Carolina is Rice* . . . and they reckon it as much their staple commodity as *sugar* is to *Barbados* and *Jamaica*, or *Tobacco* to *Virginia* and *Maryland*" (Morgan 1998, 147–48). Rice production accounted for 50 to nearly 70 percent of South Carolina's total value of exports during most of the colonial era. According to another eighteenth-century ob-server, "Rice is raised as to buy more negroes, and negroes are bought as to get more rice" (Morgan 1998, 147–49).

African knowledge of rice cultivation, brought from West Africa to New World plantations, as well as their labor played key roles in the success of the Deep South economy. A long and laborious process, rice cultivation took twelve to fourteen months to complete from initial preparations to ship-ment to consumers in international trade networks. French historian Fernand Braudel compared the labor requirements of rice production with a variety of other crops, concluding that "rice holds the record for the man handling it requires." For his part, in his popular poem, *Carolina or, The Planter*, George Ogilvie likened the establishment and cultivation of rice plantations to the "rechanneling of the Euphrates and the building of the pyramids" (Berlin 1998; 146; Morgan 1998, 156–57).

In order to construct an extensive network of "banks, canals, ditches, and drains," enslaved people regularly removed some five hundred cubic yards of river swamp for each acre of rice under cultivation. In their advertisements for enslaved workers, South Carolina rice planters were emphatic in seeking labor for the special conditions of rice cultivation. The planter Pierce Butler advertised for "a gang of negroes accustomed to cultivate rice." He made it clear that he wanted "no cotton negroes"; he wanted only "people that can go in the ditch." According to historian Philip D. Morgan, "The rice cycle was the most arduous, the most unhealthy, and the most prolonged of all mainland staples" (Morgan 1998, 149). Rice planters imported 15,000 new Africans between 1734 and 1740, but the black population rose from about 26,000 to only 40,000 during the same period. This pattern resembled the Caribbean where planters often "worked slaves to death," because they could rely on cheap sources of new workers from the transatlantic slave trade. Only at a very slow rate would new births exceed death rates for South Carolinians of African descent (Wood 1974).

A similarly harsh work environment greeted enslaved African people in the sugar producing low country of Louisiana. Nearly two decades after British proprietors established South Carolina under the British Crown, the French claimed possession of the Louisiana Territory. During the 1720s, France initiated an aggressive drive to transform Louisiana into a tobacco-, indigo-, and finally a sugar-growing colony centered on New Orleans and enslaved African labor (Usner Jr. 1979; Usner Jr. 1992, 31–34, 54–56; Hall 1992, 126–27, 179). Early Africans built the levees and drainage ditches along the Mississippi River, cleared forest land and cut and hauled timber for the construction of plantation houses and other buildings, and ultimately constructed and toiled on huge sugar plantations that produced increasing volumes of sugar that greatly enriched slaveholding elites (Usner Jr. 1979, 28).

While enslaved blacks initially produced tobacco and indigo, sugar steadily rose to prominence in the Louisiana economy by the mid-eighteenth century. As early as 1731, more than one thousand Africans labored on some fifty sugar plantations across the river from indigo- and tobacco-growing Chapitoulas, just above the city of New Orleans. The rise of sugar intensified during the late eighteenth century. Between 1796 and 1800 alone, some sixty plantations converted production from tobacco and indigo to sugar. In the wake of the Haitian Revolution, between 1806 and 1810, the slaves of French refugees accounted for 25 percent of the growth of the Orleans Territory's enslaved population, which increased from 27,000 to more than 34,000. By the time the United States acquired the Louisiana Territory from the French, the colony produced more than 4.5 million pounds of sugar, valued at nearly a million dollars. By the mid-nineteenth century, an estimated fifteen hundred sugar plantations had emerged all along the Mississippi River and its bayous. In 1860, the fourteen largest sugar parishes reported 116,000 enslaved people of African descent who produced some "87,000 metric tons of sugar, along with cotton and corn." Sugar, as many commentators declared, "became king in lower Louisiana" (Berlin 1998, 86, 340–41, 343; Baptist 2014, 56; Scott 2005, 12).

From the outset of Louisiana's labor history, enslavement took a huge toll on the lives of African people. Much like the South Carolina rice region, sugar mortality rates were exceedingly high (McDonald 1993, 207; Usner Jr. 1979, 33; Scott 2005, 12). The suffering of overworked, ill, and tortured sugar workers sometimes reached the colony's Superior Council. In 1727, one slaveowner petitioned the council against his overseer "for ruining one of his most valuable slaves" as punishment for the offense of running away. The overseer had tightly bound the runaway's hands and given him "600 rawhide lashes." In the process of administering this extreme punishment, the enslaved man "lost two fingers from his right hand and two fingertips from his left hand." The Superior Council also heard the case of another "brutish overseer" who had regularly raped and tortured slave women "in the open field," withheld essential food provisions, and caused "frequent abortion among the slave women" by severe corporal punishment during pregnancy (Usner Jr. 1979, 38). An estimated 7,000 Africans arrived in Louisiana between 1718 and 1735, but the resident African population stood at only 3,400 in 1735 (Usner Jr. 1979, 33).

Although sugar, rice, and tobacco claimed the bulk of enslaved African labor before the onset of the American Revolution, cotton dominated African American life and labor during the early nineteenth century. More than a million black people not only endured the painful forced migration from the upper to the lower South but were also put to work building the cotton plantations before they could plant, cultivate, and harvest the cotton crop. Enslaved workers carved out the cotton plantation from the earth and wilderness through backbreaking labor of "cutting trees, grubbing out and burning underbrush, constructing cabins, outbuildings, and fences" among a variety of other work ahead of cotton production (Miller 1993, 158; Berlin 1998, 345).

Cotton required extensive plowing, hoeing, and picking. Under the strict supervision of overseers, men, women, and children worked the cotton fields. The slave Charles Ball, sold from the tobacco growing state of Maryland into bondage in the Deep South cotton region, later recalled how cotton labor was more "excessive" and "incessant throughout the year" than tobacco (Reidy 1993, 142; Johnson 2013, 151–53, 156–59, 173–74; Baptist 2014, 128–30, 138–41).

Even as enslaved workers prepared the ground for and planted cotton seed, they also cultivated collateral fields of corn, potatoes, and even sugar cane. On one Georgia plantation, "Frank, Mat, Evans, and Peggy finished planting cotton in a field bordered on one side by a new crop of cane and on the other dryland rice. Frank led the way with his drill, Mat came next 'strew[ing] cotton seed; and Evans and Peggy brought up the rear with their hoes" (O'Donovan 2007, 28–30; see also Reidy 1993, 138–43; and Miller 1993, 155–66).

Cotton production and profits soared. Between 1790 and 1800 alone, for example, South Carolina's annual exports of cotton rose from less than 10,000 pounds to an estimated 6.0 million pounds. In the United States as a whole, cotton production soared from 1.5 million pounds in 1790 (three years ahead of Whitney's cotton gin) to 167.5 million pounds by 1820. By 1860, cotton made in the United States had increased to more than 1,500 million pounds (O'Donovan 2007, 25–32; Reidy 1993, 138–54; Miller 1993, 155–69; Berlin 1998, 307; Baptist 2014, 114; Beckert 2014, 104).

Whether plantations specialized in rice, tobacco, sugar, or cotton, large slave-owners hired overseers to supervise the day-to-day details of the plantation labor force. Overseers, usually poor whites, worked on annual contracts, with an annual income that ranged from as low as $100 to a high of $1,200, plus a house, food, and a slave as a personal servant. In 1853, one overseer signed a contract with significant benefits beyond the salary: "I am to have a woman exclusively devoted to washing and cooking for me, she being the only person belonging to the plantation that I am to give any call or occupation to whatever for any of my household affairs, she never to be a field hand. I am also to be provided with a boy to wait on me and to go to the new ground to cut wood from any logs or stumps for my fire wood" (Scarborough 1984, 25–29).

The "gang" system of labor placed large numbers of workers in one group under close supervision of an overseer or driver. Most overseers and drivers used a narrow strip of tough cowhide, whipcord, or cat-o'-nine-tails, which left deep gashes in the skin. In his pioneering study, *Medicine and Slavery*, historian Todd L. Savitt declared, "From a medical point of view, whipping inflicted cruel and often permanent injuries upon its victims. Laying stripes across the bare back or buttocks caused indescribable pain, especially when each stroke dug deeper into previously opened wounds" (Savitt 1978, 111–12; Baptist 2014, 120–21). More recently, Edward Baptist describes how severe floggings undermined the capacity of people to "speak in sentences or think coherently. They 'danced,' trembled, babbled, [and] lost control of their bodies." Nonetheless, driven by an unquenchable thirst for profits, slaveowners consistently disputed the damage inflicted by the overseer's whip. "Sure, it might etch deep gashes in the skin

of its victim, make them 'tremble' or 'dance' . . . but it did not disable them."
Henry Bibb, an ex-slave on a plantation along the Red River, later recalled
how cotton planters produced large "quantities of cotton" and "extorted" their
wealth "by the lash" (Baptist 2014, 121).

Although male field hands endured the most brutal torture through whip-
pings, women and household workers were not immune. The whipping of slave
women, as historian Deborah Gray White notes, carried sharp "sexual over-
tones." An escaped slave living in Canada, Christopher Nichols, "remembered
how his master laid a woman on a bench, threw her clothes over her head,
and whipped her." Another ex-slave described a whipping where the woman's
naked "quivering" body was "tied up" and put on display for "the public gaze of
all" (White 1985, 33).

Poor housing, improper clothing, and unsanitary living conditions reinforced the health hazards of work environments. Whereas planters, small farmers, and poor whites lived in widely scattered rural households, blacks often
occupied dense three-, ten-, or thirty-family communities. Although planters
clothed their personal servants and household workers in the best garments,
they usually cut costs in dressing the field hands. Inadequate disposal of human
waste and contaminated water also led to epidemics of cholera, dysentery, di-
arrhea, typhoid, and hepatitis as well as influenza, pneumonia, tuberculosis, and diphtheria (Savitt 1978, 49–50, 57–73 [especially 57–58 and 60–61],
80–82, 115–29).

The enslavement of African people was by no means limited to the plantation and farms of the agricultural South. African people also faced enslavement
in colonial and early American cities of the North and South. Moreover, by the
onset of the Civil War, nearly a half million enslaved people had gained their
freedom and moved to cities in rising numbers. Free blacks became the most
urbanized component of the nation's population. Black urbanites, enslaved and
free, lived and labored under even more congested and unsanitary conditions
than their rural brothers and sisters. When one Virginia slave owner moved
his family and enslaved blacks from the farm to a house in town, more than
twenty blacks died as well as a few of his own family members. According to a
report of the man's friend, crowded and unsanitary conditions precipitated the
epidemic: "The lot was small, and back yard so much crowded with outhouses,
and trees, as to exclude the sun almost entirely. The cellars of course must have
been exceedingly damp, and in them the negroes lodged" (Savitt 1978, 80). Specific occupational hazards compounded the medical difficulties of industrial
bondsmen: lung disease afflicted tobacco workers; rock falls, deadly gases, and

explosions injured and killed miners; and hot molten metal burned and damaged the skin and eyes of iron workers (Savitt 1978, 80–82, 106–10, 226–40; Wade 1964, 33–43; Lewis 1979, 154–55; Whitman 1997, 37–39, 48, 53).

African Americans were not solely dependent on slaveowners and their hired doctors for medical treatment. Enslaved people developed their own trusted medicine men and medicine women. Historian Todd Savitt documents the emergence of what he describes as a "dual system" of medical care. Some enslaved people received treatment from both their masters and their own "black practitioners" (Savitt 1978, 149–50). In some cases, European physicians took instructions from enslaved people to help remedy certain ailments. In colonial Louisiana, an African doctor taught one French physician (referred to as Le Page) his "secret cure for yaws and scurvy." Le Page later credited the black doctor with imparting this knowledge, "The negro who taught me those remedies, observing the great care I took of both the negro men and negro women, taught me likewise the cure of all distempers to which the women are subject; for the negro women are as liable to disease as the white women" (Usner Jr. 1979, 33).

Bondsmen and women developed a keen sense of property ownership and insisted on access to their own plots of land. Most plantation owners relented and allowed enslaved people to plant their own gardens and produce subsistence crops for their own use as well as for local markets. Early on, a Virginia colonist declared, "There is no master almost [who] will [not] allow his servant a parcel of clear ground to plant some tobacco for himself." The pattern persisted into the nineteenth century. One South Carolina slave recalled how his owner limited enslaved people's access to interplantation visitations, church building, and literacy, but relented and allotted bondsmen and women acreage to till on their own behalf. He gave every one of his plantation families "so much land to plant for dey garden, and den he give em evey Saturday for day time to tend dat garden" (Schweninger 1990, 13–14, 30–31; Walker 2009, 81–82; Olwell 1998, 149–50).

Enslaved people not only helped themselves through a variety of day-to-day strategies for improving the conditions of their lives. They also helped to forge liberation movements that demolished the institution of slavery itself. Emancipation of some four million people of African descent following the Civil War was partly a product of the self-activities of enslaved black rural and urban people before the Civil War. While slavery itself for black people was much like a persistent COVID-19 type of crisis, they refused to succumb to the brutal impact of enslavement on their lives.

Emancipation

In the wake of the Civil War and emancipation, people of African descent entered a new and more hopeful phase of their history in North America. But their initial feelings of jubilee and liberation were short-lived. In his book *Sick from Freedom*, medical historian Jim Downs describes how the Civil War resulted in the "largest biological crisis" of the nineteenth century United States. It produced enormous suffering on and off the battlefields. Yet, despite the 600,000 casualties in the war zones, emancipated people bore the brunt of the "massive epidemics that plagued" the South following the war. Inadequately clothed, housed, fed, and treated for serious ailments requiring medical attention, freed people struggled daily to survive in a region devastated by physical destruction and disease. From a health perspective, medical scholars W. Michael Byrd and Linda A. Clayton conclude that both Reconstruction and post-Reconstruction eras "were a disaster" for former slaves as "new waves of epidemics [including excessively high rates of tuberculosis], poor health, sickness and death swept through the postwar South" (Downs 2012, 4; Byrd and Clayton 2000, 322).

During the emancipation era, even as black people celebrated their freedom, US military authorities, the Freedmen's Bureau, and state and local governments helped to underwrite a new system of labor coercion that undermined the health and well-being of newly emancipated slaves. Rather than even a modicum of concern with the general health of enslaved people, they focused almost exclusively on what they termed "able bodied" men and "their ability to work" and provide productive labor. As such, they largely neglected the health needs of black women and children, who were perceived as less valuable than workers (Downs 2012, 8).

From the outset of the emancipation years, military officials aided planters to coerce black workers into signing inequitable wage labor contracts, but freedmen and freedwomen resisted these contracts. They embarked upon a relentless quest for their own land. The Virginia freedman Bayley Wyat spoke for many when he declared, "Our wives, our children, our husbands, has been sold over and over again to purchase the lands we now locates on. . . . we has a right to [that] land . . . [D]idn't we clear the land and raise de crops . . . And den didn't dem large cities in de North grow up on de cotton and de sugars and de rice dat we made?" (Hahn 2003, 135).

Despite their firm resolve to gain land, freedom, and independence following the Civil War, their hopes gradually faded under the impact of a new postbellum white supremacist regime. By the turn of the twentieth century, the new segregationist order had not only created a coercive and unequal sharecropping labor system but had also instituted a racially stratified social order—one that placed African Americans at the bottom of the body politic as well as at the bottom of the economy. Legally sanctioned mob violence, injustice before the law, and disfranchisement reinforced the confinement of black people to the land as exploited workers and second-class citizens. Their quest for their own homes and landownership yielded only modest but not insignificant results. By 1890, under 20 percent of African Americans nationwide owned their own land and homes compared to nearly 50 percent for white families. In the South, black landownership peaked between 15 and 20 percent by the onset of World War I. Thereafter, black people saw their property "taxed, taken, stolen, and frittered away" (Jones 1998, 316; US Bureau of the Census 1918, 459; 2011; Schweninger 1990, 182–84).

The Industrial Era

As their hopes for landownership, full citizenship, and social justice faded under the impact of the Jim Crow social order, African Americans embraced urban migration as an alternative to racial apartheid in southern agriculture. Beginning gradually during the late nineteenth century, the Great Migration escalated during World War I and its aftermath. Blacks also moved to a broader range of cities in the West and Midwest than they did during the prewar years. Between World War I and 1930, Detroit's black population increased most dramatically. It rose by more than 600 percent during the war years and another 200 percent during the 1920s, increasing from fewer than 6,000 in 1910 to more than 120,000 in 1920. At the same time, the black population of Los Angeles jumped from fewer than 8,000 to nearly 40,000. Nonetheless, as in the prewar era, New York City, Chicago, and Philadelphia continued to absorb disproportionately large numbers of black newcomers. Chicago's black population increased more than fivefold from 44,000 to 234,000; New York City's trebled from roughly 100,000 to 328,000; and Philadelphia's grew from 84,500 to an estimated 220,600 (Marks 1989; Grossman 1989; Thomas 1992; Trotter Jr. 1991, 1–21).

The Great Migration slowed but did not stop during the Great Depression years of the 1930s. It reignited during World War II and ran its course by the early 1970s. Over the entire period, an estimated eight million black Americans moved from the rural and urban South to the North and West. For the first time in the nation's history, black Americans became a national population spread almost equally over the urban South, North, and West (Gregory 2005, 14–15, 20–27; Wilkerson 2010, 8–15; Berlin 2010, 153–56).

The nation's expanding industrial cities opened up broader and more promising opportunities for African American life and labor than southern agriculture. Southern black workers, especially young men, took jobs at the heart of the modern urban economy. They toiled mightily in the nation's most lucrative extractive and manufacturing firms—including coal mining, the lumber industry, steel, meat-packing, and automobile production, to name only a few. Wages in northern industries ranged from $3.00 to $5.00 per eight-hour day, compared to as little as 75 cents to $1.00 per day in southern agriculture. In southern industries, black Americans earned no more than $2.50 for a nine-hour day. According to a recent study of the Great Migration, even after adjustments for higher costs of living in the industrial cities, southern black workers increased their earnings significantly from a minimum of 56 percent to as much as 130 percent. It is no wonder that they often celebrated their movement into higher wage industrial jobs as a "Flight from Egypt," the "New Jerusalem," and the "Promised Land" (Boustan 2017, 50–54).

Despite optimism and improvements over their lives as southern farm workers on rented land under oppressive conditions, African American workers powered the nation's industrial growth on a segregated and unequal basis. They worked at the bottom of the occupational hierarchy in the most hazardous and unhealthy jobs in the industrial economy. In the steel industry, they manned the blast furnaces and performed the most difficult jobs making rails for the railroads. In the meat packinghouses, rather than gaining significant access to the skilled butcher job, they spent the bulk of their working days on the killing floor, slaughtering livestock, transporting entrails, and cleaning the factory. In the coal mines, they often worked in low coal seams, where they had to crawl on their knees to make their way to the good coal through excessive water, bad air, and rock. As one miner later recalled, "I have been sick and dizzy off of that smoke many times. . . . That deadly poison is there. . . . It would knock you out too, make you weak as water." In the coke ovens of the steel industry, as historian Steven A. Reich describes, "Exposure to extreme heat quickened their heart beat, changed the pitch of their voice, gave them headaches and stomach cramps, and often left them unconscious and in need of hospitalization. . . . Fires burned their clothes, and acid spills scared their skin." These were some of the costs that black workers paid for fueling the industrial machine (Reich 2013, 67–69; Harris 1982; Dickerson 1986; Halpern 1997).

Even more so than the preindustrial age before the Civil War, racial discrimination and segregation extended well beyond the workplace into the neighborhoods, housing, and community life of the industrial city. Between World War I and 1930, the size and number of racially segregated neighborhoods increased—a phenomenon described by some historians as the making of the "first ghetto" (Trotter Jr. 1990, 106). The index of dissimilarity (a statistical tool for measuring segregation, usually by city ward before 1940 and by block thereafter) rose from 67 to 85 percent in Chicago; 61 to 85 percent in Cleveland; 64 to 78 percent in Boston; and from 46 to 63 percent in Philadelphia. In Chicago, well over 35 percent of the city's blacks lived in census tracts that were more than 75 percent black (Taeuber and Taeuber 1965, 119; Massey and Denton 1993, 20–22; Lieberson 1980, 265–67; Nightingale 2012, 307–17)

Several southern cities—including Atlanta, Baltimore, Richmond, Norfolk, and Louisville—entered the war years with housing segregation statutes on the books. Although the US Supreme Court ruled housing segregation laws unconstitutional in 1917, it did little to halt the customary segregation of blacks in the city's housing market (Nieman 1991, 128–29; McGruder 2015, 94, 231–32, n52; Gonda 2015, 4, 134; Nightingale 2012, 306–07).

Residential segregation meant overcrowded, unsanitary, deteriorating, and overpriced housing for African Americans. Landlords, real estate brokers, and financial institutions took advantage of the desperate housing needs of black migrants, forcing them to pay higher rents for housing of substantially less quality than that of their white counterparts. Real estate speculators took over large mansions in older sections of cities, subdivided them into small one- or two-room apartments, and charged exorbitant rents to desperate black tenants. In order to pay rent, tenants took in large numbers of boarders, which led to overcrowding. The Cincinnati Better Housing League reported cases of extreme overcrowding: twenty blacks inhabited one three-room flat, while another twelve-room tenement housed ninety-four blacks. Among urban blacks, heart disease, pneumonia, and tuberculosis (TB) represented the three most common causes of death, but TB was the number one killer of black Americans nationally. As housing and health conditions deteriorated for the urban black population, one public official exclaimed that, "You could not produce a prize hog to show at the fair under conditions that you allow negroes to live in this city" (Fairbanks 1993, 197).[1]

Beginning with the rise of the New Deal social welfare state during the Great Depression, the federal government helped to underwrite a system of racially segregated and unequal public and private housing across urban America. Federal lawmakers enacted a series of measures to improve the housing and living conditions of white citizens but steadfastly refused to guarantee mortgages or erect public housing that admitted blacks and whites on a nonsegregated basis. Federal housing programs included the Home Owners Loan Corporation (1933), the Federal Housing Administration (1934), the US Housing Authority

(1937), and the Federal Housing Act of 1949, among others. A plethora of home-owners' associations, banks, real estate agencies, municipalities, corporate elites, and violent grassroots white activists had fueled the rise of racially segregated urban communities before the onset of the Great Depression. Thereafter, federal financial support played a commanding role in segregating black and white residents between World War II and the early 1970s. In his pioneering study of segregation in Chicago's housing market from World War II through 1960, historian Arnold Hirsch forcefully concludes that "government support and sanction" distinguished what he dubbed the "second ghetto," a pattern of residential segregation that extended well beyond the geographical boundaries of the predepression "first ghetto" (Flamming 2005, 351–52; Connolly 2014, 94–98; Rothstein 2017, 63–64).

Urban renewal programs reinforced the racially divided urban housing market. Between the early 1950s and 1973, urban renewal programs, called "Negro Removal" by black residents, demolished some 2,500 neighborhoods and extended housing segregation in nearly one thousand US municipalities (Self 2003, 137). Projects included Pittsburgh's the Lower Hill District, Detroit's Paradise Valley, and the Bay Area's West Oakland neighborhood. In August 1949, black Bay Area resident Lola Bell Sims wrote to President Harry Truman expressing fear of displacement. A decade later, the Oakland City Council and Redevelopment Agency devised a plan for renewal, listing the West Oakland neighborhood among the first sites scheduled for the bulldozer (Fullilove 2005, 4–5; Sides 2003, 118–20; Trotter Jr. and Day 2010, 69–73; Sugrue 1996, 47–50).

Black Americans did not take discrimination in the industrial city sitting down. From the outset of the Great Migration, they built their own Black Metropolis. Across urban industrial America, southern black migrants, alone and in concert with old residents, helped to establish a rich infrastructure of independent African American religious, fraternal, civic, social welfare, civil rights, labor, and political organizations. The Black Metropolis established the institutional springboard for the rise of the modern Black Freedom Movement, which demolished the old Jim Crow order and established a new equal opportunity regime by the late 1960s and early 1970s (Weems and Chambers 2017, 1–22; Drake and Cayton [1945] 1993, 61; Baldwin 2007, 25; Higham 1997, 1–30; Fuchs 1997, 59–85; Moreno 1997; Delton 2009; Horton 2005).

In addition to dismantling the legal underpinnings of Jim Crow's economic, labor, and housing policies and practices, industrial-age black workers and their communities channeled considerable energy into demolishing the effects of medical apartheid. During the early twentieth century, TB took the lives of black Americans at three times the rate of their white counterparts, but the medical establishment treated TB largely as a white disease before the onset of the Civil War and the emancipation of some four million people of African descent. Between 1900 and the beginning of the Great Migration during World War I, however, when it became clear that TB claimed rising numbers of both whites and blacks, racist portraits of the disease treated white TB sufferers as "victims," while maligning blacks, especially black women household workers, as "perpetrators" or "carriers" of the disease (Hunter 1997).

African Americans not only challenged racist interpretations of TB, but also mobilized to combat this and other diseases that plagued the black community. In 1915, when Booker T. Washington and the Negro Business League spearheaded the establishment of Negro Health Week, the widespread incidence of TB represented a major impetus for the organization. The Negro Business League mounted pressure on the US Public Health Service to address the health inequities among black Americans. The agency instituted National Negro Health Week and launched a vigorous campaign to improve their health; National Negro Health Week campaigns engaged a broad cross section of African American organizations, including the Urban League, churches, and black public-health nurses. The movement soon produced the *National Negro Health News*, a publication of the US Public Health Services (Washington 2006, 326; Hine 1989, 89–90; Trotter Jr. 2020).

In schools, churches, fraternal order meetings, and elsewhere, movement activists pushed to improve the health conditions of black people. In April 1918, during what appears to have been the League's earliest Negro Health Education Campaign, ministers of black churches added healthcare issues to their regular Sunday services and distributed over twenty-thousand copies of public-health literature provided by government agencies. School children participated in Negro Health Week parades. The popular black weekly *Pittsburgh Courier* regularly published a schedule of times and places of health events, including health education parades through different parts of the African American community. Pittsburghers also launched campaigns to hire black public-health nurses and build a hospital to serve the city's expanding black population. While the hospital campaign in Pittsburgh faltered, similar efforts in Philadelphia, Chicago, and New York succeeded (Gamble 1995, 3–34; Trotter Jr. 2020).[2]

Conclusion

Twentieth-century blacks did not carve out a dynamic world of activism and social struggle solely from their own experiences within the segregated and unequal modern urban industrial order. They also built upon a legacy of struggle bequeathed to them by their enslaved staple-producing agricultural forbears. In turn, their fight would soon animate protests against the ravages of deindustrialization; the persistence of inequality during the emergence of the digital age; and the epidemic of lethal policing of young black people and their communities by the turn of the new millennium. The social and political struggles of the industrial age also laid the groundwork for the rise of black mayoral regimes across the country during the closing years of the twentieth century. These grassroots electoral victories, in turn, buoyed the election of Barack Obama as the first US President of African descent—whose crowning achievement was the passage of the Affordable Care Act—to address historic patterns of class and racial inequality in the US healthcare system.

Nonetheless, on the eve of COVID-19's arrival in the United States, a variety of forces had already predisposed black Americans to the ravages of the virus: notably, the painful collapse of the industrial economy, the war on drugs, mass incarceration, and the dismantling of the New Deal social welfare state. These recent phenomena built upon long-standing factors such as inadequate housing, poor nutrition, and unhealthy living environments that exacerbated the effects of COVID-19 on the health and well-being of black people. But black Americans did not quietly endure the destructive impact of these conditions on their lives. They built upon the social struggles of the industrial age; launched a second wave of the Black Lives Matter movement; and continued to challenge the twenty-first century system of racial and class inequality. A historical perspective on these issues, hopefully, will advance the long-term struggle to eradicate entrenched racial inequality not only from the healthcare system but also from all facets of the politics, culture, and institutional life of the nation.

Perhaps most important, a historical perspective provides much needed socioeconomic, structural, and political context for addressing accelerating grassroots demands for reparations in our own times. Contemporary calls for material, cultural, and societal redress not only target big federal and regional bureaucracies but also identify specific localities as perhaps the most promising space for redistributive policy-making efforts moving forward. Whether local, regional, or federal in scope, successful reparations solutions must reach the bottommost rungs of the racialized postindustrial capitalist hierarchy of jobs, housing, and access to health, social, and human services.

Equally significant, in addition to underscoring how inequities emerged from prevailing conditions at particular moments in time and space, history also makes clear how the seeds of inequality sown at one point in time help to shape inequities that emerge in the new age. As such, the age of COVID-19, like other challenging moments in African American, US, and global history, mirrors earlier forms of injustice.

NOTES

1. For specific cities, see Lewis 1993, 80–81; Thomas 1992, 104–5; Greenberg 1991, 31–32, 186–87, 192; Hunter 2013, 80–81; Dickerson 1986, 59.

2. For an emblematic perspective on the ways that poor and working-class black people confronted recurring health crises during the industrial age with determination to survive and ultimately to thrive as a people, see also Trotter 2015.

REFERENCES

Baldwin, Davarian L. 2007. *Chicago's New Negroes: Modernity, the Great Migration, and Black Urban Life*. Chapel Hill: University of North Carolina Press.

Baptist, Edward E. 2014. *Half Has Never Been Told: Slavery and the Making of American Capitalism*. New York: Basic Books.

Beckert, Sven. 2014. *Empire of Cotton: A Global History*. New York: Vintage.

Berlin, Ira. 1998. *Many Thousands Gone: The First Two Centuries of Slavery in North America*. Cambridge, MA: Harvard University Press.

Berlin, Ira. 2010. *The Making of African America: The Four Great Migrations*. New York: Viking.

Berlin, Ira, and Philip D. Morgan, eds. 1993. *Cultivation and Culture: Labor and the Shaping of Slave Life in the Americas*. Charlottesville: University Press of Virginia.

Boustan, Leah Platt. 2017. *Competition in the Promised Land: Black Migrants in Northern Cities and Labor Markets*. Princeton, NJ: Princeton University Press.

Byrd, Alexander X. 2008. *Captives and Voyagers: Black Migrants across the Eighteenth-Century British Atlantic World*. Baton Rouge: Louisiana State University Press.

Byrd, W. Michael, and Linda A. Clayton. 2000. *An American Health Dilemma: A Medical History of African Americans and the Problem of Race—Beginnings to 1900*. New York: Routledge.

Charles, Nick. 2020. "Race Rises to the Forefront for Activists in the Coronavirus Pandemic." NBC *News*. April 10. https://www.nbcnews.com/news/nbcblk/race-rises -forefront-activists-coronavirus-pandemic-n1181336.

Clark, Christopher, Nancy A. Hewitt, Stephen Brier, and Joshua Brown. 2008. *Who Built America? Working People and the Nation's History*. 3rd ed. Boston: Bedford/St. Martins.

Connolly, N. D. B. 2014. *A World More Concrete: Real Estate and the Remaking of Jim Crow South Florida*. Chicago: University of Chicago Press.

Delton, Jennifer A. 2009. *Racial Integration in Corporate America, 1940–1990*. Cambridge: Cambridge University Press.

Dickerson, Dennis C. 1986. *Out of the Crucible: Black Steelworkers in Western Pennsylvania, 1875–1980*. Albany: State University of New York Press.

Downs, Jim. 2012. *Sick from Freedom: African American Illness and Suffering during the Civil War and Reconstruction*. New York: Oxford University Press.

Drake, St Clair, and Horace R. Cayton. (1945) 1993. *Black Metropolis: A Study of Negro Life in a Northern City*. Vols. 1 and 2. Chicago: The University of Chicago Press.

Fairbanks, Robert B. 1993. "Cincinnati Blacks and the Irony of Low-Income Housing Reform, 1900–1950." In *Race and the City: Work, Community and Protest in Cincinnati 1820–1970*, edited by Henry Louis Taylor, 193–208. Champaign: University of Illinois Press.

Flamming, Douglas. 2005. *Bound for Freedom: Black Los Angeles in Jim Crow America*. Berkeley: University of California Press.

Fuchs, Lawrence H. 1997. "The Changing Meaning of Civil Rights, 1954–1994." In *Civil Rights and Social Wrongs: Black-White Relations since World War II*, edited by John Higham, 59–85. University Park: Pennsylvania State University Press.

Fullilove, Mindy T. 2005. *Root Shock: How Tearing Up City Neighborhoods Hurts America, and What We Can Do about It*. New York: Ballantine Books.

Gamble, Vanessa N. 1995. *Making a Place for Ourselves: The Black Hospital Movement, 1920–1945*. New York: Oxford University Press.

Gonda, Jeffrey D. 2015. *Unjust Deeds: The Restrictive Covenant Cases and the Making of the Civil Rights Movement*. Chapel Hill: University Of North Carolina Press.

Greenberg, Cheryl L. 1991. *"Or Does It Explode?": Black Harlem in the Great Depression*. New York: Oxford University Press.

Gregory, James N. 2005. *The Southern Diaspora: How the Great Migrations of Black and White Southerners Transformed America*. Chapel Hill: University of North Carolina Press.

Grossman, James R. 1989. *Land of Hope: Chicago, Black Southerners, and the Great Migration*. Chicago: University of Chicago Press.

Hahn, Steven. 2003. *A Nation under Our Feet: Black Political Struggles in the Rural South, from Slavery to the Great Migration*. Cambridge, MA: Belknap Press of Harvard University Press.

Hall, Gwendolyn Midlo. 1992. *Africans in Colonial Louisiana: The Development of Afro-Creole Culture in the Eighteenth Century*. Baton Rouge: Louisiana State University Press.

Halpern, Rick. 1997. *Down on the Killing Floor: Black and White Workers in Chicago's Packinghouses; 1904–1954*. Champaign: University of Illinois Press.

Harris, William H. 1982. *The Harder We Run: Black Workers since the Civil War*. New York: Oxford University Press.

Higham, John. 1997. "Introduction: A Historical Perspective." In *Civil Rights and Social Wrongs: Black-White Relations since World War II*, edited by John Higham, 1–30. University Park: Pennsylvania State University Press.

Hine, Darlene Clark. 1989. *Black Women in White: Racial Conflict and Cooperation in the Nursing Profession, 1890–1950*. Bloomington: Indiana University Press.

Horton, Carol A. 2005. *Race and the Making of American Liberalism*. New York: Oxford University Press.

Hunter, Marcus A. 2013. *Black Citymakers: How the Philadelphia Negro Changed Urban America*. New York: Oxford University Press.

Hunter, Tera W. 1997. "Tuberculosis as the 'Negro Servants Disease.'" In *To 'Joy My Freedom: Southern Black Women's Lives and Labors after the Civil War*. Cambridge, MA: Harvard University Press.

Johnson, Walter. 2013. *River of Dark Dreams: Slavery and Empire in the Cotton Kingdom*. Cambridge, MA: Harvard University Press.

Jones, Jacqueline. 1998. *American Work: Four Centuries of Black and White Labor*. New York: W. W. Norton.

Lewis, Earl. 1993. *In Their Own Interests: Race, Class, and Power in Twentieth-Century Norfolk, Virginia*. Berkeley: University of California Press.

Lewis, Ronald L. 1979. *Coal, Iron, and Slaves: Industrial Slavery in Maryland and Virginia, 1715–1865*. Westport, CT: Greenwood Press.

Lieberson, Stanley. 1980. *A Piece of the Pie: Blacks and White Immigrants since 1880*. Berkeley: University of California Press.

Marks, Carole. 1989. *Farewell, We're Good and Gone: The Great Black Migration*. Bloomington: Indiana University Press.

Massey, Douglas S., and Nancy Denton. 1993. *American Apartheid: Segregation and the Making of the Underclass*. Cambridge, MA: Harvard University Press.

McDonald, Roderick A. 1993. "Independent Economic Production by Slaves on Antebellum Louisiana Sugar Plantations." In *Cultivation and Culture: Labor and the Shaping of Slave Life in the Americas*, edited by Ira Berlin and Philip D. Morgan, 275–302. Charlottesville: University Press of Virginia.

McGruder, Kevin. 2015. *Race and Real Estate Conflict and Cooperation in Harlem, 1890–1920*. New York: Columbia University Press.

Miller, Steven F. 1993. "Plantation Labor Organization and Slave Life on the Cotton Frontier: The Alabama Mississippi Black Belt, 1815–1840." In *Cultivation and Culture: Labor and the Shaping of Slave Life in the Americas*, edited by Ira Berlin and Philip D. Morgan, 155–69. Charlottesville: University Press of Virginia.

Moreno, Paul D. 1997. *From Direct Action to Affirmative Action: Fair Employment Law and Policy in America, 1933–1972*. Baton Rouge: Louisiana State University Press.

Morgan, Philip D. 1998. *Slave Counterpoint: Black Culture in the Eighteenth-Century Chesapeake and Lowcountry*. Chapel Hill: The University of North Carolina Press.

Nieman, Donald G. 1991. *Promises to Keep: African Americans and the Constitutional Order, 1776 to the Present*. New York: Oxford University Press.

Nightingale, Carl H. 2012. *Segregation: A Global History of Divided Cities*. Chicago: University of Chicago Press.

O'Donovan, Susan E. 2007. *Becoming Free in the Cotton South*. Cambridge, MA: Harvard University Press.

Olwell, Robert. 1998. *Masters, Slaves and Subjects: The Culture of Power in the South Carolina Low Country, 1740–1790*. Ithaca, NY: Cornell University Press.

Rediker, Marcus. 2007. *The Slave Ship: A Human History*. London: Penguin Books.

Reich, Steven A. 2013. *Working People: A History of African American Workers since Emancipation*. Lanham, MA: Rowman and Littlefield Publishers.

Reidy, Joseph P. 1993. "Obligation and Right: Patterns of Labor, Subsistence, and Exchange in the Cotton Belt of Georgia, 1790–1860." In *Cultivation and Culture: Labor and the*

Shaping of Slave Life in the Americas, edited by Ira Berlin and Philip D. Morgan, 138–54. Charlottesville: University Press of Virginia.

Rothstein, Richard. 2017. *The Color of Law: A Forgotten History of How Our Government Segregated America*. New York: Liveright.

Savitt, Todd L. 1978. *Medicine and Slavery: The Diseases and Health Care of Blacks in Antebellum Virginia*. Champaign: University of Illinois Press.

Scarborough, William Kauffman. 1984. *The Overseer: Plantation Management in the Old South*. Athens: University of Georgia Press.

Schweninger, Loren L. 1990. *Black Property Owners in the South, 1790–1915*. Champaign: University of Illinois Press.

Scott, Rebecca J. 2005. *Degrees of Freedom: Louisiana and Cuba after Slavery*. Cambridge, MA: Belknap Press of Harvard University Press.

Self, Robert O. 2003. *American Babylon: Race and the Struggle for Postwar Oakland*. Princeton, NJ: Princeton University Press.

Sides, Josh. 2003. *L.A. City Limits: African American Los Angeles from the Great Depression to the Present*. Berkeley: University of California Press.

Smallwood, Stephanie E. 2007. *Saltwater Slavery: A Middle Passage from Africa to American Diaspora*. Cambridge, MA: Harvard University Press.

Sugrue, Thomas J. 1996. *The Origins of the Urban Crisis: Race and Inequality in Postwar Detroit*. Princeton, NJ: Princeton University Press.

Taeuber, Karl E., and Alma F. Taeuber. 1965. *Negroes in Cities: Residential Segregation and Neighborhood Change*. Chicago: Aldine Publishing.

Thomas, Richard Walter. 1992. *Life for Us Is What We Make It: Building Black Community in Detroit, 1915–1945*. Bloomington: Indiana University Press.

Trotter, Joe William, Jr. 1990. *Coal, Class, and Color: Blacks in Southern West Virginia, 1915–32*. Champaign: University of Illinois Press.

Trotter, Joe William, Jr., ed. 1991. *The Great Migration in Historical Perspective: New Dimensions of Race, Class, and Gender*. Bloomington: Indiana University Press.

Trotter, Joe William, Jr. 2020. *Pittsburgh and the Urban League Movement A Century of Social Service and Activism*. Lexington: University Press of Kentucky.

Trotter, Joe William, Jr., and Jared N. Day. 2010. *Race and Renaissance: African Americans in Pittsburgh since World War II*. Pittsburgh, PA: University of Pittsburgh Press.

Trotter, Otis. 2015. *Keeping Heart: A Memoir of Family Struggle, Race, and Medicine*. Athens: Ohio University Press.

US Bureau of the Census. 1918. "Negro Population, 1790–1915." Washington, DC: Department of Commerce, Bureau of the Census. https://www.census.gov/library/publications/1918/dec/negro-population-1790-1915.html.

US Bureau of the Census, rev. 2011. "Historical Census of Housing Tables." US Census, Housing and Household Economic Statistics Division. https://www.census.gov/data/tables/time-series/dec/coh-owner.html.

Usner, Daniel H., Jr. 1979. "From African Captivity to American Slavery: The Introduction of Black Laborers to Colonial Louisiana." *Louisiana History: The Journal of the Louisiana Historical Association* 20, no. 1: 25–48.

Usner, Daniel H., Jr. 1992. *Indians, Settlers, and Slaves in a Frontier Exchange Economy: The Lower Mississippi Valley Before 1783*. Chapel Hill: University of North Carolina Press.

Wade, Richard C. 1964. *Slavery in the Cities: The South 1820–1860*. London: Oxford University Press.

Walker, Juliet E. K. 2009. *The History of Black Business in America: Capitalism, Race, Entrepreneurship, Volume 1, to 1865*. 2nd ed. Chapel Hill: University of North Carolina Press.

Walsh, Colleen. 2020. "Health Care Disparities in the Age of Coronavirus." *Harvard Gazette*. April 16. https://news.harvard.edu/gazette/story/2020/04/health-care-disparities-in-the-age-of-coronavirus/.

Walsh, Lorena, and Philip D. Morgan. 1993. "Slave Life, Slave Society, and Tobacco Production in the Tidewater Chesapeake, 1620–1820." In *Cultivation and Culture: Labor and the Shaping of Slave Life in the Americas*, edited by Ira Berlin, 170–99. Charlottesville: University Press of Virginia.

Washington, Harriet A. 2006. *Medical Apartheid: The Dark History of Medical Experimentation on Black Americans from Colonial Times to the Present*. New York: Doubleday.

Weems, Robert E., and Jason Chambers, eds. 2017. *Building the Black Metropolis: African American Entrepreneurship in Chicago*. Champaign: University of Illinois Press.

White, Deborah Gray. 1985. *Ar 'n't I a Woman? Female Slaves in the Plantation South*. New York: W. W. Norton.

Whitman, T. Stephen. 1997. *The Price of Freedom: Slavery and Manumission in Baltimore and Early National Maryland*. Lexington: University Press of Kentucky.

Wilkerson, Isabel. 2010. *The Warmth of Other Suns: The Epic Story of America's Great Migration*. New York: Random House.

Wood, Peter H. 1974. *Black Majority: Negroes in Colonial South Carolina from 1670 through the Stono Rebellion*. New York: W. W. Norton.

COVID-19 and Institutions

3. "God Is in Control": Race, Religion, Family, and Community during the COVID-19 Pandemic

SANDRA L. BARNES

Most research on COVID-19 and the black community focuses on health disparities (Dorn, Cooney, and Sabin 2020; Laster Pirtle 2020; Poteat et al. 2020; Yancy 2020). Fewer studies, however, consider how COVID-19 influences other aspects of their lives. This study examines the pandemic through the lens of race and religion.

Literature suggests the indelible role of religion for blacks (Barnes 2012; Du Bois [1903] 2003; Frazier 1964; Lincoln and Mamiya 1990). Often differing in theologies and intensity, religion is also important to whites (Chaves 2004; Chaves et al. 1999; Pew Research Center 2014). Yet the COVID-19 pandemic has upended regular religious practices that are intrinsically and extrinsically important to adherents. This mixed-methodological, multigenerational case study is informed by a socioecological lens (Bronfenbrenner 1977, 1979, 1986), in-depth interviews, empirical data, and bivariate and content analyses. I focus on Christianity as the prevalent faith tradition in the United States (Chaves 2004) as well as on blacks and whites given their diverse histories of religious expression. Moreover, given the paucity of research on the black experience, the lives of a specific black family, the Marshalls (a pseudonym), are referenced to contextualize the following queries: How is COVID-19 influencing religion for white and black Christians? What are religious concerns and responses to the pandemic and do they vary by race? Findings will have scholarly and practical import to better understand how these two groups are navigating the pandemic.

COVID-19 and Comparisons between Blacks and Whites

As a result of COVID-19, blacks are more likely to lose both their lives and their livelihoods (Boesler and Pickert 2020; CDC 2020a, 2020b, 2020c, 2020d; McNicholas and Poydock 2020). Findings by Yancy (2020) show that for majority-black counties in the United States, the infection and death rates are more than three- and six-times higher, respectively, than in predominantly white counties. Laster Pirtle (2020) details how racial capitalism fuels the pandemic by exacerbating existing racial inequities including historic, unaddressed inequality; homelessness; residential segregation; coexisting medical conditions; medical bias; and lack of access to requisite resources. Blacks who are poor, female, and/or disabled are even more vulnerable (American Psychological Association 2020; Gordon et al. 2020; Laurencin and McClinton 2020). Hardeman et al. (2020, n.p.) succinctly charge the following:

> Black communities bear the physical burdens of centuries of injustice, toxic exposures, racism, and white supremacist violence. . . . Racism is productive. . . . Any solution to racial health inequities must be rooted in the material conditions in which those inequities thrive. Therefore, we must insist that for the health of the black community and, in turn, the health of the nation, we address the social, economic, political, legal, educational, and healthcare systems that maintain structural racism. Because as the COVID-19 pandemic so expeditiously illustrated, all policy is health policy.

This summary suggests differential prevalence and effects of COVID-19 based on race and related factors (Poteat et al. 2020). However, religion has mitigated the full impact of certain negative outcomes for blacks in the past. Is this the case when COVID-19 is considered, and will outcomes and experiences differ for whites?

Socioecological Framework

A socioecological theoretical framework combines aspects of sociology and ecology to examine environmental factors that are historic and structural across time. Ecological theory suggests that individual and collective histories, social institutions, societal values, norms, systemic forces, and social networks influence individual behavior (Bronfenbrenner 1977, 1979, 1986). Ecology helps frame the pandemic's context and the Marshalls' place in it. A sociological lens is employed to consider the influence of religion, broadly defined, on beliefs and behavior based on race (Barnes 2005, 2012; Billingsley 1992; Chaves 2004; Du Bois [1903] 2003; Lincoln and Mamiya 1990). This multidisciplinary framework provides a lens to assess whether and how space and place matter when assessing religion and race during the COVID-19 pandemic [see Barnes and Blanford-Jones (2019) for details on this framework].

Data Collection

This project reflects a multigenerational case study about the effects of COVID-19 on three generations of a thirteen-person black family. A case study design is intentionally used rather than a survey or larger sample to perform an in-depth analysis about a specific black family, the Marshalls. The objective is not generalizability, but rather to allow this family's experiences to provide the ecological context for a broader study of race and religion during the pandemic (Yin 2017). The Marshalls consist of a matriarch (a widow), her children (four daughters and a son), and their seven children (two of whom are minors). Six of the seven grandchildren currently reside with their parents. This specific black family was chosen because multiple generations exist; each family member resides in a pandemic hotspot (i.e., a densely populated city in New York, Indiana, Georgia, and Illinois with a disproportionate percentage of COVID-19 cases and deaths among blacks); their profiles are diverse in terms of age, place of residence, education, and occupation; and, as these results suggest, many of their experiences illumine ways COVID-19 can be understood through the lens of race, religion, family, and community. The Marshalls were identified and recruited by community partners of the researcher. Individuals were not provided a monetary incentive to participate in this study.

Findings are based on quantitative and qualitative data. National statistics on the pandemic's effects by race as well as secondary academic and mainstream sources provide the backdrop for an examination of the virus' impact on the Marshalls. The qualitative analysis is based on in-depth interviews captured during May–June 2020. The sample (n = 11) consists of six females (ages 20–78 years old) and five males (ages 22–39 years old) (mean age of 41.5 years old). The family's educational portrait is as follows: some college (four persons); associate's degree (one person); bachelor's degree (one person); master's degree (four persons); and doctor of education degree (one person). Each person lives in a COVID-19 hotspot: Georgia (five persons); Indiana (four persons); Illinois (one person); and New York (one person). The rapidity of the pandemic's effects in the United States fostered the relatively short data collection period. Interviews lasted between thirty and ninety minutes and were audiotaped and transcribed by this researcher. Second interviews were performed with two family members to clarify several responses. In addition to individual and family demographics, a total of ten questions were posed to gather data about life before and during COVID-19; religious, academic, and employment experiences; beliefs about COVID-19; and strategies to navigate the pandemic.

Analytical Approach

During the qualitative phase, content analysis was used to identify the most common themes in the Marshalls' comments (Krippendorf 1980; Neuendorf 2002). Interview results were reviewed by hand by this researcher using two primary processes: open-coding, in which broad concepts were labeled and categorized, and axial coding, in which connections between common words were made and possible themes were determined. Line-by-line coding was used to identify frequently used language across family members (for example, pandemic-related experiences). This step differs from the earlier stage in its focus on longer phrases rather than on individual words. This process was continued in order to capture and confirm the most common patterns in these phrases. Representative quotes were also identified during this phase. Validity and reliability are not common criteria for qualitative analyses, yet the multiple analytical steps provide confidence in the recurring concepts and themes. The quantitative analysis (table 3.1) was based on national data by race collected from the *Atlantic*'s Racial Data Tracker (RDT) on May 21, 2020, which had been last updated at 3:13 p.m. that day (COVID Tracking Project 2020). The table compares percentages of infections and deaths for blacks and whites in select states where the Marshalls reside. The RDT also indicates when a percentage likely represents a racial/ethnic disparity. The RDT tracker flags a group's case or death proportion as suggestive of racial/ethnic disparity when it meets three criteria: (1) is at least 33 percent higher than the census percentage of the population; (2) remains elevated whether cases/deaths with unknown race/ethnicity are included or excluded; and (3) is based on at least thirty actual cases or deaths. I include these specific COVID-19 statistics because they provide the actual ecological context in which the Marshalls were living during their interviews. Statistical results, emergent themes, thick descriptions, and representative quotes are provided next (pseudonyms are used).

Contemporary COVID-19 Statistics in the United States by Race

Table 3.1 shows that blacks make up 14 percent of the population in Illinois but represent 27 percent of COVID-19 cases and 31 percent of COVID-19 deaths. Thus, blacks in Illinois experience almost twice as many cases and more than twice as many deaths compared to their population presence. Indiana reports

TABLE 3.1: Selected states and the percentage of cases and deaths where race/ethnicity is reported

State	Cases that include race/ ethnicity data (%)	Deaths that include race/ ethnicity data (%)	Race	State population (%)	Reported cases (%)	Reported deaths (%)
Indiana	.79	.93	Black/AA	9	18*	16*
			White	84	58	70
Georgia	.74	.98	Black/AA	31	46*	49*
			White	52	34	44
New York	.0	.91	Black/AA	14	Not reported	25*
			White	55		34
Illinois	.75	.99	Black/AA	14	23*	31*
			White	61	27	43

Notes: The *Atlantic*'s Racial Data Tracker (COVID Tracking Project 2020). The tracker flags a group's case or death proportion as suggestive of racial/ethnic disparity when it meets three criteria: (1) is at least 33% higher than the census percentage of population; (2) remains elevated whether we include or exclude cases/deaths with unknown race/ethnicity; and (3) is based on at least thirty actual cases or deaths. Figures accessed at 3:13 p.m. on May 21, 2020. AA = African American.
*Percentage likely represents a racial/ethnic disparity.

that blacks make up 9 percent of the state population but represent 18 percent of COVID-19 cases and 16 percent of COVID-19 deaths, demonstrating that blacks in Indiana experience twice as many cases and almost twice as many deaths compared to their population presence. In Georgia, blacks make up 31 percent of the population but 46 percent of COVID-19 cases and 49 percent of COVID-19 deaths. New York state, which includes the onetime pandemic epicenter New York City, reports that blacks make up 14 percent of the state's population but 25 percent of COVID-19 deaths. Overall, in the states listed in table 3.1, blacks are contracting COVID-19 at disproportionately higher rates as compared to their population presence, and these patterns likely reflect racial and ethnic disparities. But how do the experiences of the Marshalls as residents in these hotspots inform us about US trends around race and religion more broadly?

Navigating the COVID-19 Pandemic: Voices and Experiences

Narratives from the Marshalls and secondary sources suggest the following three themes about race and religion during the COVID-19 pandemic: (1) To meet or not to meet: corporate worship and loss of social support during COVID-19;

(2) "It's my right": COVID-19 and heightened civil religion; and (3) This too will pass: religion as a pandemic mediator. The first theme focuses on tensions reconciling congregational gathering with social distancing edicts. The second theme considers how Christianity is being appropriated because of the pandemic in the form of civil religion. The final theme highlights usage of Christian tenets and practices to negotiate the pandemic.

THEME 1. TO MEET OR NOT TO MEET: CORPORATE WORSHIP AND LOSS OF SOCIAL SUPPORT DURING COVID-19

Corporate worship is a fundamental Christian practice (Chaves 2004; Du Bois [1903] 2003; Lincoln and Mamiya 1990). The Black Church (I capitalize this term only when referencing the collective and otherwise use *black churches*) has historically been a safe haven and the central place for communal gathering, social support, and community action for blacks (Barnes 2005, 2008; Billingsley 1992; Frazier 1964; Lincoln and Mamiya 1990). Yet the CDC reports that such congregating can trigger a chain of COVID-19 transmission (2020c). Theme 1 focuses on how some Christians have responded to being unable to congregate and differences based on race. Constance, a seventy-seven-year-old retired service provider with an AS in sociology and the Marshall family matriarch, expresses a common concern: "I can't go to church to meet other people and go to Bible study. And I help with the kids. I miss most being able to come together, just seeing people and talking to them. Now we have to take communion at home. You call them little things, but they are still important. . . . You have to look at Zoom for preaching, the Bible class and activities with the kids all happen on Zoom. You can't even go to the building."

Although the digital footprint of some black churches is low, Constance's church provides virtual worship (Carrega and Brown 2020). She notes both the possible spiritual and practical benefits of church attendance regardless of race, gender, class, and their intersection (Chaves 2004); however, online alternatives pale in comparison. Corporate worship fortifies many blacks against racial disparities and provides sanctuary against an often-unwelcoming society (Barnes and Blanford-Jones 2019; Lincoln and Mamiya 1990). From an ecological perspective, the Black Church is considered one of the most important protective mechanisms for both black families and children (Billingsley 1992). Yet they are unable to experience this same support to combat COVID-19. As Keith, a fifty-two-year-old business administrator in Illinois with an MBA, explains, "My mind races now—church used to help calm me down. I'm worried about a lot—my Mom, who's recovering from a heart attack, COVID-19, and now George Floyd. He represents all those black people who have been killed—going back to Emmett Till. . . . I've been stopped by cops too many times to remember. I pray for the protesters every day. Sometimes I think, if Rona doesn't get us, the cops will."

For Keith, church attendance helped him process the myriad challenges he faces as a black man; this loss of social support has resulted in emotional and psychological trauma. At present, he is attempting to reconcile, alone, an oppressive past (i.e., murders from Emmett Till to George Floyd) and current problems (i.e., COVID-19 and police brutality) that are disproportionately impacting the black community as well as his own family concerns (i.e., his mother's health) (Brown et al. 1990; Chen 2020; Hardeman et al. 2020; Hubler and Rojas 2020). Yet tensions exist about invisible (i.e., *Rona*, shorthand for the coronavirus COVID-19) and visible (i.e., racist police and concerns for protestors) dangers he believes blacks continually face (Gordon et al. 2020; Laster Pirtle 2020; Wells-Barnett 2014). Per members of the Marshall family, past marginalization as well as contemporary racial and political unrest mean that more is at stake for many black Christians than their white peers when members of the former race are unable to meet for sanctuary and support (Barnes and Blanford-Jones 2019; Billingsley 1992; Lincoln and Mamiya 1990).

Like Constance and her son Keith, black and white Christians value church attendance, but participation often has different meanings and motivations based on different histories and experiences (Chen 2020; Pew Research Center 2014). Greater percentages of blacks than whites attend church, pray frequently, read the Bible, and believe in God (Chaves et al. 1999; Earls 2018; Pew Research Center 2014). News sources show racial differences in how Christians rejected social distancing decrees. For example, certain church leaders, both white and black, initially downplayed the virus' severity, defied stay-at-home orders, and continued to hold church services (Woodward 2020). Black and white Pentecostals and evangelicals were more apt to defy such orders than their non-Pentecostal and nonevangelical peers (Djupe 2020; Woodward 2020). COVID-19 cases followed, particularly for blacks, some of whom believed their faith in God would protect them from infection (Boorstein 2020; Carrega and Brown 2020; Gutierrez and Helsel 2020). However, conservative white pastors were more apt to tell parishioners it was their duty to attend church despite stay-at-home edicts and to sue the state for violation of their First Amendment rights (Andone and Moshtaghian 2020; Jackson 2020; Orso 2020; Rubin 2020). Thus, underlying political motivations for whites differed from those of their black counterparts.

It appears that most churches eventually adhered to social distancing edicts; many implemented virtual services. Lauren provides pros and cons of her

Black Church experience before and since the onset of the pandemic: "To a certain degree I miss going to church and to a certain degree I don't. Our church service is extremely long. But since we've been streaming, it's exactly an hour. . . . Church will open again soon, but I won't take my family" (forty-seven-year-old teacher, MS in public administration). Two songs, announcements, and a sermon have replaced the usual three-hour worship service that Lauren does not seem to miss. Concerns about her children and elderly mother mean she won't return immediately once the church reopens (Koenig 2020). Unlike Lauren's church, when racial differences are considered, some traditional black churches do not have the virtual infrastructure that many white churches have largely because of an emphasis historically on meeting collectively and economic constraints apparent via the digital divide (Carrega and Brown 2020; Lincoln and Mamiya 1990). Levi, a twenty-four-year-old college sophomore in psychology, defines the church and corporate worship differently, saying "I work in campus ministry. . . . I know I'm making a difference. The kids need a voice. . . . The virus has showed me what church is all about. I knew it wasn't just a building. . . . It's meeting up with people and discipling. It's benefited my relationship with God. Anyone can go to church on Sunday—like on Easter Sunday when you see people you've never seen before. But now you can't just perform your faith. No one sees it 'cause you're at home. So are you really what you claim to be at home?"

The pandemic has strengthened Levi's faith. He questions the preoccupation with being present in an edifice over evangelizing, supporting younger Christians, and authentic godly living (Barnes 2005, 2008; Wimberly and Parker 2002). For Levi, failing to meet may have an unanticipated intrinsic benefit if persons use the time to fortify their Christian beliefs. Levi's comment also parallels reports that more blacks than whites note that their faith has been strengthened by the pandemic (Gecewicz 2020).

White and black Christians are attempting to reconcile the benefits of collective worship with the drawbacks of potentially contracting or spreading COVID-19 (Andone and Moshtaghian 2020; CDC 2020c; Mazzei 2020; Vigdor 2020; Wolford 2020; Woodward 2020). For seemingly different reasons, both black and white protestors of stay-at-home measures yearn for communal worship and the social support it can provide. Responses range from defying court-ordered sanctions to, for some white churches, suing their states. Moreover, reported reasons vary by race, with blacks citing the need for congregational support to help weather challenges and whites citing more political, nationalistic reasons (Jackson 2020; Orso 2020; Rubin 2020). Yet concurrent health and social disparities mean black Christians are more vulnerable to COVID-19 than their white peers (Boorstein 2020; Carrega and Brown 2020; Gutierrez and Helsel 2020; Poteat et al. 2020; Woodward 2020).

THEME 2. "IT'S MY RIGHT": COVID-19 AND
HEIGHTENED CIVIL RELIGION

This second theme documents the impact of secular-based beliefs among whites on the religious beliefs and behavior of blacks like the Marshalls. COVID-19's influence on race and religion is also manifesting in increased emphasis on civil religion among whites. Broadly defined, civil religion is an ideology that ascribes religious features to US nationalism (Bellah 1967; Demerath and Williams 1985; Woodrum and Bell 1989). Christian tenets such as prayer and the Bible are supplanted by patriotism, the American flag, and a focus on citizen's rights. According to Demerath and Williams (1985, 164–65), civil religion "has become again a religious nationalism, justifying and legitimating the status quo. Conservative Protestantism has articulated its political demands in nationalistic terms linking the a priori approval of the Almighty with the actions of the American body politic." Fueled by the current political climate, civil religion tends to manifest today in protests by heavily armed whites upset about declining national strength and white Christians similarly concerned about constitutional rights (Woodrum and Bell 1989). Donald, a twenty-three-year-old with a BS in criminal justice, describes this dynamic at his workplace:

> Customer's behavior was different at first. There were lots of arguments because everyone was trying to fend for themselves. Nowadays, they seem like they are pretty much ignoring the virus. Even though we have a six-foot rule, people ignore it and in the checkout line, people are right up on each other's backs. They've reverted back to shopping like they did before the virus. Now I'm seeing a lot of customers with no mask or gloves. Save Mart will allow you in without a mask. I've just been asking God to protect me and my family from COVID, but I was already doing that before COVID. I asked God to protect us no matter what the danger.

As an essential worker at the discount store in a predominantly white area, Donald is concerned by many white customers who ignore PPE (personal protective equipment) protocols that put him and, by extension, his family at risk (De La Garza 2020). However, he relies on prayer for protection. For Donald, this important Christian ritual fortifies him at an often racially charged workplace. His cousin Lyle, a twenty-two-year-old junior studying electrical engineering who is also an essential worker, details this phenomenon:

I miss my girlfriend a lot, but the hardest thing is getting the strength to go to work. The people that come into the store, don't really follow any rules. Some have their face masks cover their mouths, but not their noses. Most of the time, I'm there all day with people who don't follow the CDC rules. They keep saying, "It's my right as a US citizen to not wear a mask." . . . I don't want to put my family at risk. I don't want to put my girlfriend at risk because she has diabetes, so she's at higher risk.

Lyle describes nationalistic rhetoric (i.e., "it's my right") indicative of civil religion used to justify PPE noncompliance and the associated trauma he feels for himself (i.e., "getting the strength to go to work") and his girlfriend with a preexisting medical condition whom he now sees only via Facetime (American Psychological Association 2018; Blazer 2020; Gordon et al. 2020; McNicholas and Poydock 2020; Resnick 2020). Like Donald and Lyle, blacks and other minorities are more apt to hold "essential" jobs and, often for economic reasons, continue working (Alleyne 2020; De La Garza 2020; Gordon et al. 2020). And as these two young men suggest, exposure to white expressions of civil religion can necessitate reliance on Christian rituals for solace and strength.

Keith describes similar experiences: "For me social distancing is good in a way. . . . It means I don't have to physically deal with my coworkers. When something about race happens, all you hear are crickets. But when they feel offended, all hell breaks loose." Like his nephews, Keith has witnessed white privilege and entitlement in the workplace (Beckett 2020; Blumer 1958; Feagin 2008) that have caused him to welcome being sequestered. Contemporary civil religion seems to reflect an appropriation of Christianity for certain whites in both church and nonchurch spaces in ways not espoused by blacks (Demerath and Williams 1985; Woodrum and Bell 1989). This disparate pattern illustrates how factors like race can affect how biblical dictates are understood and lived out. Moreover, the exclusionary beliefs and behavior typically associated with civil religion (i.e., us vs. them) counter Christian tenets that encourage inclusivity and community building across differences.

THEME 3. THIS TOO WILL PASS: RELIGION AS A PANDEMIC MEDIATOR

The most common responses to COVID-19 among the Marshalls focus on how the pandemic has increased their faith in God, their thankfulness, and their involvement in prayer and Bible study. Their experiences also parallel literature indicating that blacks are more likely than whites to engage in such practices (Barnes 2004, 2005; Diamant 2018; Earls 2018; Pew Research Center

2014). Also, blacks are more apt than whites to say their faith has increased as a result of the pandemic (Gecewicz 2020). According to the family matriarch, Constance:

> When I go to bed, I pray. You still thank the Lord that in the middle of the pandemic, you still have a lot to be thankful for. It could be worse. It's just trying times. People have lost their jobs and people are standing in line for food that have never done that before. It's just hard on people. . . . It confines you. It feels like you aren't free. But the Bible says that God hasn't given us a spirit of fear. . . . But you have to have a sound mind and use common sense to deal with Corona. And I never did think something like this would happen in my lifetime. But my pastor preached about plagues that have killed lots of people that I had never heard of.

The above remark references economic problems exacerbated by the pandemic (Boesler and Pickert 2020; Brown 2020; Romm 2020). Despite concerns about social distancing, Constance paraphrases 2 Timothy 1:7 to encourage fearlessness and logical decisions to avoid contracting and spreading the virus. Constance's comment also suggests reliance on prayer and scriptures for solace. Moreover, evidence of God's historic provisions during similar trials (plagues) bolsters her current confidence (Ferraro and Albrecht-Jensen 1991). Lola, a fifty-six-year-old marketing analyst with an MS in business, acknowledges increased religiosity as a result of COVID-19, saying, "It has improved my religious life because we have a prayer ministry every Sunday at 8 a.m. . . . I listen to multiple churches and to Tony Evans [a popular black televangelist]. It has increased my spiritual life because I'm praying more and I read my Bible more. I've always done it, but I do it more. 'There's going to be hundreds and ten thousand that fall by my side.' I know this sounds bad, but He has me."

Lola details her religious practices (i.e., prayer, watching online church services, and Bible study) and suggests that the pandemic has stimulated an already strong Christian commitment (Earls 2018). Similar to her mother, Lola paraphrases Leviticus 26:8 that assures her of God's protection from enemies—in this instance, COVID-19. A common mediating approach among the Marshalls is referencing scriptures that assuage fears, foster confidence despite seemingly insurmountable odds, and result in unwavering faith in God (Barnes 2005; Brown et al. 1990; Wimberly and Parker 2002).

Two members of the Marshall family, Claudia and Charles, lost their jobs as a result of COVID-19. In the following two quotes, each describes corollaries between the pandemic and religion. Claudia, a twenty-year-old college sophomore studying psychology, explains that "my supervisor was trying to reassure me that I'd have a job, but I knew. . . . They didn't want to let us go. . . . I realized that I needed this time to work on my family and to work on me. In the long run, it has helped me. I realized that God is very powerful and He's with us no matter what. It's forced me to become stronger in my faith, pray more, and depend on Him. And I hadn't realized that I had stopped doing that for a while."

In the remark above, Claudia now sees benefits in being furloughed because it has provided time to improve herself and her religious practices. A recommitment to Christianity has strengthened her faith, prayer life, and reliance on God (Barnes 2008; Ecklund and Coleman 2020; Wimberly and Parker 2002) and parallels Pew findings about racial differences in religiosity for millennials: "About six-in-ten black Millennials (61 percent) say they pray at least daily, a significantly higher share than the 39 percent of nonblack Millennials. . . . [N]early two-thirds (64 percent) of black Millennials are highly religious . . . which includes belief in God and self-described importance of religion, in addition to prayer and worship attendance—compared with 39 percent of nonblack Millennials" (Diamant and Mohamed 2018).

To the degree that these patterns persist today, younger blacks like Claudia are expected to rely on such religious practices and beliefs to help navigate the pandemic. Yet her older cousin, thirty-nine-year-old Charles, a construction worker who attended college but didn't graduate, provides a contrasting view: "My religious life is the same. Everything that happens in life is spiritual if you have foresight and hindsight. If you pay attention. A personal relationship with my Creator is based on my daily building upon it, so it [the pandemic] has not affected me differently. It has just given me something else to address. I'm not three times more spiritual nor have I been shaken. It's the same because the next time it's going to be another thing. I didn't change nothing because COVID came."

Charles considers himself more spiritual than religious; his resolve has not wavered during the pandemic. He considers COVID-19 one of a plethora of challenges he and other people will face designed to foster wisdom and fortitude. Rather than become distressed (American Psychological Association 2018), Charles is using this unemployment period to earn job certification. Applying existing research on religious differences based on the intersection of race and gender suggests that Charles' female family members would tend to be more religious than he; yet he is likely more religious than white men and women (Cox and Diamant 2018; Pew Research Center 2014). As noted by most of the Marshalls, like many other black Christians, their religious faith has been strengthened during the pandemic (Gecewicz 2020).

Discussion and Conclusion

This study examines the implications of COVID-19 through the lens of race and religion. Informed by the experiences of the Marshalls, a multigenerational black family residing in several pandemic hotspots, this analysis considers religious life for white and black Christians. Findings illustrate the relevance of a socioecological lens for illuminating links between families, communities, and the pandemic (Billingsley 1992; Bronfenbrenner 1977, 1979, 1986). Scholarship, mainstream reports, and family narratives suggest that both white and black Christians are employing religiosity to mediate the pandemic's effects. Yet certain motivations and behavior differ by race. Literature on the relatively greater religious attitudes and behavior among blacks suggests the likelihood of greater reliance on religiosity to help negotiate COVID-19 than whites. Remarks by the Marshalls illustrate both COVID-19-related problems and religious responses. These findings do not mean that religion isn't important among whites but rather highlight how it is intricately embedded in the lives and lifestyles of blacks (Barnes 2005, 2012; Chaves 2004; Du Bois [1903] 2003; Ecklund and Coleman 2020; Lincoln and Mamiya 1990; Pew Research Center 2014).

It seems that many conservative black and white church leaders behaved similarly when defying social distancing orders. Moreover, evangelicals, both white and black, were more supportive of defying social distancing than non-evangelicals (Djupe 2020). Such church leaders often assured congregants that God was more powerful than the virus (Nexstar Media Wire 2020; Woodward 2020). However, white church leaders were more apt to sue their states to remain open (Andone and Moshtaghian 2020). Yet more cases and deaths among black Christians than white Christians have been reported (CDC 2020a, 2020d; Boorstein 2020; Garg et al. 2020; Laster Pirtle 2020; Pilkington 2020; Raifman and Raifman 2020; Severino 2020). There is also evidence of heightened civil religion among whites who deify nationalism, claim violations of their First or Second Amendment rights, and often refuse to adhere to pandemic mitigating steps (Bellah 1967; Woodrum and Bell 1989). Other studies suggest such sentiments are driven by white privilege and entitlement linked to systemic racism (Beckett 2020; Blumer 1958; Demerath and Williams 1985; Feagin 2008). A failure to comply in workplaces puts essential workers, like several Marshall family members, at high risk of contracting COVID-19; moreover, several mid-career members of the Marshall family describe social distancing as a respite from workplace racism with religious, emotional, and psychological benefits (Chen 2020; Resnick 2020).

Churches have historically been sanctuaries in the black community to help negotiate disparities; ordinarily, they would likely have played an important role as blacks navigated the pandemic and protests about police violence. Thus, for some blacks, closed churches may be just as damaging as opened ones (Ecklund and Coleman 2020; Hubler and Rojas 2020). Ways in which today's churches may help combat health issues, foster activism against social problems, and placate followers should be examined (Barnes and Blanford-Jones 2019; Ferraro and Albrecht-Jensen 1991). Studies must also consider the implications of COVID-19 on the aging populace in mainline white and black denominations (Chaves 2004; Ferraro and Albrecht-Jensen 1991; Lincoln and Mamiya 1990) and ways to protect them in such spaces (Koenig 2020). The current endeavor focuses on black and white religious dynamics. It will be important to extend this work to include other ethnic groups, other religious and/or spiritual groups, and to confirm mainstream reports on this subject. This research illustrates how race, space (i.e., hotspots), and place (i.e., churches) can affect adherents' abilities to negotiate the COVID-19 pandemic as well as how religion can inform, equip, and empower individuals during such challenging times.

REFERENCES

Alleyne, Kenneth R. 2020. "How COVID-19 Is a Perfect Storm for Black Americans." *Washington Post.* April 26. https://www.washingtonpost.com/opinions/2020/04/26/we -must-address-social-determinants-affecting-black-community-defeat-covid-19/.

American Psychological Association. 2018. *Black Male Millennial: Unemployment and Mental Health.* Accessed May 29, 2020. https://www.apa.org/advocacy/health -disparities/black-male-unemployment.pdf.

American Psychological Association. 2020. "How COVID-19 Impacts People with Disabilities." Accessed May 18, 2020. https://www.apa.org/topics/covid-19/research -disabilities.

Andone, Dakin, and Artemis Moshtaghian. 2020. "A Person in California Who Was COVID-19 Positive Attended a Church Service and Exposed 180 People, Officials Say." CNN. May 17. https://www.cnn.com/2020/05/17/us/covid-19-mothers-day-church -exposure/index.html.

Barnes, Sandra L. 2004. "Priestly and Prophetic Influences on Black Church Social Services." *Social Problems* 51, no. 2: 202–21.

Barnes, Sandra L. 2005. "Black Church Culture and Community Action." *Social Forces* 84, no. 2: 967–94.

Barnes, Sandra L. 2008. "'The Least of These': Black Church Children's and Youth Outreach Efforts." *Journal of African American Studies* 12, no. 2: 97–119.

Barnes, Sandra L. 2012. *Live Long and Prosper: How Black Megachurches Address HIV/AIDS and Poverty in the Age of Prosperity Theology.* New York: Fordham University Press.

Barnes, Sandra Lynn, and Benita Blanford-Jones. 2019. *Kings of Mississippi: Race, Religious Education, and the Making of a Middle-Class Black Family in the Segregated South.* New York: Cambridge University Press.

Beckett, Lois. 2020. "Armed Protesters Demonstrate against COVID-19 Lockdown at Michigan Capitol." *Guardian*. April 30. https://www.theguardian.com/us-news/2020 /apr/30/michigan-protests-coronavirus-lockdown-armed-capitol.

Bellah, Robert N. 1967. "Civil Religion in America." *Journal of the American Academy of Arts and Sciences* 96, no. 1: 1–21.

Billingsley, Andrew. 1992. *Climbing Jacob's Ladder: The Enduring Legacy of African-American Families*. New York: Touchstone Books.

Blazer, Deborah. 2020. "COVID-19: How Much Protection Do Face Masks Offer?" *News-Network*. May 19. https://newsnetwork.mayoclinic.org/discussion/covid-19-how-much -protection-do-face-masks-offer/.

Blumer, Herbert. 1958. "Race Prejudice as a Sense of Group Position." *Pacific Sociological Review* 1, no. 1 (Spring): 3–7.

Boesler, Matthew, and Reade Pickert. 2020. "Salaries Get Chopped for Many Americans Who Manage to Keep Jobs." *Bloomberg*. May 27. https://www.bloomberg.com/news /articles/2020-05-27/salaries-get-chopped-for-many-americans-who-manage-to-keep -jobs.

Boorstein, Michelle. 2020. "COVID-19 Has Killed Multiple Bishops and Pastors within the Nation's Largest Black Pentecostal Denomination." *Washington Post*. April 19. https://www.washingtonpost.com/religion/2020/04/19/church-of-god-in-christ -pentecostal-coronavirus-kills-bishops/.

Bronfenbrenner, Urie. 1977. "Toward an Experimental Ecology of Human Development." *American Psychologist* 32, no. 7: 513–31.

Bronfenbrenner, Urie. 1979. *The Ecology of Human Development: Experiments by Nature and Design*. Cambridge, MA: Harvard University Press.

Bronfenbrenner, Urie. 1986. "Ecology of the Family as a Context for Human Development: Research Perspectives." *Developmental Psychology* 22, no. 6: 723–42.

Brown, Diane R., Samuel C. Ndubuisi, and Lawrence E. Gary. 1990. "Religiosity and Psychological Distress among Blacks." *Journal of Religion and Health* 29, no. 1 (Spring): 55–68.

Brown, Steven. 2020. "How COVID-19 Is Affecting Black and Latino Families' Employment and Financial Well-Being." Urban Institute. May 6. https://www.urban.org/urban -wire/how-covid-19-affecting-black-and-latino-families-employment-and-financial -well-being.

Carrega, Christina, and Lakeia Brown. 2020. "'Sorrowful': Black Clergy Members and Churches Reeling from COVID-19 Losses." *ABC News*. May 21. https://abcnews.go.com /US/sorrowful-black-clergy-members-churches-reeling-covid-19/story?id=70434181.

CDC (Centers for Disease Control and Prevention). 2020a. "Coronavirus Disease 2019 (COVID-19)—Symptoms." Accessed May 22, 2020. https://www.cdc.gov/coronavirus /2019-ncov/symptoms-testing/symptoms.html.

CDC (Centers for Disease Control and Prevention). 2020b. "Community Transmission of SARS-CoV-2 at Two Family Gatherings—Chicago, Illinois, February–March 2020." *Morbidity and Mortality Weekly Report* 69, no. 15 (April 17): 446–50. https://www.cdc .gov/mmwr/volumes/69/wr/mm6915e1.htm?s_cid=mm6915e1_w.

CDC (Centers for Disease Control and Prevention). 2020c. "Daily Updates of Totals by Week and State." Accessed June 1, 2020. https://www.cdc.gov/nchs/nvss/vsrr/covid19 /index.htm.

CDC (Centers for Disease Control and Prevention). 2020d. "Social Distancing." Accessed May 27, 2020. https://www.cdc.gov/coronavirus/2019-ncov/prevent-getting-sick/social -distancing.html.

Chaves, Mark. 2004. *Congregations in America*. Cambridge, MA: Harvard University Press.

Chaves, Mark, Mary E. Konieczny, Kraig Beyerlein, and Emily Barman. 1999. "The National Congregations Study: Background, Methods, and Selected Results." *Journal for the Scientific Study of Religion* 38, no. 4: 458–76.

Chen, Te-Ping. 2020. "For Black Professionals, Unrest Lays Bare a Balancing Act at Work." *Wall Street Journal*. June 3. https://www.wsj.com/articles/for-black-professionals -unrest-lays-bare-a-balancing-act-at-work-11591202955.

COVID Tracking Project. 2020. "Racial Data Dashboard." Accessed May 22, 2020. https:// covidtracking.com/race/dashboard.

Cox, Kiana, and Jeff Diamant. 2018. "Black Men are Less Religious Than Black Women, but More Religious Than White Women and Men." Pew Research Center. September 26. https://www.pewresearch.org/fact-tank/2018/09/26/black-men-are-less -religious-than-black-women-but-more-religious-than-White-women-and-men/.

De La Garza, Alejandro. 2020. "'We All Worry about It.' Grocery Workers Fear Confrontations with Shoppers over Mask Rules." *Time*. May 26. https://time.com/5841124 /grocery-workers-masks/.

Demerath, Nicholas, and Rhys Williams. 1985. "Civil Religion in an Uncivil Society." *Annals of the American Academy of Political and Social Science* 480, no. 1 (July): 154–66.

Diamant, Jeff. 2018. "Blacks More Likely Than Others in US to Read the Bible Regularly, See It as God's Word." Pew Research Center. May 7. https://www.pewresearch.org/fact -tank/2018/05/07/blacks-more-likely-than-others-in-u-s-to-read-the-bible-regularly -see-it-as-gods-word/.

Diamant, Jeff, and Besheer Mohamed. 2018. "Black Millennials are More Religious Than Other Millennials." Pew Research Center. July 20. https://www.pewresearch.org/fact -tank/2018/07/20/black-millennials-are-more-religious-than-other-millennials/.

Djupe, Paul A. 2020. "Survey Numbers Chart Evangelical Defiance against the States." *Religion News Service*. April 17. https://religionnews.com/2020/04/17/survey-numbers -chart-evangelical-defiance-against-the-states/.

Dorn, Aaron van, Rebecca E. Cooney, and Miriam L. Sabin. 2020. "COVID-19 Exacerbating Inequalities in the US." *Lancet* 395, no. 10232 (April): 1243–44.

Du Bois, W. E. B. (1903) 2003. *The Negro Church*. Walnut Creek: Alta Mira Press.

Earls, Aaron. 2018. "Black Americans are the Most Bible-Engaged Ethnic Group." *Lifeway Facts and Trends*. May 16. https://factsandtrends.net/2018/05/16/black-americans-most -bible-engaged-ethnic-group/.

Feagin, Joe. 2008. "The Continuing Significance of Race: Anti-Black Discrimination in Public Places." In *Social Stratification: Class, Race, and Gender in Sociological Perspective*, edited by David Grusky, 703–8. Boulder, CO: Westview Press.

Ferraro, Kenneth F., and Cynthia M. Albrecht-Jensen. 1991. "Does Religion Influence Adult Health?" *Journal for the Scientific Study of Religion* 39, no. 2: 193–202.

Frazier, Franklin E. 1964. *The Negro Church in America*. New York: Schocken Books.

Garg, Shikha, Lindsay Kim, Michael Whitaker, Alissa O'Halloran, Charisse Cummings, Rachel Holstein, Mila Prill, et al. 2020. "Hospitalization Rates and Characteristics of Patients Hospitalized with Laboratory-Confirmed Coronavirus Disease 2019—COVID-NET, 14 states, March 1–30, 2020." *Morbidity and Mortality Weekly Report* 69, no. 15: 458–64.

Gecewicz, Claire. 2020. "Few Americans Say Their House of Worship Is Open, but a Quarter Say Their Faith Has Grown amid Pandemic." Pew Research Center. April 30. https://www.pewresearch.org/fact-tank/2020/04/30/few-americans-say -their-house-of-worship-is-open-but-a-quarter-say-their-religious-faith-has-grown -amid-pandemic/.

Gordon, Colin, Walter Johnson, Jason Q. Purnell, and Jamala Rogers. 2020. "COVID-19 and the Color Line." *Boston Review.* May 1. http://bostonreview.net/race/colin-gordon -walter-johnson-jason-q-purnell-jamala-rogers-covid-19-and-the-color-line.

Gutierrez, Gabe, and Phil Helsel. 2020. "Harlem Church Mourning 11 Members Who Died from COVID-19." *NBC News.* April 22. https://www.nbcnews.com/news/us-news /harlem-church-mourning-11-members-who-died-covid-19-n1189276.

Hardeman, Rachel, Eduardo M. Medina, and Rhea W. Boyd. 2020. "Stolen Breaths." *New England Journal of Medicine* 383: 197–99. https://doi.org/10.1056/NEJMp2021072.

Hubler, Shawn, and Rick Rojas. 2020. "Amid Riots and a Pandemic, Church Attendance Resumes in 'a Very Broken World.'" *New York Times.* May 31. https://www.nytimes .com/2020/05/31/us/churches-return-coronavirus-protests.html.

Jackson, Danielle. 2020. "NC Churches Sue Gov. Roy Cooper over Coronavirus Restrictions on Church Service." *FOX News.* May 15. https://myfox8.com/news /coronavirus/nc-churches-sue-gov-roy-cooper-over-coronavirus-restrictions-on-church -services/.

Koenig, Harold G. 2020. "Ways of Protecting Religious Older Adults from the Conse-quences of COVID-19." *American Journal of Geriatric Psychiatry* 28, no. 7 (July): 776–79. https://doi.org/10.1016/j.jagp.2020.04.004.

Krippendorf, Klaus. 1980. *Content Analysis: An Introduction to Its Methodology.* Beverly Hills, CA: SAGE.

Laster Pirtle, Whitney N. 2020. "Racial Capitalism: A Fundamental Cause of Novel Coro-navirus (COVID-19) Pandemic Inequities in the United States." *Health Education and Behavior.* April 26. https://doi.org/10.1177/1090198120922942.

Laurencin, Cato T., and Aneesah McClinton. 2020. "The COVID-19 Pandemic: A Call to Action to Identify and Address Racial and Ethnic Disparities." *Journal of Racial and Ethnic Health Disparities* 7, no. 3: 398–402.

Lincoln, C. Eric, and Lawrence H. Mamiya. 1990. *The Black Church in the African-American Experience.* Durham, NC: Duke University Press.

McNicholas, Celine, and Margaret Poydock. 2020. "Who Are Essential Workers?: A Comprehensive Look at Their Wages, Demographics, and Unionization Rates." *Economic Policy Institute.* May 19. https://www.epi.org/blog/who-are-essential-workers-a -comprehensive-look-at-their-wages-demographics-and-unionization-rates/.

Neuendorf, K. A. 2002. *The Content Analysis Guidebook.* Thousand Oaks, CA: SAGE.

Nexstar Media Wire. 2020. "Louisiana Church Hosts More Than 1,800 People amid COVID-19 Outbreak." *WGN-TV.* March 23. https://wgntv.com/news/coronavirus /louisiana-church-hosts-more-than-1800-people-amid-covid-19-outbreak/.

Orso, Anna. 2020. "NJ Churches Sue Gov. Murphy, Wish to be Deemed 'Essential.'" *Phil-adelphia Inquirer*. May 30. https://www.inquirer.com/health/coronavirus/new-jersey -churches-sue-murphy-pandemic-closure-policy-alliance-20200530.html.

Pew Research Center. 2014. *Religious Landscape Study*. https://www.pewforum.org /religious-landscape-study/.

Pilkington, Ed. 2020. "Black Americans Dying of COVID-19 at Three Times the Rate of White People." *Guardian*. May 22. http://www.theguardian.com/world/2020/may/20 /black-americans-death-rate-covid-19-coronavirus.

Poteat, Tonia, Greg Millett, LaRon E. Nelson, and Chris Beyrer. 2020. "Understanding COVID-19 Risks and Vulnerabilities among Black Communities in America: The Lethal Force of Syndemics." *Annals of Epidemiology* 47 (May 14): 1–3. https://doi.org/10 .1016/j.annepidem.2020.05.004.

Raifman, Matthew, and Julia Raifman. 2020. "Disparities in the Population at Risk of Severe Illness from COVID-19 by Race/Ethnicity and Income." *American Journal of Preventive Medicine* 59, no. 1: 137–39.

Resnick, Brian. 2020. "A Third of Americans Report Anxiety or Depression Symptoms during the Pandemic. " *Vox*. May 29. https://www.vox.com/science-and-health/2020/5 /29/21274495/pandemic-cdc-mental-health.

Romm, Tony. 2020. "Americans Have Filed More Than 40 Million Jobless Claims in Past 10 Weeks." *Washington Post*. May 28. https://www.adn.com/nation-world/2020/05/28 /americans-have-filed-more-than-40-million-jobless-claims-in-past-10-weeks/.

Rubin, Alicia. 2020. "Churches and Individuals Sue Gov. Brown, Arguing Executive Orders are Unconstitutional." KDRV.com. May 13. https://www.kdrv.com/content /news/Churches-and-individuals-sue-Gov-Brown-arguing-Stay-home-save-lives -executive-orderis-unconstitutional-570457001.html.

Severino, Joe. 2020. "COVID-19 Tore through a Black Baptist Church Community in WV. Nobody Said a Word about It." *Charleston Gazette-Mail*. May 2. https://www.wvgazettemail .com/coronavirus/covid-19-tore-through-a-black-baptist-church-community-in-wv-nobody -said-a-word/article_a84c0bbb-7433-54db-b228-85188cbef726.html.

Wells-Barnett, Ida B. 2014. *On Lynchings*. Mineola, NY: Dover Books.

Wimberly, Anne Streaty, and Evelyn L. Parker, eds. 2002. *In Search of Wisdom: Faith Formation in the Black Church*. Nashville, TN: Abingdon.

Woodrum, Eric, and Arnold Bell. 1989. "Race, Politics, and Religion in Civil Religion among Blacks." *Sociological Analysis* 49, no. 4: 353–67.

Woodward, Alex. 2020. "America's Bible Belt Played Down the Pandemic and Even Cashed In. Now Dozens of Pastors Are Dead." *Independent*. April 24. https://www.independent.co .uk/news/world/americas/bible-belt-us-coronavirus-pandemic-pastors-church-a9481226 .html.

Yancy, Clyde W. 2020. "COVID-19 and African Americans." JAMA 323, no. 19: 1891–92. https://doi.org/10.1001/jama.2020.6548

Yin, Robert. 2017. *Case Study Research and Applications: Design and Methods*. 6th ed. Thousand Oaks, CA: SAGE.

4. COVID-19, Race, and Mass Incarceration

ARVIND KRISHNAMURTHY

In March 2020, the jail in Marion County, Ohio, became one of the first carceral facilities in America to test all its occupants and workers for COVID-19. When the results were returned from the lab, 73 percent of residents tested positive for COVID-19 (Chappell and Pfleger 2020). Soon thereafter Ohio began increasing COVID 19 testing in prisons, and within weeks, 20 percent of the state's cases were in prisons and jails. Such a finding was no coincidence but rather a harbinger of things to come.

As of June 2021, the United States accounted for 4 percent of the world's population, 18 percent of worldwide COVID-19 cases, and 21 percent of worldwide prisoners. Outside of college campuses, the largest outbreaks in the United States have occurred in jails or prisons (see *New York Times* 2020). American correctional facilities are, by design, packed as full as possible, making social distancing nearly impossible (Warmsley 2005). Within prisons, access to medical treatment and personal protective equipment like masks is limited, increasing the likelihood of infection even further. And prisons are indoor facilities, where residents mostly share locales like sleeping quarters, dining halls, and recreation areas. With a powerful, infectious virus, this arrangement is a recipe for disaster.

As of January 2022, reports indicate that 716,546 incarcerated people and carceral staffers had tested positive for the virus (UCLA Law 2021). If the US prison population were its own country, it would rank sixty-third in confirmed cases, above nations like Greece, Egypt, Kenya, and Finland (Worldometer

2022). This disparity is especially problematic given that incarcerated populations have elevated rates of serious health conditions, placing many in the high-risk population for COVID-19 (Maruschak, Berzofsky, and Unangst 2015).

Importantly, this crisis of COVID-19 in prisons has contributed to the racial inequality in COVID-19's impact across America: the racialized carceral state in America has helped amplify the racialized effects of COVID-19 across the country. As described on page 8 of the introduction to this volume, Centers for Disease Control and Prevention (CDC) estimations in late November 2021 suggested Latinos and blacks were, respectively, 90 and 70 percent more likely than non-Hispanic whites to die of COVID-19 (CDC 2021). Given black and Hispanic residents are over three times as likely to be incarcerated as white residents (Gottschalk 2016) the increased likelihood of contracting COVID-19 in prison and America's racialized punishment regime serve as a critical driver for the racial disparities in COVID-19 contraction.

In this chapter I show how the COVID-19 spread in America is driven in part by our mass incarceration. To do so I collect county-level data on coronavirus spread from the *New York Times* and data on coronavirus spread among people incarcerated in all state and federal prisons, as well as the staff in those facilities, from the Marshall Project.[1] Using these data I first present rough estimates of how jail and prison populations changed in response to COVID-19. Next, I present rough estimates of the likelihood of infection outside of jail or prison versus the likelihood of infection inside of jail or prison and show that detained residents are far more likely to contract COVID-19. Finally, I explain how America's racialized carceral state causes racial inequality in COVID-19 impact.

How Incarceration Is Affected by COVID-19

One of the first documented influenza outbreaks occurred in California's San Quentin prison during the 1918 influenza pandemic. Historical accounts note that nearly half of the nineteen hundred inmates actually contracted the disease during the first wave of the epidemic, but most of the ill were kept in the general prison population because the hospital wards were already overpopulated (Mills, Robins, and Lipsitch 2004). The same pattern emerged when COVID-19 burst on the scene in early 2020. On February 29, 2020, 40 percent of COVID-19 cases reported in Wuhan, China, were from the city's prison system (Liu and Saltman 2020). But despite the tragedies of 1918, it is not clear that the United States incorporated the lessons learned into its COVID-19 response. Carceral facilities like state prisons and local jails remain hotspots for the virus.

Theoretically, there are strong reasons to believe that COVID-19 is more likely to spread in a detention facility than elsewhere. First, historically, detained and incarcerated populations have been shown to have increased prevalence of infectious diseases like HIV, hepatitis C, and tuberculosis (Akiyama, Spaulding, and Rich 2020). This pattern was, and is, a strong indicator that the conditions of an American detention facility are likely to allow an infection to spread more widely and faster than among the general population. Next, prisons share a number of characteristics with other key "super-spreader" sites such as college dormitories, nursing homes, and meat-packing plants. They are all high–population density areas with shared living quarters, shared sanitation, and limited air circulation. The primary public policy strategies of social distancing and self-isolation are largely unavailable in detention facilities.

These factors alone suggest that it was always likely COVID-19 would wreak havoc on carceral facilities. However, structural and institutional design features also increased the likelihood of COVID-19's spread and heightened death tolls. Half of all incarcerated persons have at least one chronic disease, meaning any infections within the prison are more likely to be fatal than infections among the general population (Maruschak, Berzofsky, and Unangst 2015). Next, detention facilities have a high level of population turnover, or churn. Jails or other pretrial detention facilities are designed for short-term, sometimes only nightly, spells of detention and often have hundreds of new residents on a daily basis. Even longer-term facilities like prisons frequently have shuffling in and out on a weekly basis. This high level of turnover means new potential pathogen carriers regularly are entering shared spaces. And American prisons are often overcrowded, so much so that in 2011 the US Supreme Court ruled that overcrowding undermined healthcare in California's prisons, causing avoidable deaths (*Brown v. Plata*). That is, in a time without a pandemic, overcrowding can cause death. During a pandemic, it is certain to create mass casualties with an airborne virus.

Experts noted these facts early on. In peer-reviewed journals like the *New England Journal of Medicine* (Akiyama, Spaulding, and Rich 2020) and journalistic outlets like the *Atlantic* (Friedersdorf 2020), epidemiologists, doctors, and virologists argued for reducing the prison population immediately. But to what extent were those calls for change followed by the sheriffs, judges, and district attorneys with authority to make changes to our criminal justice system?

I answer this question by looking at two distinct kinds of facilities where the number of incarcerated individuals can be reduced. The first are jails, which are primarily filled by pretrial detainees. These detainees are legally innocent but usually have bail set at an amount they cannot afford to pay, or have no bail set because they are deemed to be a safety or flight risk. For that reason jails are shorter-term warehouses with higher levels of churn and turnover. The second are prisons, which are primarily filled by postconviction detainees. These detainees have been found guilty, and usually a sentence has already been issued in their case. As a result, prisons are longer-term residence facilities, with less churn and turnover. I look at how each of these facilities was affected by COVID-19.

How Was Jail Population Affected by COVID-19?

To evaluate whether the number of individuals incarcerated in jails decreased during COVID-19, I use data gathered from the NYU Public Safety Lab Jail Data Initiative (JDI). The JDI scours daily county jail rosters and criminal case records in over eleven hundred counties to provide facility-level data on detainee counts. I use a time series of the JDI data set to show how the total number of detainees changed from February 1, 2020, to March 31, 2021, across 186 county facilities.

Figure 4.1 displays weekly rolling-average jail population counts for 186 counties with jail data throughout the full time series of the sample. Jails in this

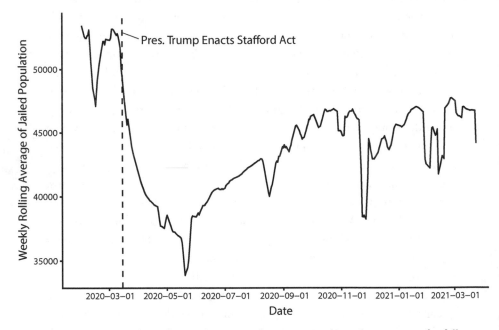

FIGURE 4.1. Sampling of 186 jails nationwide reporting jail population counts for full time-series period (February 1, 2020–April 1, 2021). Data courtesy of the NYU Public Safety Lab Jail Data Initiative.

sample began decreasing their detained populations soon after COVID-19 outbreaks began spreading across the country. This decrease was relatively monotonic across jails in our sample from the March 1, 2020, peak jail population of 53,986, until it reached its low point of 30,675 detainees on May 25, 2020, a 43 percent decrease in jail population. While we do not have data from these same jails in past years, historically there is an uptick in incarcerated individuals between March and June because of the seasonal trends in crime (McDowall, Loftin, and Pate 2012). Following that low point, we've seen a linear increase in jailed populations. As of March 31, 2021, the jailed population among our sample sits at 46,804, or 87 percent of the pre-COVID-19 jailed population.

Importantly, though, this data compilation is only a sampling of all jails in the United States, and it is not a representative or random sampling. Still, it can tell us something about what was happening across jails in the United States at the height of the COVID-19 pandemic. Journalistic accounts using alternate data sources have observed a similar pattern of initial rapid decreases in jail populations followed by a slow and steady increase back toward the pre-COVID-19 jail population (Sharma et al. 2020).

Why Did the Jail Population Fall?

What caused the decrease in jail population for these few months? There are three key policy changes that drove these decreases. First, magistrates, judges, prosecutors, and sheriffs began changing their pretrial detention practices to reduce the number of *new* detainees entering facilities. For example, on April 6, 2020, California set a statewide emergency bail schedule that reduced bail to $0 for most misdemeanor and some low-level felony offenses; and survey data from the National Association of Pretrial Services Agency (NAPSA) conducted in June 2020 showed that in nonviolent cases surveyed agencies reported a 65.17 percent increase in cite and release and a 67.98 percent increase in release on personal recognizance, two policies that don't involve pretrial detention unless there is a failure to pay or appear in court (Smith 2020; NAPSA 2020).

Next, some jurisdictions began releasing previously detained individuals who were awaiting trial. The same NAPSA survey had responding jurisdictions also reporting an 81.46 percent increase in releases from jail for persons awaiting trial (NAPSA 2020). Many major cities like Philadelphia and St. Louis convened special court hearings to handle petitions for release upon recognizance petitions among those already detained (Vargas 2020; Cardinale 2020). Other states like Kentucky and Kansas enacted legislative or judicial orders issuing emergency administrative release schedules that expanded the use of release on recognizance for some already detained (National Center for State Courts 2020; National Conference of State Legislators 2020).

Finally, a number of jurisdictions began depolicing during the initial COVID-19 surge when states were in complete lockdown. These approaches generally involved police officers simply not arresting individuals for nonviolent offenses, or limiting the number of police-citizen interactions to citizen initiated contact. For example, police departments in Los Angeles County, California; Denver, Colorado; and Philadelphia, Pennsylvania, all made explicit pronouncements that they would reduce arrests by increasing the frequency of cite and release practices, delaying arrests, and issuing summons for later appearances in court (Hernandez 2020; Schmelzer 2020; Melamed and Newall 2020). These approaches, coupled with prosecutors often simply dismissing any low-level charges, meant the actual amount of cases making their way to the courts system was likely decreased during this period.[2]

However, as cities and states opened up, these policies halted. Police returned to previous levels of contact, courts began to reopen and hold pretrial detention hearings, and a glut of delayed summons and citations finally made their way to the court system to handle. Relatedly, because most cities and states were hesitant to release individuals convicted of "violent" offenses, a substantial number of individuals remained detained throughout this period of time.

How Was the Prison Population Affected by COVID-19?

To evaluate whether the number of individuals incarcerated in prisons decreased during COVID-19, I use data gathered from the Marshall Project's prison population database. This database contacts state and federal department of corrections facilities to receive monthly prison counts. Because this database only receives counts monthly, rather than daily, it is not possible to look at a more granular variation in prison populations. This data set contains all individuals imprisoned in the United States. I use a time series of this data set to show how the total number of prisoners has changed from March 31, 2020, to January 31, 2021. Because this data set contains only prison population counts through January 2021, our time series ends there.

Figure 4.2 shows that the prison population monotonically decreased from March 2020 to January 2021. In total, the number of prisoners in state and federal facilities fell from 1.34 million to 1.12 million across those ten months of COVID-19, a decrease of about 222,000 prisoners or 16.6 percent of the total prison population. To put this amount in context, between 2018 and 2019, the

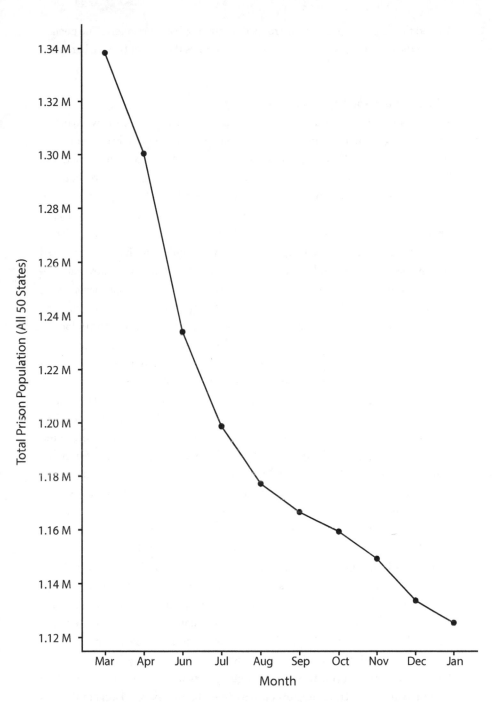

FIGURE 4.2. Monthly counts of total prison population (March 31, 2020–January 31, 2021). Data courtesy of the Marshall Project Prison Population database. Data for May 2020 were not collected and thus that month does not appear on the graph. Each state population was sampled between the 27th and 31st of the month.

United States prison population dropped by about 33,000 prisoners. The decline during the COVID-19 pandemic is about seven times the size of that earlier drop.

Why Did the Prison Population Fall?

Prison populations fell during COVID-19 in large part because of two types of policy changes. First, a number of states released prisoners early or commuted ongoing sentences. There are two types of prisons in America: state and federal. The vast majority of prisoners are in these state facilities, giving governors the authority to change the composition of the state facilities. Many governors used this authority to either commute sentences or sign executive orders to release prisoners. In New Jersey, Governor Phil Murphy passed an executive order allowing the temporary release of more than seven hundred individuals convicted of nonviolent offenses, and he most recently passed a bill that will allow early releases to continue for nonviolent offenders (O'Dea 2020). Similar orders were passed in Michigan, California, and New York, among others (van Wagtendonk 2020; California Department of Corrections and Rehabilitation 2021; Taddeo 2020). Importantly though, these orders were not all meant to create permanent changes to the prison populations. For example, similar orders in Pennsylvania and New Jersey temporarily suspended the sentences of incarceration for qualifying inmates (Prison Policy Institute 2021). Other states commuted sentences entirely, like Kentucky, where Governor Andy Beshear commuted more than one thousand sentences for medically vulnerable prisoners who were often imprisoned on technical parole violations (Ragusa 2020). Governors in many states issued executive orders that blocked new transfers into state prisons, and many states began holding mass hearings among their parole boards (Crime and Justice Institute 2021). Versions of these approaches have been adopted relatively uniformly across the country and are the primary reason that prison populations began to fall soon after COVID-19 began spreading.

Next, prison populations remained lower because of changes in the functioning of courts and prosecutors, akin to the changes that occurred in jail populations discussed above. Most states implemented a moratorium on statewide jury trials during the COVID-19 pandemic, and many more implemented citations in lieu of arrest policing, each of which reduces the inflow of potential new prisoners through the criminal justice system (Prison Policy Institute 2021). Some locales went even further, with governors in sixteen states, including Colorado and Florida, issuing executive orders halting new prison admissions for at least some period of time (Crime and Justice Institute 2021). Coupled with statewide lockdown orders that left individuals inside more often and closed businesses, criminal activity is likely to have fallen, though it is difficult to render any conclusions about crime rates given changes in the policing style during the COVID-19 pandemic.

But Was This Enough?

In many respects these changes to the incarcerated and detained population in America are remarkable. These decreases are substantively and historically significant, and they appear to be the largest decrease in prison and jail populations across a single year in the past fifty years. But that does not mean they are sufficient to handle the public-health crisis that COVID-19 poses. In response to COVID-19, schools closed to reduce face-to-face contact, businesses were temporarily shut down, and shelter-in-place orders were issued across the country. These are actions that dramatically altered the way of living for most of the population, but government officials viewed them as necessary steps to mitigate the spread of the virus and to limit fatalities. While the operation of jails and prisons in our criminal justice system certainly changed, a 16 percent reduction in prison populations and a temporary decrease in our jail population (that was quickly met with an increase close to normal levels) was not sufficient in scope to effectively mitigate the spread of COVID-19 both within prisons and jails and in our communities.

Importantly, even when states did reduce their prison populations, they often did little to ensure that released or deferred individuals were economically and medically secured. COVID-19 saw an economic downturn and high levels of contraction among employers, placing formerly incarcerated individuals—already at a disadvantage in the job market—in the position of choosing between economic precarity or taking up employment at frontline positions that carried a higher risk of COVID-19 contraction. Additionally, released or deferred individuals were likely to be placed directly into crowded family living arrangements that increased their likelihood of contracting disease, a cycle that appeared to contribute to COVID-19's community spread (Reinhart and Chen 2020).

In April 2020, the American Civil Liberties Union (ACLU) wrote that COVID-19 epidemiological models were underestimating the potential death count in America because our mass incarceration was likely to accelerate the virus. Because many of these models were trained on data from countries that do not have jail and prison populations anywhere near the United States', like South Korea and Italy, the ACLU analysts argued that these estimates were greatly underestimating the potential spread of COVID-19. With the privilege of hindsight, it is clear that those analysts were right, as the COVID-19 death count in America is far above what initial projections estimated. Epidemiological models suggested that a 90 percent decrease in all incarcerations and discontinuing incarceration for low-level offenses would result in a 60 percent decrease in COVID-19 deaths within the jails (Lofgren et al. 2020). Polling suggested that these mitigation strategies had broad support. A Data for Progress survey showed that in order to dramatically reduce jail and prison populations to slow the spread of COVID-19, a majority of likely voters supported releasing people who were within six months of completing their sentence (Ganz 2021). The decision to only marginally reduce prison and jail populations was a choice made by political operatives and criminal justice officials, and this choice cost lives.

How COVID-19 Is Affected by Mass Incarceration

Certainly, the American government and criminal justice officials could have done more to prevent COVID-19. But given that they did not, what were the consequences? Put another way, how much more likely were incarcerated individuals to contract COVID-19 than nonincarcerated individuals? In this section I estimate the differences in the likelihood of contracting COVID-19 in prison or jail versus in the general community.

To provide evidence on this claim, I rely on publicly available data sets. However, these numbers are not official or verified by any governmental authority, because currently no central government reporting and collection agency, such as the Centers for Disease Control and Prevention (CDC) or the Bureau of Justice Statistics, tracks data on COVID-19 in correctional facilities. Nonprofits and universities have taken it upon themselves to provide some form of data to the public, although these data are not necessarily accurate or comprehensive. This deficiency has been a substantial limitation on the ability of scholars to conduct research on incarceration, detention, and COVID-19 spread. In fact, one of the major nonprofits that has gathered data on COVID-19 in prisons is the Marshall Project. The Marshall Project requests these data every week from state departments of corrections and the federal Bureau of Prisons; however, not all departments provide data for the date requested, leading to occasionally missing and incomplete data.

To overcome these weaknesses, I built a data set of state-by-state and county-by-county COVID-19 infections by merging two publicly available sources of data: the Marshall Project's efforts and the UCLA Prison Law and Policy Program's COVID-19 Behind Bars Data Project.[3] I then merged these data sets with the *New York Times* county-by-county and state-by-state COVID-19 infection data sets. Finally, I folded in Marshall Project state-by-state and county-by-county monthly prison population counts.

This combined data set allowed me to measure the likelihood of contracting COVID-19 outside of prison (general population) and the likelihood of contracting COVID-19 within state or federal prisons (among prisoners). Specifically, I calculated three measures. The first measure is the likelihood of contracting COVID-19 in prison. This metric is calculated by looking at the number of COVID-19 cases in each jail or prison and looking at the total population in the jail or prison. I calculated the ratio of positive tests to total number of incarcerated individuals using only snapshots of jail and prison populations. This approach meant that I had total incarcerated individuals at a moment in time, but I did not have the daily individual-level counts that would have allowed me to measure the daily churn in and out of jails and prisons.

Instead I was left with an approximate ratio of positive tests to approximate population. Next, I calculated the ratio of the positive tests among nonincarcerated individuals to the total nonincarcerated population in a given county or state. Finally, I calculated a third metric, the difference in likelihood of a positive COVID-19 test among incarcerated individuals in a state or county relative to the likelihood of a positive COVID-19 test among nonincarcerated individuals.

Maps 4.1 and 4.2 display the number of COVID-19 cases in US prisons (excluding jails) and the number of COVID-19 cases in American counties, respectively,

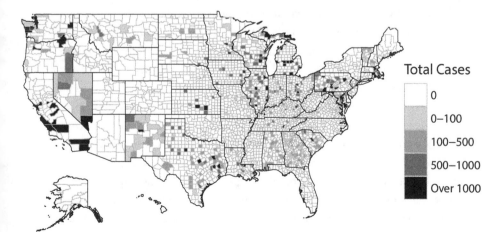

MAP 4.1. Number of COVID-19 cases in US prisons as of October 20, 2020.

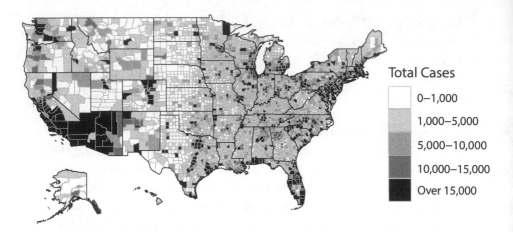

MAP 4.2. Number of COVID-19 cases in US counties as of October 20, 2020.

as of October 20, 2020. While many counties have jails, there are only about eighteen hundred state and federal correctional facilities across the country—meaning most counties do not have any state or federal prisons (Stephan 2008). Relatedly, many individual facilities were not reporting COVID-19 data in states like Delaware, Idaho, and Rhode Island. Still, the counties with the five highest counts of COVID-19 positive tests are Los Angeles County, California; Miami Dade County, Florida; Cook County, Illinois; Harris County, Texas; and Maricopa County, Arizona. Each of these five counties rank among the one hundred counties with the highest number of COVID-19 cases in state or federal prisons.

Finally, Map 4.3 presents differences in the likelihood of contracting COVID-19 inside a state or federal prison facility versus the likelihood of contracting COVID-19 outside of a state or federal prison facility. These numbers can be interpreted as odds ratios, or increased odds of contracting COVID-19 in a state or federal prison facility versus outside the prison facility. I use the state as the unit of analysis here because the data set is more complete than at the county level.

Forty-seven out of fifty states had a higher likelihood of contracting COVID-19 in a state or federal prison than outside a state or federal prison. As of June 2021, the crude estimated rate of contracting COVID-19 inside state or federal prisons appears to be around 33.4 percent, while the crude estimated rate outside of state or federal prisons appears to be 9.1 percent. Put substantively, these estimations suggest that the likelihood of contracting COVID-19 inside of prison are about 3.67 times higher than the likelihood of contracting COVID-19 outside of prison. This finding fits with existing research, conducted

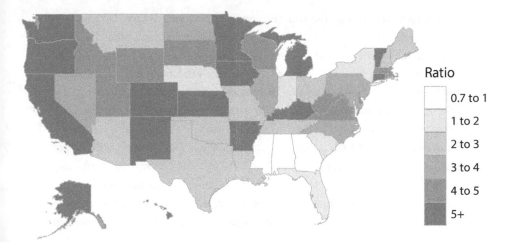

MAP 4.3. Odds ratios of likelihood of COVID-19 contraction in a state or federal prison facility versus outside the prison facility (between March 2020 and November 2020).

in June of 2020, that estimated that the COVID-19 case rate for prisoners was 5.5 times higher than among the US population at large (Saloner et al. 2020). The median state in my data set had a ratio of 4.18, meaning federal and state prisoners were 4.18 times more likely to contract COVID-19 than the general population.

Differences in death rates are less pronounced. The likelihood of a prisoner dying from COVID-19 is about 213 per 100,000, and the COVID-19 death rate for a nonincarcerated individual is 183 per 100,000. This comparison means that prisoners are actually 1.16 times more likely to die from COVID-19 than nonincarcerated individuals, a substantially lower ratio than the 3.67 times higher case rate for incarcerated individuals than for nonincarcerated individuals. This lower death ratio is likely driven by differences in the composition of the general population and the incarcerated population. Specifically, the incarcerated population is more male and younger than the nonincarcerated population. Analysis in the *Journal of the American Medical Association* (JAMA) that estimates demographic adjusted mortality rates found that the adjusted death rate in the prison population was 3.0 times higher than would be expected if the age and sex distributions of the US and prison populations were equal (Saloner et al. 2020).

These increased death rates (3.0 times, when demographic adjusted) and increased contraction rates (4.23 times) do not merely affect those within prison. They also are likely to affect those outside of prison. According to the Marshall Project's estimates, 28,721 prison staffers have contracted COVID-19.

These staffers live among the community, risking spread to their families and friends. Research in the *Health Affairs* journal analyzed data from the Cook County Jail, showing that jail-to-community cycling was a significant predictor of cases at the zip-code level, and it even seems likely to have accounted for about 16 percent of all cases in the state of Illinois (Reinhart and Chen 2020). Additional work focused on Milwaukee, Wisconsin, came to similar conclusions (Escobar and Taheri 2020). Even well-intentioned policies aiming to reduce the size of prison and jail populations may increase risk. Unless facilities are mass testing their incarcerated population, many virus-carrying residents may return to their communities. Reflecting these concerns, an analysis from the ACLU in August 2020 estimated that the American mass imprisonment could increase the number of COVID-19 deaths in the United States by 99,000 to 190,000 people.

Limits to This Analysis

There are important limits to this analysis. First, these are crude estimates of COVID-19 case rates and fatality rates in prisons. Because no publicly available data sets of individual-level inflow and outflow through jails and prisons exist, there is no way to measure jail and prison churn. This churn means that I do not know the "true" number of prisoners but rather only the counts at a moment in time. Relatedly, I have no ability to identify individuals who contracted the virus while incarcerated but who only tested positive after they left the prison or jail. Finally, these estimates are limited by the availability of testing in prison facilities. Because many facilities do not engage in surveillance or mass-population testing, they severely underestimate the number of positive cases present in their locations. For example, a report published in the *Morbidity and Mortality Weekly Report* analyzed data from sixteen prisons and jails in six jurisdictions that engaged in mass testing (testing all inmates). These scholars found a median 12.1-fold increase in the number of cases that had been identified by earlier symptom-based testing alone (Hagan et al. 2020). As of July 2020, researchers at the COVID Prison project estimate that only around 40 percent of incarcerated individuals in prisons received a COVID-19 test (Macmadu et al. 2020; Lemasters et al. 2020). This shortcoming indicates that the number of positive tests may reflect testing capacity across facilities within a state.

Alabama, Georgia, and Mississippi each stand out for being the only states with substantial prison populations that maintained a lower likelihood of contraction of COVID-19 while incarcerated. However, these lower relative rates may have been driven by high likelihood (generally) of contraction within the state. Alabama, Georgia, and Mississippi were three of the twelve states with the highest rates of contraction *outside* of a state or federal prison. Still, many other states used similar measures but were not as effectively able to combat the virus among their general populations. Future work should seek to explain variation in COVID-19 spread across jurisdictions based on prison and jail policies in response to the virus.

Incarceration Contributes to Racial Disparities in COVID-19

One striking feature of COVID-19 has been its racially disparate impact across rates of infection, hospitalization, and death. Some have attributed these disparities to simply the product of economic inequality that is *correlated* with race. But in line with Whitney Laster Pirtle (2020), I argue that racism and capitalism together are the fundamental causes (Link and Phelan 1995) of racial and socioeconomic inequality in COVID-19. Specifically, these disparities are the product of deep structural racial inequality in the United States. Racial inequality in access to healthcare (Williams and Sternthal 2010), employment in essential jobs (McClure et al. 2020), and economic resources (Darity and Myers Jr. 1998; Oliver and Shapiro 2006) leaves racial and ethnic minorities more at risk of contracting COVID-19. Residential segregation (Massey and Denton 1993; Williams and Collins 2016), lower water quality (Jones and Rainey 2006), limited access to healthy food (Odoms-Young, Zenk, and Mason 2009), increased exposure to police violence (Ang 2021; Legewie and Fagan 2019) and to environmental pollutants (Mikati et al. 2018), and day-to-day discrimination (Geronimus et al. 2006) leave racial and ethnic minorities more likely to have comorbidities that increase the fatality rate of COVID-19 (Gravlee 2020). Racism within the medical field means that, often, even if patients do access and receive medical treatment, patients of color have their symptoms, claims, and self-reports dismissed or minimized by medical personnel (Porter 1993). These layers of inequality in access, resources, and treatment come together to produce stark racial inequality in COVID-19 contraction and fatality rates, despite survey data suggesting white residents are less likely than racial and ethnic minorities to follow key COVID-19 transmission protocols like mask wearing (Igielnik 2020).

In this chapter I put forward one more key structural determinant of racial inequality in COVID-19 impact: the racialized American carceral state (Alexander 2020; Gilmore 2007; Gottschalk 2016). As outlined above, COVID-19 is more likely to be spread within prisons and jails. But American carceral facilities are sites of deep racial inequality because of the same racial capitalism

(Robinson 2000) that defines the racial inequality in COVID-19. The carceral state is used to reduce the political power of minority groups (Eubank and Fresh 2022); to raise funds for fiscally distressed municipalities (Goldstein, Sances, and You 2020); and to warehouse individuals for whom the state fails to secure necessary financial, medical, and housing security (Subramanian et al. 2015). This political project leaves blacks, Native Americans, and Latinos dramatically overrepresented, with incarceration rates over 2.5 times higher than that for whites in the United States (Gottschalk 2016).

This overrepresentation in a high-risk location means these groups are far more likely to contract COVID-19 simply because of their being more likely to reside in a facility like a jail or prison. But in fact, many people of color who were not incarcerated at all during the COVID-19 pandemic also faced increased risks of contraction due to the racialized carceral state, because of the deep residential racial segregation in America (Massey and Denton 1993). When residents leave carceral facilities and return to their communities, they usually return to communities and neighborhoods that consist of members of their own racial group. And because these carceral facilities seldom provide adequate personal protective equipment (PPE) or testing to their residents, oftentimes these individuals return to their neighborhoods as active carriers or spreaders of the virus without knowing it. In Chicago, for example, black residents represent only 30 percent of the population but make up about 75 percent of detainees at the Cook County Jail. Analysts found that 60 percent of COVID-19 cases associated with cycling through Cook County Jail were in majority-black zip codes (Reinhart and Chen 2020).

In fact, there are real incentives for political officials and criminal justice operatives to leave prisons and jails full. Roughly half of the 1.4 million people incarcerated in state and federal prisons work behind bars, and throughout COVID-19 they served in essential roles for the state at pay rates unavailable outside of a carceral facility. For example, in California, during the rampant forest fires in fall 2020, prisoners served as firefighters at wages of $1 per hour, saving the state tens of millions of dollars. The nonprofit advocacy organization Worth Rises has found that more than forty states have used prisoners to make hand sanitizer and protective equipment despite often not having access to the same PPE and hand sanitizer themselves (Kamisher 2020). This reliance on prison labor may explain why levels of arrests remained high throughout COVID-19 and why carceral facilities did not engage in mass decarceration across the country despite evidence that high levels of arrests and mass incarceration negated the positive benefits of social distancing and stay-at-home orders (Reinhart and Chen 2020).

Conclusion

This chapter provided a brief overview of the relationship between COVID-19 and mass incarceration in three parts. First, I explained how COVID-19 affected pretrial detention policies and prison release policies across the United States. Using data from the NYU Public Safety Lab Jail Data Initiative and the Marshall Project's COVID in Prisons data sets, I showed how pretrial detention (jail) populations and state prison populations changed during COVID-19. These data show that while there were meaningful decreases in the prison and jail population, these decreases were generally small in magnitude. Next, I showed how mass incarceration affected COVID-19 spread in the United States. I estimate the differences in likelihood of contracting COVID-19 in state or federal prisons as compared to the likelihood of contracting COVID-19 outside of prison, demonstrating that inmates were far more likely to contract COVID-19. Finally, I explained how America's racialized mass incarceration contributes to the racial inequality in the effects of COVID-19.

The choices made by America's political officials and criminal justice operatives have consequences. The choice of mass incarceration for nonwhite people in America has consequences. And as COVID-19 arrived in the United States, the choice to not decarcerate en masse also had consequences: tens of thousands of lost American lives. As researchers begin to reckon with the inadequate American institutional response to the coronavirus pandemic, mass incarceration should not be overlooked. Future research should continue to study the public-health consequences of the political project of mass incarceration in America.

NOTES

1. *New York Times* data can be found at https://github.com/nytimes/covid-19-data, and the Marshall Project data can be found at https://github.com/themarshallproject/COVIDprisondata.

2. Baltimore, Maryland, State's Attorney Marilyn Mosby dismissed pending criminal charges against anyone arrested for drug offenses, trespassing, and minor traffic offenses, among other nonviolent offenses; see Prudente and Jackson 2020.

3. The UCLA *COVID-19 behind Bars* data can be found at https://uclacovidbehindbars.org/.

REFERENCES

Akiyama, Matthew J., Anne C. Spaulding, and Josiah D. Rich. 2020. "Flattening the Curve for Incarcerated Populations—COVID-19 in Jails and Prisons." *New England Journal of Medicine* 382, no. 22 (May): 2075–77.

Alexander, Michelle. 2020. *The New Jim Crow: Mass Incarceration in the Age of Colorblind-ness*. New York: New Press.

American Civil Liberties Union (ACLU). 2020. *COVID-19 Model Finds Nearly 100,000 More Deaths Than Current Estimates, Due to Failures to Reduce Jails*. https://www.aclu.org /sites/default/files/field_document/aclu_covid19-jail-report_2020-8_1.pdf.

Ang, Desmond. 2021. "The Effects of Police Violence on Inner-City Students." *Quarterly Journal of Economics* 136, no. 1: 115–68.

California Department of Corrections and Rehabilitation. 2021. "Additional Actions to Reduce Population and Maximize Space." COVID-19 Information. April 2. https://www .cdcr.ca.gov/covid19/frequently-asked-questions-expedited-releases/.

Cardinale, John. 2020. "St. Louis County Jail Releases Low-Level Inmates to Prevent the Spread of COVID-19." KBJR. April 2. https://kbjr6.com/2020/04/01/st-louis-county-jail -releases-low-level-inmates-to-prevent-the-spread-of-covid-19/.

CDC (Centers for Disease Control and Prevention). 2021. "Risk for COVID-19 Infection, Hospitalization, and Death By Race/Ethnicity." November 22. https://www.cdc.gov/ coronavirus/2019-ncov/covid-data/investigations-discovery/hospitalization-death-by- race-ethnicity.html.

Chappell, Bill, and Paige Pfleger. 2020. "73 percent of Inmates at an Ohio Prison Test Positive for Coronavirus." NPR. April 20. https://www.npr.org/sections/coronavirus -live-updates/2020/04/20/838943211/73-of-inmates-at- an-ohio-prison-test-positive -for-coronavirus.

Crime and Justice Institute. 2021. "How Criminal Justice Systems are Responding to the Coronavirus Outbreak." https://www.cjinstitute.org/corona/.

Darity, William A., Jr., and Samuel L. Myers Jr. 1998. *Persistent Disparity*. Cheltenham, UK: Edward Elgar Publishing.

Escobar, Gipsy, and Sema Taheri. 2020. "Incarceration Weakens a Community's Immune System: Mass Incarceration and COVID-19 Cases in Milwaukee." *Measures for Justice*, Prison Policy Initiative report. https://www.prisonpolicy.org/scans/measuresforjustice /Incarceration_Weakens_Community_Immune_System_Preliminary_Results.pdf.

Eubank, Nicholas, and Adriane Fresh. 2022. "Enfranchisement and Incarceration after the 1965 Voting Rights Act." *American Political Science Review* (January 20): 1–16. https://doi.org/10.1017/S0003055421001337.

Friedersdorf, Conor. 2020. "Let People Out of Jail." *Atlantic*. March 31. https://www .theatlantic.com/ideas/archive/2020/03/public-safety-case-more-jail-releases /609166/.

Ganz, Jason. 2021. "Memo: Fighting the Coronavirus with Decarceration: Policies and Polling." *Data for Progress*. June 29. https://www.dataforprogress.org/memos/fighting -coronavirus-with-decarceration.

Geronimus, Arline T., Margaret Hicken, Danya Keene, and John Bound. 2006. "'Weath-ering' and Age Patterns of Allostatic Load Scores among Blacks and Whites in the United States." *American Journal of Public Health* 96, no. 5 (May): 826–33.

Gilmore, Ruth Wilson. 2007. *Golden Gulag: Prisons, Surplus, Crisis, and Opposition in Globalizing California*. Berkeley: University of California Press.

Goldstein, Rebecca, Michael W. Sances, and Hye Young You. 2020. "Exploitative Revenues, Law Enforcement, and the Quality of Government Service." *Urban Affairs Review*
56, no. 1: 5–31.

Gottschalk, Marie. 2016. *Caught: The Prison State and the Lockdown of American Politics.*
Princeton, NJ: Princeton University Press.

Gravlee, Clarence C. 2020. "Systemic Racism, Chronic Health Inequities, and COVID-19:
A Syndemic in the Making?" *American Journal of Human Biology* 32, no. 5 (September–
October): e23482.

Hagan, Liesl M., Samantha P. Williams, Anne C. Spaulding, Robin L. Toblin, Jessica
Figlenski, Jeanne Ocampo, Tara Ross, Heidi Bauer, Justine Hutchinson, and
Kimberley D. Lucas. 2020. "Mass Testing for SARS-CoV-2 in 16 Prisons and Jails—Six
Jurisdictions, United States, April–May 2020." *Morbidity and Mortality Weekly Report*
69, no. 33: 1139–43.

Hernandez, Salvador. 2020. "Los Angeles Is Releasing Inmates Early and Arresting Fewer
People over Fears of the Coronavirus in Jails." *BuzzFeed News*. March 17. https://www
.buzzfeednews.com/article/salvadorhernandez/los-angeles-coronavirus-inmates-early
-release.

Igielnik, Ruth. 2020. "Most Americans Say They Regularly Wore a Mask in Stores in the
Past Month; Fewer See Others Doing It." Pew Research Center. June 23. https://www
.pewresearch.org/fact-tank/2020/06/23/most-americans-say-they-regularly-wore-a
-mask-in-stores-in-the-past-month-fewer-see-others-doing-it/.

Jones, Robert Emmet, and Shirley A. Rainey. 2006. "Examining Linkages between Race,
Environmental Concern, Health, and Justice in a Highly Polluted Community of
Color." *Black Studies* 36, no. 4: 473–96.

Kamisher, Eliyahu. 2020. "Prison Labor Is on the Frontlines of the COVID-19 Pandemic."
Appeal. October 5. https://theappeal.org/prison-labor-is-on-the-frontlines-of-the-covid
-19-pandemic/.

Laster Pirtle, Whitney N. 2020. "Racial Capitalism: A Fundamental Cause of Novel Coronavirus (COVID-19) Pandemic Inequities in the United States." *Health Education and
Behavior* 47, no. 4: 504–8.

Legewie, Joscha, and Jeffrey Fagan. 2019. "Aggressive Policing and the Educational Performance of Minority Youth." *American Sociological Review* 84, no. 2: 220–47.

Lemasters, Katherine, Erin McCauley, Kathryn Nowotny, and Lauren Brinkley-
Rubinstein. 2020. "COVID-19 Cases and Testing in 53 Prison Systems." *Health and
Justice* 8, no. 24: 1–6.

Link, Bruce G., and Jo Phelan. 1995. "Social Conditions as Fundamental Causes of Disease." *Journal of Health and Social Behavior* (Extra issue): 80–94.

Liu, Yu, and Richard B. Saltman. 2020. "Policy Lessons from Early Reactions to the
COVID-19 Virus in China." *American Journal of Public Health* 110, no. 8: 1145–48.

Lofgren, Eric, Kristian Lum, Aaron Horowitz, Brooke Madubuowu, and Nina Feffer-
man. 2020. "The Epidemiological Implications of Incarceration Dynamics in Jails for
Community, Corrections Officer, and Incarcerated Population Risks from COVID-19."
medRxiv. https://doi.org/10.1101/2020.04.08.20058842.

Macmadu, Alexandria, Justin Berk, Eliana Kaplowitz, Marquisele Mercedes, Josiah D. Rich, and Lauren Brinkley-Rubinstein. 2020. "COVID-19 and Mass Incarceration: A Call for Urgent Action." *Lancet Public Health* 5, no. 11 (November): e571–e572. https://doi.org/10.1016/S2468-2667(20)30231-0.

Maruschak, Laura M., Marcus Berzofsky, and Jennifer Unangst. 2015. *Medical Problems of State and Federal Prisoners and Jail Inmates, 2011–2012*. US Department of Justice, Office of Justice Programs, Bureau of Justice. https://bjs.ojp.gov/library/publications/medical-problems-state-and-federal-prisoners-and-jail-inmates-2011-12.

Massey, Douglas, and Nancy A. Denton. 1993. *American Apartheid: Segregation and the Making of the Underclass*. Cambridge, MA: Harvard University Press.

McClure, Elizabeth S., Pavithra Vasudevan, Zinzi Bailey, Snehal Patel, and Whitney R. Robinson. 2020. "Racial Capitalism within Public Health—How Occupational Settings Drive COVID-19 Disparities." *American Journal of Epidemiology* 189, no. 11 (November): 1244–53.

McDowall, David, Colin Loftin, and Matthew Pate. 2012. "Seasonal Cycles in Crime, and Their Variability." *Journal of Quantitative Criminology* 28, no. 3: 389–410.

Melamed, Samantha, and Mike Newall. 2020. "With Courts Closed by Pandemic, Philly Police Stop Low-Level Arrests to Manage Jail Crowding." *Philadelphia Inquirer*. April 9. https://www.inquirer.com/health/coronavirus/philadelphia-police-coronavirus-covid-pandemic-arrests-jail-overcrowding-larry-krasner-20200317.html.

Mikati, Ihab, Adam F. Benson, Thomas J. Luben, Jason D. Sacks, and Jennifer Richmond-Bryant. 2018. "Disparities in Distribution of Particulate Matter Emission Sources by Race and Poverty Status." *American Journal of Public Health* 108, no. 4 (April): 480–85.

Mills, Christina E., James M. Robins, and Marc Lipsitch. 2004. "Transmissibility of 1918 Pandemic Influenza." *Nature* 432: 904–6.

NAPSA (National Association of Pretrial Services Agencies). 2020. "COVID-19 Sparks 'Unprecedented' Pretrial Reforms, Survey Shows." *Arnold Foundation*. July 17. https://www.arnoldventures.org/stories/covid-19-sparks-unprecedented-pretrial-reforms-survey-shows/.

National Center for State Courts. 2020. "Coronavirus and the Courts." April 24. https://www.ncsc.org/newsroom/public-health-emergency.

National Conference of State Legislators. 2020. *COVID-19 and the Criminal Justice System: A Guide for State Lawmakers*. August 19. https://www.ncsl.org/research/civil-and-criminal-justice/covid-19-and-the-criminal-justice-system-a-guide-for-state-lawmakers.aspx.

New York Times. 2020."Coronavirus in the US: Latest Map and Case Count." March 3. https://www.nytimes.com/interactive/2021/us/covid-cases.html.

O'Dea, Colleen. 2020. "DOC Commissioner Defends COVID-19 Care in State Prisons, Murphy Orders Release of Some Inmates." *NJ Spotlight News*. May 20. https://www.njspotlight.com/2020/04/doc-commissioner-defends-covid-19-care-in-state-prisons-murphy-orders-release-of-some-inmates/.

Odoms-Young, Angela M., Shannon Zenk, and Maryann Mason. 2009. "Measuring Food Availability and Access in African-American Communities: Implications for Intervention and Policy." *American Journal of Preventive Medicine* 36, no. 4: S145–S150.

Oliver, Melvin L., and Thomas M. Shapiro. 2006. *Black Wealth / White Wealth: A New Perspective on Racial Inequality.* New York: Routledge.

Porter, Sam. 1993. "Critical Realist Ethnography: The Case of Racism and Professionalism in a Medical Setting." *Sociology* 27, no. 4 (November): 591–609.

Prison Policy Institute. 2021. "Prison Policy Initiative Virus Response Tracker." https://www.prisonpolicy.org/virus/virusresponse.html.

Prudente, Tim, and Phillip Jackson. 2020. "Baltimore State's Attorney Mosby to Stop Prosecuting Drug Possession, Prostitution, Other Crimes amid Coronavirus." *Baltimore Sun.* March 19. https://www.baltimoresun.com/coronavirus/bs-md-ci-cr-mosby-prisoner-release-20200318-u7knneb605gqvnqmtpejftavia-story.html.

Ragusa, Joe. 2020. "Governor Plans More Commutations Because of Coronavirus." *Spectrum News.* July 30. https://spectrumnews1.com/ky/lexington/news/2020/07/30/governor-considers-700-more-commutations.

Reinhart, Eric, and Daniel Chen. 2020. "Incarceration and Its Disseminations: COVID-19 Pandemic Lessons from Chicago's Cook County Jail: Study Examines How Arrest and Pre-trial Detention Practices May Be Contributing to the Spread of COVID-19." *Health Affairs* 39, no. 8: 1412–18.

Robinson, Cedric J. 2000. *Black Marxism: The Making of the Black Radical Tradition.* Chapel Hill: University of North Carolina Press.

Saloner, Brendan, Kalind Parish, Julie A. Ward, Grace DiLaura, and Sharon Dolovich. 2020. "COVID-19 Cases and Deaths in Federal and State Prisons." *JAMA* 324, no. 6: 602–3.

Schmelzer, Elise. 2020. "Denver, Boulder Law Enforcement Arresting Fewer People to Avoid Introducing Coronavirus to Jails." *Denver Post.* May 7. https://www.denverpost.com/2020/03/16/colorado-coronavirus-jails-arrests/.

Sharma, Damini, Weihua Li, Denise Lavoie, and Claudia Lauer. 2020. "Prison Populations Drop by 100,000 during Pandemic." Marshall Project. July 16. https://www.themarshallproject.org/2020/07/16/prison-populations-drop-by-100-000-during-pandemic.

Smith, Darrell. 2020. "Judicial Council of California Approves $0 Bail for Low-Level Suspects." *Sacramento Bee.* April 6. https://www.sacbee.com/news/coronavirus/article241817606.html.

Stephan, James J. 2008. *Census of State and Federal Correctional Facilities, 2005.* Washington, DC: Bureau of Justice Statistics.

Subramanian, Ram, Ruth Delaney, Stephen Roberts, Nancy Fishman, and Peggy McGarry. 2015. *Incarceration's Front Door: The Misuse of Jails in America.* Brooklyn: Vera Institute of Justice.

Taddeo, Sarah. 2020. "NY to Release up to 1,100 Low-Level Parole Violators from Jails to Stop Coronavirus Spread." *Democrat and Chronicle.* March 28. https://www.democratandchronicle.com/story/news/2020/03/28/new-york-release-up-1-100-low-level-parole-violators-jails/2933262001/.

UCLA Law. 2021. *COVID behind Bars Data Project.* https://uclacovidbehindbars.org/.

van Wagtendonk, Anya. 2020. "Amid Spike in Prison Coronavirus Cases, Gov. Whitmer Orders Testing and Safety Protocols." *Mlive*. August 15. https://www.mlive.com/news/2020/08/amid-spike-in-prison-coronavirus-cases-gov-whitmer-orders-testing-and-safety-protocols.html.

Vargas, Claudia. 2020. "Prisoners Being Released from City, State Prisons Are Not Being Tested for COVID-19." NBC10 Philadelphia. April 17. https://www.nbcphiladelphia.com/investigators/prisoners-being-released-from-city-state-prisons-are-not-being-tested-for-covid-19/2365885/.

Warmsley, Roy. 2005. "Prison Health Care and the Extent of Prison Overcrowding." *International Journal of Prisoner Health* 1, no. 1: 3–12.

Williams, David R., and Chiquita Collins. 2016. "Racial Residential Segregation: A Fundamental Cause of Racial Disparities in Health." Public Health Reports. Los Angeles: SAGE.

Williams, David R., and Michelle Sternthal. 2010. "Understanding Racial-Ethnic Disparities in Health: Sociological Contributions." *Journal of Health and Social Behavior* 51, no. S1: S15–S27.

Worldometers. 2022. "Coronavirus Cases." https://www.worldometers.info/coronavirus/.

COVID-19 and Financial Disparities

5. Housing, Student Debt, and Labor Market Inequality: COVID-19, Black Families/Households, and Financial Insecurity

FENABA R. ADDO AND ADAM HOLLOWELL

When the economy shut down in March 2020 to curtail the spread of the COVID-19 pandemic, it created a severe income crisis and financial shock to most US households who relied on earned income for financial support and stability. It only took a few weeks for scholars, academics, and the media to recognize that the negative financial impacts of COVID-19 would be unevenly distributed across racial groups. (This is not to ignore the racialized distribution of negative health impacts, discussed elsewhere in this volume.)

Pre-COVID-19 economic conditions primed black households to have smaller financial buffers and greater labor vulnerability to economic crisis than their white counterparts. In February 2020, just before the pandemic arrived, McIntosh and colleagues reported for the Brookings Institution that the median net worth of white families in the United States was ten times higher than the median net worth of black families (2020). This is known as the racial wealth gap, a term that describes persistent and substantial wealth disparities between families of different racial and ethnic groups across a variety of measures (Addo and Darity 2021). Additionally, black families faced lower levels of prepandemic income, higher rates of unemployment, and greater levels of food and housing insecurity, as Hardy and Logan have observed (2020, 2).

This chapter explores how prepandemic economic inequality shaped the financial lives of black families during the pandemic and how it will continue to shape them in the decades to follow. In particular, we consider black household vulnerability across three areas of economic inequality: housing, student debt, and the labor market. We conclude with a brief outline of ameliorative policy responses that should be a national priority in the years ahead.

Housing Insecurity

Prior to the pandemic, the primary source of wealth for most US households was their homes: for households in the three middle-income quintiles in 2015, home equity was the largest single financial asset, representing between 50 percent and 70 percent of net wealth (Schuetz 2020). Although less fungible than liquid savings, the ability to draw upon home equity as a financial source is an active practice among US homeowners. It is therefore an anchoring source of financial stability in both the short term and the long term.

Among racial groups in the United States, black Americans are the least likely to be homeowners, even after controlling for education, age, and geographic location. The black-white home ownership gap is even more pronounced in low-income households because of a higher likelihood of intergenerational wealth transfer among white families (Choi et al. 2019). Before the pandemic began, rates of black homeownership in the United States hit their lowest point since 1970 (Gopal 2019).

Housing-related inequality is not only a difference between homeowners and everyone else; there are also disparities within the finances of home ownership. As Keeanga-Yamahtta Taylor notes, "Even when the terms were created to make home ownership possible for poor and working-class black people, this did not change the fact that those homes and the neighborhoods black people resided in were valued differently" (2019). When black households do own homes, the costs are disproportionately higher. Because of systematic over-assessment, black homeowners pay, on average, 10 percent more in property taxes than white homeowners and contribute a greater share of their income to housing costs than their white counterparts (Hardy and Logan 2020, 3). In 2018, Gallup and the Brookings Institution released findings that homes in majority-black neighborhoods were likely to be appraised at values 23 percent less than near-identical homes in majority-white neighborhoods. The same report estimated a cumulative loss of $156 billion to black homeowners due to devalued appraisals (Kamin 2020).

There are racial disparities in rates and implications of mortgage debt, too. Black and Latino borrowers are frequently charged higher rates for mortgage loans than white borrowers in similar financial situations (Steil et al. 2018). The share of homeowners with a mortgage—those homeowners who have not completed payments on their home loan—declined in the decade before the pandemic, dropping from 68.4 percent to 62.9 percent between 2008 and 2017 (Neal 2019). But this drop was largely due to "baby boomers" paying off their mortgages; among homeowners over 65, black homeowners were more likely to hold mortgage debt than white homeowners (Lee, Lown, and Sharpe 2007).

Then there is rent. Rental costs send money out of the home—money that does not get reinvested into the household for future consumption or wealth accumulation. Renters are also more likely to be economically vulnerable. Even before the pandemic, eviction was far too common and disproportionately concentrated in black and low-income communities—e.g., black households are more than twice as likely as white households to be evicted (Benfer et al. 2020, 3). Renters were also disproportionately cost burdened before the pandemic— in 2018, for example, 48 percent of all renter households paid over 30 percent of their income toward rent, and in March 2020, at the start of the pandemic, 25 percent of all renter households were spending more than 50 percent of their income on rent each month (Benfer et al. 2020, 2).

These existing realities created conditions for the racially disparate impacts of unemployment on housing during the height of economic losses in 2020.[1] For black households whose main source of financial resources was earned income, with little savings or only a few months of emergency savings, the unemployment crisis due to COVID-19 was especially burdensome. More than six in ten black adults with a 2019 household income of less than $35,000 reported losing labor income in 2020 during the economic recession (Sanchez Cumming and Kopparam 2021).

The CARES Act, signed into federal law on March 27, 2020, made borrowers with mortgage loans backed by the federal government eligible to apply for a forbearance period of 180 days if they experienced financial hardship due to COVID-19. Federally backed home loans include those issued by the Federal Housing Administration, the Department of Veterans Affairs, the Department of Agriculture, and Fannie Mae and Freddie Mac (Smith and Henricks 2020). But roughly 30 percent of US mortgages—14.5 million loans—are held privately and are not federally backed, and black homeowners are more likely than white homeowners to hold subprime or predatory housing loans (Smith and Henricks 2020; Aalbers 2016). The CARES Act also included provisions for renters, including housing vouchers and an eviction moratorium that lasted until July 24, 2020. It covered renters whose landlords had federally backed mortgages or who otherwise receive federal assistance, but it failed to cover about 72 percent of the rental housing market (Thomas 2020).

By directing more aid toward homeowners than toward renters and by fortifying federally backed properties, the CARES Act effectively provided more help to white households than to black households. Cashauna Hill, executive director of the Louisiana Fair Housing Action Center, described in August 2020 the effect of federal aid on New Orleans residents: "We've got the majority of black homes in the city who are going to be left out of any programs that are geared toward homeowners. And then the majority of white folks, who make up the minority of city residents, will be eligible for those programs" (Thomas 2020).

In August 2020, reports indicated that 44 percent of black households already deferred rent payments or lacked confidence that they would be able to make their next rent payment, almost double the number of white households (24 percent) with the same vulnerabilities (Kapadia 2020). In September 2020, Pew Research reported that 43 percent of black adults said they were having trouble paying their bills, including mortgage payments, since the beginning of the COVID-19 pandemic, more than any other racial or ethnic group (Parker, Minkin, and Bennett 2020; Greene and McCargo 2020). By December 2020, according to a survey conducted by the Social Policy Institute at Washington University in St. Louis, the eviction/foreclosure rate of black and Hispanic survey respondents increased by 7 percent as compared to only 2 percent among white respondents (Chun and Grinstein-Weiss 2020).

Prepandemic economic inequality left black households in the United States with fewer cushions to absorb the financial shocks of 2020. The CARES Act provided short-term, largely ineffective solutions that did little to address underlying racial economic inequality. We propose more equitable solutions to addressing housing insecurity and evictions in the conclusion. For now, we turn to education.

Student Debt and Household Economic Vulnerability

The COVID-19 crisis left higher-education students and their families facing a plethora of outstanding concerns related to their educational and financial futures. Perhaps chief among those concerns was student debt. While postsecondary education can have a positive impact on household wealth through the earning power associated with credentials, negative wealth through student loan debt is a growing crisis at the household level and, in aggregate, at the national level (Addo 2021). Education debt reinforces inequalities in enrollment and rising costs, with Americans holding, in total, more than $1.5 trillion in student debt (Zimmerman 2020).

Enrolling in or returning to school for most students and their families is a costly endeavor. Even with access to federal Pell grants and institutional financial aid, low-income students have a higher likelihood of borrowing money to pay for college than their peers (Mitchell, Leachman, and Saenz 2019). Rising student debt among students and their families reflects the increasing costs of higher education and minimal economic growth at the household level. In 1988, tuition accounted for roughly one-quarter of revenue for public colleges and universities, while state and local governments provided the remaining three-quarters. With rising tuition and drastically reduced government funding, the split today is close to fifty-fifty (Mitchell et al. 2019). Public colleges and universities increased tuition more than 37 percent from 2009 to 2019 (Friga 2020). And in recent decades, household income has not kept up with college and university tuition inflation (Maurer 2020).

Education debt is particularly prevalent among black students and their families. Prior to the crisis, black students enrolled at institutions of higher education disproportionately took on student debt to cover the costs of college, accumulated more debt, and took longer to repay those debts upon leaving school. Low-income and low-wealth black families with Parental PLUS loans have more average debt than white families (Fishman 2018). Black-white disparities in wealth are related to black-white differences in student debt accumulation, and disparities in student accumulation and repayment contribute to black-white wealth gaps (Addo, Houle, and Simon 2016; Houle and Addo 2018). In 2016, 85 percent of black graduates across all higher-education institution types graduated with debt, compared to just under 70 percent of their white peers (Mitchell et al. 2019).

Among recent cohorts of college attendees, there is growing concern that the financial risks associated with pursuing a college degree for black borrowers are beginning to outweigh the returns of that education. In 2018 young college graduates faced an underemployment rate of 11.1 percent, as compared with 9.4 percent in 2007 and 6.9 percent in 2000 (Gould et al. 2018). Additionally, black college graduates in 2018 faced a wage penalty of more than 16 percent relative to their white counterparts (Gould et al. 2018; Nzinga 2020). Underemployment and wage penalties are particularly acute for black PhD graduates. A 2012 report from the National Center for Education Statistics indicated a 42 percent increase in the award of PhDs to black students in the years between 2000 and 2010, yet the average increase in black faculty appointments at predominantly white institutions during the same years was only 1.3 percent (Nzinga 2020, 59).

Each vector of household and education vulnerability will have disparate impacts on women, and on black women, in particular. Women have been going to school and completing their degrees at higher rates than men but do not have the same economic outcomes (Addo and Zhang 2019). Although black borrowers carry higher levels of student debt than other borrowers, women across all races carry more student debt than men (Wakamo 2020). Over $900 billion of the $1.6 trillion dollars in national student loan debt are carried by women (Miller 2017; AAUW 2020). Black women are the least likely among their peers to receive institutional funding for graduate education and, relatedly, most likely use private funding for education (Nzinga 2020, 13). At both the graduate and undergraduate level, black women carry the largest higher-education loan debt in the nation (Nzinga 2020, 13). For example, among millennials, black women completed college (22.76 percent) at almost twice the rate of black men (13.36 percent). Yet the median wealth of black male millennials ($8,105) was 2.5 times greater than black female graduates ($3,316) (Bhattacharya, Price, and Addo 2019).

Despite these cautionary factors, during previous economic recessions when the labor market tanked and unemployment rates rose, a common trend was to return to institutions of higher education to bolster one's skills. The Great Recession was no exception as total postsecondary enrollment increased from 17.2 million students in 2006 to 20.4 million students in 2011 (Schmidt 2018), and aggregate student debt levels also increased. In fact, student debt was the only consumer debt that continued to rise throughout the recessionary period (Garriga, Noeth, and Schlagenhauf 2017). However, the benefits of education in a recession are unevenly distributed—for example, the black-white unemployment rate among college graduates widened during the Great Recession (Reddy 2010; Scott-Clayton and Li 2016).[2]

The CARES Act had some ameliorative effects during the height of the COVID-19 pandemic. Once passed, federal student loan debt payments were suspended from March 27, 2020, through September 30, 2020, and the suspension was later extended through January 31, 2021, and then again through September 30, 2021. The CARES Act also set interest rates at 0 percent during this period and halted collections on defaulted loans. At the time of this writing, President Joe Biden has continued the federal loan payment suspension through September 1, 2022, and he seems unlikely to issue a proposed $50,000 student debt cancellation through executive order. "I will not make that happen," Biden said shortly after taking office (Hale 2021; Berman 2022).

Given these pauses in federal repayment for all borrowers, it will be difficult to tell in the short term how the economic downturn associated with the COVID-19 pandemic will impact student loan repayment and default. Even before the pandemic began, nearly two-thirds of student loan borrowers were unable to pay down the principal of the full monthly interest on their student loans, adding to rising debt balances (Calhoun and Harrington 2020). Additional data indicate that one in seven student loan borrowers in loan repayment was more than ninety days delinquent or in deeper default on their payments at the outset of the pandemic (Calhoun and Harrington 2020). This will be especially true if, as expected, wage growth in the years ahead does not match the rising costs of debt, despite job growth in sectors that require postsecondary credentials.

The ability to pay student loans will, of course, be closely tied to employment status. This intertwining brings us to the precarity of the labor market during the height of economic losses in 2020 and, in particular, to the precarity of women's employment during this period. Indeed, some commentators called the economic impacts of COVID-19 the country's first "female recession," because unemployment rates were higher among women than among men in the summer of 2020 (Carrazana 2020; Tappe 2020). Here, as elsewhere in this chapter, the precarity is particularly acute for black families.

Labor Market Inequality

While gender gaps in unemployment had closed in the run-up to 2020, it quickly became clear that women would fare much worse than men in the pandemic economy. The US economy lost nearly eleven million jobs held by women between February and May 2020, and female unemployment reached double digits for the first time since 1948 (Carrazana 2020). By June 2020 the unemployment rate was 15.3 percent for Latinas and 14 percent for black women, while the rate for white men held at 9 percent (Carrazana 2020). Even before the pandemic the gender pay gap remained acute: the National Partnership for Women and Families reported in March 2020 that among full-time year-round workers, for every dollar paid to non-Hispanic white men, non-Hispanic white women are paid 79 cents; Asian women are paid 90 cents; black women are paid 62 cents; Native American women are paid 57 cents; and Latinas are paid 54 cents (2020, 1).

Alon and colleagues suggest that sharper employment losses for women during the downturn of 2020 were due to two factors, the first of which was a concentrated loss of jobs in high-contact service sectors such as restaurants, hospitality, and travel, where women are a large share of the workforce (2020, 1–2). Albanesi and colleagues find that in occupations that are considered "high in personal contact," women account for 74 percent of employment (2020). This overrepresentation may also be a function of a higher concentration of women in jobs with fewer opportunities to telecommute, which suffered larger unemployment during the pandemic (Papanikolaou and Schmidt 2020).

The second factor in gender disparities in unemployment that Alon and colleagues identify is the increase in childcare needs due to school closures, which prevented some women from working or drove dual-earner heterosexual households to prioritize men's labor (2020, 1–2). Collins and colleagues (2021) found that working mothers of young children reduced their work hours four-to-five times more than working fathers of young children during the first three months of the pandemic. To call it a reduction of "work hours" is, of course, a misnomer, since those same working mothers were "taking on a larger burden of childcare and homeschooling at the expense of paid work time" (Collins et al. 2021, 9). In dual-earner, heterosexual married couples, where both partners were able to work remotely through telecommuting-capable jobs, the increased level of visibility of childcare and other domestic responsibilities "did not result in fathers' increased participation in caregiving" (Collins et al. 2021, 10).

Both "high contact" occupational vulnerability and disparities in childcare access hit black women especially hard. Black workers were overrepresented, relative to their share of the population, in "essential" front-line jobs: grocery, convenience, and drug stores; public transit; trucking; warehouse; postal service; and healthcare, childcare, and social services (Gould and Wilson 2020). In particular, black women were overrepresented among front-line industry workers who were required to work outside of the home during the spring and summer of 2020, escalating the pressure to maintain health safety and serve as a "proxy educator" while schools remained closed (Kapadia 2020). According to Gould and Wilson (2020), more than one in six black workers lost a job between February and April 2020. Nearly 19 percent of black women workers lost their jobs in that same window.

Once state and federal governments began to sort jobs and businesses as essential and nonessential, a divide grew between those who were able to keep working remotely and earn a living and those who had to report physically to a work site and interact with people, increasing their risks of transmission. Workers deemed essential may not have lost their income, but frontline employees encountered customer interactions and increased health risks. For instance, black Americans were more likely than white Americans to be employed in assisted living facilities and nursing homes, food preparation and meatpacking, and personal care and service positions (Hardy and Logan 2020, 4).[3]

As the pandemic created structural barriers to providing and receiving care, it also raised awareness regarding the hypocrisies related to the essential nature of formal and informal care work in our society and how it remains undervalued in terms of compensation. Working remotely may not necessarily be correlated with increased productivity, especially for adult caregivers. Gould and Wilson (2020) found that black workers are twice as likely as white workers to live in households with residents that span three or more generations, for example, a child living in a household with parents and grandparents. Care for children was relatively less affordable for black families than for white families prior to the pandemic, a problem that was compounded because of the widespread closure of daycare centers, afterschool programs, and public schools across the country (Hardy and Logan 2020, 6). For example, black and Hispanic Americans were disproportionately impacted by the prohibitive costs of childcare services and the shortage of available services due to pandemic closures (Grooms, Ortega, and Rubalcaba 2020).

In July 2020, 57 percent of black adults reported on a Census Bureau survey that someone in their household had experienced loss of income during the pandemic (Brenson, Fulton, and Overton 2020). In April 2020 Ganong and colleagues reported that when experiencing an "income shock" of the same magnitude, black families, as compared to white families, experience more severe and more prolonged declines in household consumption (2020). In other words, the cost of an income shock to consumption in black households is 50 percent higher than it is for white households.

But job loss is so much more than simply an exit from the labor market. As noted throughout this chapter, black workers had relatively fewer financial resources to survive the economic impact of the pandemic, including fewer earners per household, lower incomes, and lower liquid wealth than white workers (Gould and Wilson 2020). Ultimately, precarity in the labor market also meant cascading and compounding vulnerabilities. Consider these three consequences of job loss, in brief: loss of health insurance, onset of food insecurity, and discrimination in receipt of benefits.

Black workers were 60 percent more likely to be in jobs without health insurance than white workers during the pandemic (Gould and Wilson 2020). The Kaiser Family Foundation estimated as early as July 2020 that 27 million Americans had already lost health insurance coverage during the pandemic (Stolberg 2020). Data collected from Grooms and colleagues between March and July 2020 indicated that black and Hispanic essential non-healthcare workers reported working without health insurance coverage at rates four times higher than white essential non-healthcare workers (2020).

Black families disproportionately lacked the savings and wealth cushion necessary to handle an unexpected expense, such as emergency medical expenses in the face of a COVID diagnosis or emergency transportation expenses with the closure of public transportation services (Hardy and Logan 2020). Nearly four in ten black and Hispanic households with children experienced food insecurity and trouble feeding their families during the pandemic, almost double the rate of food insecurity among white households (Evich 2020). The numbers from the pandemic summer are staggering. In a July 2020 survey conducted by the Hamilton Project, 29 percent of black households with children reported that the children did not have enough food to eat the previous week (Evich 2020). Golla and colleagues examined food requests to 2-1-1 helplines across twenty-three states: requests at least doubled in every state, rose 500 percent in half of the states, and increased by 2,200 percent in New Jersey (2020). In June 2020, a survey by the Census Bureau indicated that fourteen million children in the United States experienced hunger because of financial strain—more than five times the number in 2018. One in three black households and one in five Hispanic households with children reported some food insecurity for children (Darville 2020).

When benefits were available to workers who lost jobs, those benefits were distributed unequally. As of July 2020, nearly fifty million Americans filed for unemployment insurance (Benfer et al. 2020). The federal government paid $600 per week to jobless workers between April and June 2020, supplying over $200 billion to the economy, almost 5 percent of total household income (Cohen and Hsu 2020). Data from Grooms and colleagues collected between March and July 2020 revealed that after filing for benefits, unemployed black Americans waited, on average, seven to eight days longer than white Americans to receive those benefits (2020). The average wait time between application and benefits was twenty-three days (Grooms et al. 2020). Among unemployed black Americans, only 29 percent had received unemployment benefits by mid to late March (Grooms et al. 2020).

Conclusion: Policy Responses to Housing, Education, and Labor Market Precarity

The negative financial impacts of the pandemic were unquestionably unevenly distributed across racial and ethnic groups. We must now ask how federal and state interventions might improve outcomes in the years ahead, with particular focus accorded to the areas of housing, student debt, and the labor market. We conclude by offering several avenues of public policy that would address the vulnerabilities of black families in these areas.

A federal jobs guarantee would avert state-level vulnerabilities and discrimination against black workers. Black workers receive lower average earnings, face less-predictable work hours, experience less overall employment stability, and reside disproportionately in states where the federal minimum wage for low-wage workers is binding (Hardy and Logan 2020, 2). As proposed by Darity (2010) and Paul and colleagues (2018), a federal jobs guarantee could eliminate economic insecurity produced by fluctuations in the stock market and create an avenue for a federal health insurance program to eliminate recession-related widespread uninsurance. It could also be a direct response to mass unemployment in the wake of the COVID-19 pandemic, as argued by Pavlina Tcherneva in *The Case for a Job Guarantee* (2020).

Federal and state aid should directly support black-owned businesses, which were more likely to have been operating in COVID-19 hotspots and were twice as likely to have closed during summer 2020 (Kapadia 2020). The Small Business Association's (SBA) two main lending programs for small businesses in the United States distributed $1.52 billion between 2014–2019: black-owned businesses received just 2.5 percent of those funds, and the SBA was tapped to oversee federal loans for small businesses during COVID-19 (Frank 2020). More direct oversight of the SBA to eliminate racial discrimination and provide for the health and thriving of black businesses is essential in the future.

A national program to alleviate or cancel student debt would improve the financial position of black families and may have a significant effect in bolstering the black middle class (Houle and Addo 2018). Calhoun and Harrington have noted that debt cancellation proposals must account for the financial hardships that plague all borrowers, even those who are employed and current on their loans (2020). Miller and colleagues have indicated that prioritizing equity in student debt forgiveness must include targeted relief for black borrowers (n.d.). A federal loan forgiveness plan proposed by Senator Elizabeth Warren designates a set amount for each borrower rather than the value of the full loan for each borrower, which may lessen the impact of the legislation on black borrowers (Berman 2022).

According to New America, Hispanic borrowers occupy a disproportionate share of low-balance student loan debts, while black borrowers are overrepresented among those with balances between $40,000 and $100,000 (Miller et al. n.d.).

A first step to addressing black housing precarity would be federal reimplementation of the Obama-era policy Affirmatively Furthering Fair Housing (AFFH), which required municipalities to take meaningful actions to combat housing discrimination (Kahlenberg and Quick 2019). Housing and Urban Development should use fair housing testers through the Fair Housing Initiatives Program (FHIP) to identify FHA violations and support programs of redress and repair to communities with documented discrimination (Kahlenberg and Quick 2019). Richard D. Kahlenberg (2017) has called upon federal lawmakers to pass an Economic Fair Housing Act that parallels the Fair Housing Act of 1968, curbing exclusionary zoning laws and making it illegal for municipalities to discriminate in housing policy on the basis of income.

Renters will need policy solutions, too. Matthew Desmond (2016) has proposed a universal housing voucher program that would cap eligible families' spending on rent at 30 percent of their income. Blumgart (2016) outlines additional housing policy proposals, including a nationwide ban on source-of-income discrimination against voucher-holding renters, an expansion of the earned income tax credit to act similarly to Section 8 vouchers, a state-administered renters' tax credit similar to a property tax deduction, and an expansion of housing vouchers that does not reach "universal" access.

Prepandemic racial inequalities in housing, student, and the labor market continue to render black families disproportionately vulnerable to economic recovery efforts. In the years ahead, targeted policies will be needed to end discriminatory practices; close persistent gaps in economic outcomes; and guarantee access to healthy, financially stable household outcomes.

NOTES

1. Approximately one quarter of US households spend more than half of their monthly income on rent, making any loss of income a threat to their housing (*New York Times* Editorial Board 2020).

2. In April 2010, the nationwide jobless rate for white college graduates ages 25 and older was 4 percent, while the rate for college graduates in the same age bracket who identify themselves as black or African-American was 7.4 percent (Reddy 2010).

3. Just prior to the pandemic, Sekile Nzinga highlighted evidence that black women are less likely to benefit from institutional family leave policies due to forces of racialized gender bias, employment vulnerability, and workplace exploitation (2020, 107–38).

REFERENCES

Aalbers, Manuel B. 2016. "Housing Finance as Harm." *Crime, Law and Social Change* 66, no. 2 (September): 115–29. https://doi.org/10.1007/s10611-016-9614-x.

AAUW (American Association of University Women). 2020. "Deeper in Debt: 2020 Update." Washington, DC. https://www.aauw.org/app/uploads/2020/05/Deeper_In _Debt_FINAL.pdf.

Addo, Fenaba R. 2021. *Ensuring a More Equitable Future: Exploring and Measuring the Relationship between Family Wealth, Education Debt, and Wealth Accumulation.* Postsecondary Value Commission. https://www.postsecondaryvalue.org/wp-content/uploads /2021/05/PVC-Addo-FINAL.pdf.

Addo, Fenaba R., and William A. Darity Jr. 2021. "Disparate Recoveries: Wealth, Race, and the Working Class after the Great Recession." ANNALS *of the American Academy of Political and Social Science* 695, no. 1 (May): 173–92.

Addo, Fenaba R., Jason N. Houle, and Daniel Simon. 2016. "Young, Black, and (Still) in the Red: Parental Wealth, Race, and Student Loan Debt." *Race and Social Problems* 8, no. 1: 64–76. https://doi.org/10.1007/s12552-016-9162-0.

Addo, Fenaba R., and Yiling Zhang. 2019. "The Millennial Racial Wealth Gap." In *The Emerging Millennial Wealth Gap: Divergent Trajectories, Weak Balance Sheets, and Implications for Social Policy,* edited by Reid Cramer. Washington, DC: New America.

Albanesi, Stefania, Rania Gihleb, Jialin Huo, and Jiyeon Kim. 2020. "VMACS—Household Insurance and the Macroeconomic Impact of the Novel Corona Virus." Paper presented at the Virtual Macro Seminar, University of Pittsburgh. June 4. https://www.youtube .com/watch?v=vEVoLdMeDsg.

Alon, Titan, Matthias Doepke, Jane Olmstead-Rumsey, and Michèle Tertilt. 2020. "This Time It's Different: The Role of Women's Employment in a Pandemic Recession." Working Paper w27660, National Bureau of Economic Research, Cambridge, MA. https://doi.org/10.3386/w27660.

Benfer, Emily, David Bloom Robinson, Stacy Butler, Lavar Edmonds, Sam Gilman, Katherine Lucas McKay, Zach Neumann, Lisa Owens, Neil Steinkamp, and Diane Yentel. 2020. "The COVID-19 Election Crisis: An Estimated 30–40 Million People in America Are at Risk." Aspen Institute. https://www.aspeninstitute.org/blog-posts /the-covid-19-eviction-crisis-an-estimated-30–40-million-people-in-america-are-at -risk/.

Berman, Russell. 2022. "The Bold Economic Move Joe Biden Refuses to Make." *Atlantic.* January 12. https://www.theatlantic.com/politics/archive/2022/01/biden-student-loan -debt-cancellation/621224/.

Bhattacharya, Jhumpa, Anne Price, and Fenaba R. Addo. 2019. *Clipped Wings: Closing the Wealth Gap for Millennial Women.* Asset Funders Network. Accessed September 13, 2020. https://insightcced.org/wp-content/uploads/2019/03/AFN_2019_Clipped-Wings _BOOKLET_WEB_final-3.4.19.pdf.

Blumgart, Jake. 2016. "Too Many Americans Live on the Edge of Eviction. Here's How to Fix the Problem." *Slate Magazine.* July 1. https://slate.com/business/2016/07/its-time -for-universal-housing-vouchers.html.

Brenson, LaShonda, Jessica Fulton, and Spencer Overton. 2020. "Pandemic Relief Priorities for Black Communities." Joint Center. August 4. https://jointcenter.org/pandemic-relief-priorities-for-black-communities/.

Calhoun, Michael, and Ashley Harrington. 2020. "The Next COVID-19 Relief Bill Must Include Student Debt Cancellation." Brookings. June 3. https://www.brookings.edu/research/the-next-covid-19-relief-bill-must-include-student-debt-cancellation/.

Carrazana, Chabeli. 2020. "America's First Female Recession." *The 19th**. August 2. https://19thnews.org/2020/08/americas-first-female-recession/.

Choi, Jung Hyun, Alanna McCargo, Michael Neal, Laurie Goodman, and Caitlin Young. 2019. "Explaining the Black-White Homeownership Gap: A Closer Look at Disparities across Local Markets." Urban Institute. October 10. https://www.urban.org/research/publication/explaining-black-white-homeownership-gap-closer-look-disparities-across-local-markets.

Chun, Yung, and Michal Grinstein-Weiss. 2020. "Housing Inequality Gets Worse as the COVID-19 Pandemic Is Prolonged." Brookings. December 18. https://www.brookings.edu/blog/up-front/2020/12/18/housing-inequality-gets-worse-as-the-covid-19-pandemic-is-prolonged/.

Cohen, Patricia, and Tiffany Hsu. 2020. "$300 Unemployment Benefit: Who Will Get It and When?" *New York Times*. August 26. https://www.nytimes.com/article/stimulus-unemployment-payment-benefit.html.

Collins, Caitlyn, Liana Christin Landivar, Leah Ruppanner, and William J. Scarborough. 2021. "COVID-19 and the Gender Gap in Work Hours." *Gender, Work, and Organization* 28, no. S1: 101–12. https://doi.org/10.1111/gwao.12506.

Darity, William A., Jr. 2010. "A Direct Route to Full Employment." *Review of Black Political Economy* 37, no. 3: 179–81. https://doi.org/10.1007/s12114-010-9075-x.

Darville, Sarah. 2020. "Reopening Schools Is Way Harder Than It Should Be." *New York Times*. July 23. https://www.nytimes.com/2020/07/23/sunday-review/reopening-schools-coronavirus.html.

Desmond, Matthew. 2016. "The Eviction Economy." *New York Times*. March 5. https://www.nytimes.com/2016/03/06/opinion/sunday/the-eviction-economy.html.

Evich, Helena Bottemiller. 2020. "Stark Racial Disparities Emerge as Families Struggle to Get Enough Food." *Politico*. July 6. https://www.politico.com/news/2020/07/06/racial-disparities-families-struggle-food-348810.

Fishman, Rachel. 2018. "The Wealth Gap PLUS Debt." New America. http://newamerica.org/education-policy/reports/wealth-gap-plus-debt/.

Frank, Thomas. 2020. "Disaster Loans Entrench Disparities in Black Communities." *Scientific American*. July 2. https://www.scientificamerican.com/article/disaster-loans-entrench-disparities-in-black-communities/.

Friga, Paul N. 2020. "The Great Recession Was Bad for Higher Education. Coronavirus Could Be Worse." *Chronicle of Higher Education*. March 24. https://www.chronicle.com/article/The-Great-Recession-Was-Bad/248317.

Ganong, Peter, Damon Jones, Pascal Noel, Diana Farrell, Fiona Greig, and Chris Wheat. 2020. "Wealth, Race, and Consumption Smoothing of Typical Income Shocks." *Becker Friedman Institute* (blog). April 21. https://bfi.uchicago.edu/working-paper/wealth-race -and-consumption-smoothing-of-typical-income-shocks/.

Garriga, Carlos, Bryan Noeth, and Don E. Schlagenhauf. 2017. "Household Debt and the Great Recession." *Review* (Federal Reserve Bank of St. Louis) 99, no. 2: 183–205.

Golla, Balaji, Irum Javed, and Matthew Kreuter. 2020. "Food Pantries—UPDATED." Health Communication Research Laboratory. https://hcrl.wustl.edu/items/food -pantries-updated/.

Gopal, Prashant. 2019. "Black Homeownership Falls to Record Low as Affordability Worsens." *Bloomberg*. July 25. https://www.bloomberg.com/news/articles/2019-07-25 /black-homeownership-falls-to-record-low-as-affordability-worsens.

Gould, Elise, Zane Mokhiber, and Julia Wolfe. 2018. "Class of 2018: College Edition." Economic Policy Institute. https://www.epi.org/publication/class-of-2018-college -edition/.

Gould, Elise, and Valerie Wilson. 2020. "Black Workers Face Two of the Most Lethal Preexisting Conditions for Coronavirus—Racism and Economic Inequality." *Economic Policy Institute* (blog). June 1. https://www.epi.org/publication/black-workers-covid/.

Greene, Solomon, and Alanna McCargo. 2020. "New Data Suggest COVID-19 Is Widening Housing Disparities by Race and Income." Urban Institute. https://www.urban .org/urban-wire/new-data-suggest-covid-19-widening-housing-disparities-race-and -income.

Grooms, Jevay, Alberto Ortega, and Joaquín Alfredo-Angel Rubalcaba. 2020. "The COVID-19 Public Health and Economic Crises Leave Vulnerable Populations Exposed." Hamilton Project. https://www.hamiltonproject.org/blog/the_covid_19_public_health _and_economic_crises_leave_vulnerable_populations_exposed.

Hale, Kori. 2021. "Here's How $50,000 in Student Loan Forgiveness Will Impact the Racial Wealth Gap." *Forbes*. April 21. https://www.forbes.com/sites/korihale/2021 /04/21/heres-how-50000-in-student-loan-forgiveness-will-impact-the-racial-wealth -gap/.

Hardy, Bradley L., and Trevon D. Logan. 2020. "Racial Economic Inequality amid the COVID-19 Crisis." Hamilton Project, Brookings. https://www.brookings.edu/research /racial-economic-inequality-amid-the-covid-19-crisis/.

Houle, Jason N., and Fenaba R. Addo. 2018. "Racial Disparities in Student Debt and the Reproduction of the Fragile Black Middle Class." *Sociology of Race and Ethnicity* 5, no. 4: 562–77. https://doi.org/10.1177/2332649218790989.

Kahlenberg, Richard D. 2017. "An Economic Fair Housing Act." The Century Foundation. https://tcf.org/content/report/economic-fair-housing-act/.

Kahlenberg, Richard D., and Kimberly Quick. 2019. "The Government Created Housing Segregation. Here's How the Government Can End It." *American Prospect*. July 2. https://prospect.org/api/content/7fff016a-4652-599e-84c7 -968697d9aba7/.

Kamin, Debra. 2020. "Black Homeowners Face Discrimination in Appraisals." *New York Times*. August 25. https://www.nytimes.com/2020/08/25/realestate/blacks-minorities-appraisals-discrimination.html.

Kapadia, Reshma. 2020. "More Signs Coronavirus Exacerbates Economic Inequality. Here's How." *Barron's*. August 14. https://www.barrons.com/articles/more-signs-coronavirus-exacerbates-economic-inequality-heres-how-51597442418.

Lee, Yoon G., Jean M. Lown, and Deanna L. Sharpe. 2007. "Predictors of Holding Consumer and Mortgage Debt among Older Americans." *Journal of Family and Economic Issues* 28, no. 2: 305–20. https://doi.org/10.1007/s10834-007-9055-x.

Maurer, Tim. 2020. "Is COVID-19 Creating an Education Planning Crisis?" *Forbes*. April 24. https://www.forbes.com/sites/timmaurer/2020/04/24/is-covid-19-creating-an-education-planning-crisis/.

McIntosh, Kriston, Emily Moss, Ryan Nunn, and Jay Shambaugh. 2020. "Examining the Black-White Wealth Gap." Brookings. February 27. https://www.brookings.edu/blog/up-front/2020/02/27/examining-the-black-white-wealth-gap/.

Miller, Ben, Colleen Campbell, Brent J. Cohen, and Charlotte Hancock. n.d. "Addressing the $1.5 Trillion in Federal Student Loan Debt." NewAmerica. Accessed September 13, 2020. http://newamerica.org/millennials/reports/emerging-millennial-wealth-gap/.

Miller, Kevin. 2017. *Deeper in Debt*. Washington, DC: American Association of University Women. https://www.aauw.org/app/uploads/2020/03/DeeperinDebt-nsa.pdf.

Mitchell, Michael, Michael Leachman, and Matt Saenz. 2019. "State Higher Education Funding Cuts Have Pushed Costs to Students, Worsened Inequality." Center on Budget and Policy Priorities. https://www.cbpp.org/research/state-budget-and-tax/state-higher-education-funding-cuts-have-pushed-costs-to-students.

National Partnership for Women and Families. 2020. "America's Women and the Wage Gap: Fact Sheet." National Partnership. https://www.nationalpartnership.org/our-work/resources/economic-justice/fair-pay/americas-women-and-the-wage-gap.pdf.

Neal, Michael. 2019. "Mortgage Debt Has Peaked. Why Has the Share of Homeowners with a Mortgage Fallen to a 13-Year Low?" Urban Institute. https://www.urban.org/urban-wire/mortgage-debt-has-peaked-why-has-share-homeowners-mortgage-fallen-13-year-low.

New York Times Editorial Board. 2020. "Opinion: Millions of Americans Are about to Lose Their Homes. Congress Must Help Them." *New York Times*. https://www.nytimes.com/2020/07/23/opinion/coronavirus-evictions-rent.html.

Nzinga, Sekile M. 2020. *Lean Semesters: How Higher Education Reproduces Inequity*. Baltimore, MD: Johns Hopkins University Press.

Papanikolaou, Dimitris, and Lawrence D. W. Schmidt. 2020. "Working Remotely and the Supply-Side Impact of COVID-19." Working Paper w27330, National Bureau of Economic Research, Cambridge, MA. https://doi.org/10.3386/w27330.

Parker, Kim, Rachel Minkin, and Jesse Bennett. 2020. "Economic Fallout from COVID-19 Continues to Hit Lower-Income Americans the Hardest." Pew Research Center.

https://www.pewresearch.org/social-trends/2020/09/24/economic-fallout-from-covid
-19-continues-to-hit-lower-income-americans-the-hardest/.

Paul, Mark, William A. Darity Jr., Darrick Hamilton, and Khaing Zaw. 2018. "A Path to
Ending Poverty by Way of Ending Unemployment: A Federal Job Guarantee." RSF:
Russell Sage Foundation Journal of the Social Sciences 4, no. 3: 44–63. https://doi.org/10
.7758/rsf.2018.4.3.03.

Reddy, Sudeep. 2010. "Recession Exacerbates Race Gap." Wall Street Journal. https://www
.wsj.com/articles/SB10001424052748704292004575230543067586002.

Sanchez Cumming, Carmen, and Raksha Kopparam. 2021. "What the US Census Household Pulse Survey Reveals about the First Year of the Coronavirus Recession, in Six
Charts." Washington Center for Equitable Growth. https://equitablegrowth.org/what
-the-u-s-census-household-pulse-survey-reveals-about-the-first-year-of-the-coronavirus
-recession-in-six-charts/.

Scott-Clayton, Judith, and Jing Li. 2016. "Black-White Disparity in Student Loan Debt
More Than Triples after Graduation." Brookings. https://www.brookings.edu/research
/black-white-disparity-in-student-loan-debt-more-than-triples-after-graduation/.

Schmidt, Erik P. 2018. Postsecondary Enrollment before, during, and since the Great Recession. Washington, DC: US Census Bureau. https://www.census.gov/content/dam
/Census/library/publications/2018/demo/P20-580.pdf.

Schuetz, Jenny. 2020. "Rethinking Homeownership Incentives to Improve Household Financial Security and Shrink the Racial Wealth Gap." Brookings. https://www
.brookings.edu/research/rethinking-homeownership-incentives-to-improve-household
-financial-security-and-shrink-the-racial-wealth-gap/.

Smith, Kelly Anne, and Mark Henricks. 2020. "Mortgage Payments Interrupted by
covid-19? The Federal and State Response." Forbes. April 20. https://www.forbes.com
/sites/advisor/2020/04/20/mortgage-payments-interrupted-by-covid-19-the-federal
-and-state-response/.

Steil, Justin P., Len Albright, Jacob S. Rugh, and Douglas S. Massey. 2018. "The Social
Structure of Mortgage Discrimination." Housing Studies 33, no. 5: 759–76. https://doi
.org/10.1080/02673037.2017.1390076.

Stolberg, Sheryl Gay. 2020. "Millions Have Lost Health Insurance in Pandemic-Driven
Recession." New York Times. July 13. https://www.nytimes.com/2020/07/13/us/politics
/coronavirus-health-insurance-trump.html.

Tappe, Anneken. 2020. "Women Are Hit Harder by This Recession, and Governments
Need to Act Now, IMF Warns." CNN. July 21. https://www.cnn.com/2020/07/21
/economy/imf-covid-inequality-women/index.html.

Taylor, Keeanga-Yamahtta. 2019. "Against Black Homeownership." Boston Review.
November 15. http://bostonreview.net/race/keeanga-yamahtta-taylor-against-black
-homeownership.

Tcherneva, Pavlina R. 2020. The Case for a Job Guarantee. Cambridge: Polity.

Thomas, Taylor Miller. 2020. "Coronavirus Relief Favors White Households, Leaving
Many People of Color at Risk of Being Evicted." Politico. August 7. https://www.politico
.com/news/2020/08/07/coronavirus-relief-racial-eviction-392570.

Wakamo, Brian. 2020. "Instead of Bailing Out For-Profit Colleges, Congress Should Cancel Student Debt." Inequality.org. https://inequality.org/great-divide/private-colleges-student-debt/.

Zimmerman, Jonathan. 2020. "What Is College Worth?" *New York Review of Books.* July 2. https://www.nybooks.com/articles/2020/07/02/what-is-college-worth/.

6. Race, Entrepreneurship, and COVID-19: Black Small-Business Survival in Prepandemic and Postpandemic America

HENRY CLAY MCKOY JR.

By now the data are clear. With the exception of the Great Depression, the COVID-19-induced recession will be recorded as the worst economic downturn in modern history. Shuttered stores. Massive unemployment. Empty buildings. Bankruptcies. Unlike past economic fallouts, which happen routinely as markets heat up and cool down, this was driven not by a business crisis but by a health crisis. As a result, the economy entered into a forced and extended shutdown. Though much of the American economy eventually reopened, albeit at different levels depending on local and state politics, until the health crisis is solved, mitigated, or at least contained, the business crisis will remain a threat to a full recovery.

Though the cause of this recession is a historical anomaly, what remains consistent with past economic downturns is the relatively disparate negative impacts to various communities—as well as the identity of those communities. According to research conducted early in the pandemic by Robert Fairlie at the University of California at Santa Cruz, while small businesses owned by whites, Asians, and Latinos dropped by 17 percent, 26 percent, and 32 percent, respectively, no racial group saw a decline as significant as that of black-owned businesses (Fairlie 2020). Black-owned businesses, where the operations of the firm were the primary means of income and employment for the owner, plummeted from an estimated 1.1 million in February 2020 to just 640,000 by April 2020—a drop of 41 percent.

This rapid and dramatic loss of black business from the American landscape is not the only notable statistic from the pandemic. Very little of the federal government's economic response to this crisis made its way to black-owned firms. More than $2.2 trillion in initial direct aid to the economy was ushered through the halls of Congress in record time in March 2020. As part of this early legislation, the US Treasury's Paycheck Protection Program (PPP) was granted a total of $660 billion to assist small businesses (US Department of the Treasury 2020). The PPP was designed as a loan under the Coronavirus Aid, Relief, and Economic Security (CARES) Act to provide a direct incentive for small businesses to keep their workers on the payroll through the pandemic. Provided at an interest rate of 1 percent, with a maturity of two to five years and deferred payments for six months, these loans—which came with no fees and no collateral or personal guarantee obligations—are fully forgivable if used for approved purposes, specifically maintaining payroll (SBA 2020b).

The US Small Business Administration (SBA) launched the PPP on April 3, 2020, just a week after the CARES Act was passed (SBA 2020a). Within two weeks, more than 1,661,000 loans totaling nearly $342.3 billion had been approved. By early May 2020, those figures had risen to 4,102,736 loans totaling $525.8 billion. In just thirty-three days, this dollar figure represented more than twenty times the largest previous lending year in the history of the SBA.

Though early signs of the PPP pointed to anecdotal evidence that minority businesses, especially black firms, were being left out of this unprecedented capital program, such a hunch was difficult to quantify statistically. In the several months following the program's launch, the SBA downplayed the importance of providing any such demographic data, choosing instead to direct attention to the overall program's universal goals. Others continued to press for these data. Compelled by lawsuits from several news agencies and pressure from Congress, in July 2020 the SBA finally released data on PPP borrowers who received loans above $150,000 (Kranhold and Zubak-Sees 2020).

Though the PPP demographic data contained in the released report (see table 6.1) were limited because of the fact that just 14 percent of businesses chose to identify race in their loan applications (the SBA didn't require it), clear patterns emerged across ethnic and racial groups in terms of beneficiaries (SBA Office of Capital Access 2020). More specifically, when comparing PPP loan data across America's five major race/ethnic groups—white, black, Asian, American Indian, and Hispanic—there are sharp disparities. Matching racial

TABLE 6.1. Firm-level Paycheck Protection Program (PPP) racial analysis

	Loan Count[1]	Loans received[2] (%)	Population[3] (%)	Underrepresented or overrepresented loan count	Equity (%)
White	551,233	83.4	60.1	153,841	138.7
Black or African American	12,783	1.9	13.4	(75,820)	14.4
Hispanic	43,396	6.6	18.5	(78,929)	35.5
American Indian or Alaska Native	3,855	0.6	1.3	(4,741)	44.8
Asian	49,951	7.6	5.9	10,939	128.0
Total PPP loans	661,218				

Source: Author's analysis of data from the US Department of Treasury (2020); Small Business Association Paycheck Protection Program (US Small Business Administration 2020a); and US Census Bureau (2020b).

Note: Subsection of firms from total PPP pool: loans above $150,000 as of July 6, 2020.

1. These loan count figures by race are estimates based on data extrapolated from SBA figures of the 94,501 applicants who filled out demographic information of the 661,218 actual total loans distributed.

2. Percent of *loans received* can equal more than 100% as these figures are rounded up or down for simplicity.

3. Percent of population can equal less than 100% as multiracial populations may not be captured in this analysis. *White* captures those who responded on census survey as white only, not Hispanic or Latino, or any other nationality.

data from the US Census Bureau and the Small Business Administration offers quantitative indicators of the degree or extent to which small-business ownership in various racial/ethnic groups were either underrepresented or overrepresented given their relative population distributions.[1]

As table 6.1 reveals, both white (83.4 percent) and Asian (7.6 percent) firms were overrepresented with PPP loans compared to their shares of the overall population, while Hispanic (6.6 percent), black (1.9 percent), and American Indians (0.6 percent) were each underrepresented. Accounting for 1.9 percent (12,783) of the total loans received, black-owned firms received just 14.4 percent of the total PPP loans they should have received to be equitable to their overall population share. The black community, by far, had the most inequitable distribution share of any US business population by race. White- and Asian-owned firms both received above-equity levels of lending: white firms benefitted the most, receiving nearly 154,000 loans—38.7 percent above their equitable proportion.

Numerous national independent surveys conducted since the Paycheck Protection Program was instituted provide a glimpse into the nature of this unequitable distribution of funds across racial lines. In one such survey, a majority of black business owners reported that when they explored garnering a PPP loan, they were either outright rejected (41 percent) or were still waiting to hear back from the institution (21 percent), while only a small percentage reported ultimately receiving a loan (12 percent) (Global Strategy Group for Color of Change and UnidosUS 2020). It should be noted that this survey was conducted *after* the introduction of the second round of PPP, which by congressional statute was supposed to specifically focus on and prioritize underrepresented businesses (veterans, rural, minority-owned, women-owned, economically and socially disadvantaged, businesses less than two years old) (SBA 2020a). A May 8, 2020, report by the Small Business Administration's inspector general found that the SBA did not comply with this part of the law's guidance and did not enforce it with bank lenders.

Others argue that a primary reason for the loan disparities is that the first round of PPP required priority funding to go toward firms most at risk of laying off employees. Sole proprietorships, contractors, and gig economy workers were required to wait a week before they could apply for PPP loans (Abramson 2020). Since more than 96 percent of black businesses are sole proprietorships and have no employees, compared to 92 percent of Latinx and 82 percent of white firms, this led to exclusion by program design (US Census Bureau 2012b). In addition, qualifying for PPP as a sole proprietor required the submission of proof of income documentation—such as earnings reports, pay stubs, or invoices—that might have proven burdensome to many black business owners (US Department of the Treasury 2020). Furthermore, those sole proprietors who incorporated their business as a C corporation or S corporation, but who paid themselves through dividends instead of salary (a common practice), they were ineligible for the PPP altogether. These statutory regulations were likely disproportionately negative for black sole proprietors.

Some might argue this exclusion is not outright discrimination but rather an unintended and unfortunate byproduct of the general firm characteristics of the current US small business and entrepreneurial ecosystem. However, additional data suggest that the unequal distribution of funds might not be simply a product of the economic landscape or so benignly separated from race.

Matched-paired testing, used to detect discrimination by using a pair of testers with different races but similar profiles as a way to determine differences in treatment, was utilized by the National Community Reinvestment Coalition (NCRC) to discern whether there were any racial biases in the PPP (Lederer et al. 2020). The resulting study released by NCRC found that even with better financial profiles, black business owners were treated worse than their white counterparts and were offered fewer and different loan products. Moreover, not a single black female business owner was encouraged to apply for a PPP loan. Kanye West's apparel brand business, Yeezy, received a high-profile loan of $2–$5 million from the PPP, but he was the exception as a black-owned business, not the rule (Duffy 2020). West's success spoke more to the size of his firm at 106 employees and his personal connections than to the program's equitable execution. In the first round of PPP, 75 percent of loans went to businesses in census tracts where a majority of residents are white (Flitter 2020).

Though black-owned firms were disproportionately unsuccessful in garnering their equitable share of the PPP, others succeeded in doing so, even when they should not have. On September 1, 2020, according to a report released by members of the US House Select Committee on the Coronavirus Crisis, initial findings "suggest a high risk for fraud, waste, and abuse" within the PPP's application and distribution procedures (Select Subcommittee on the Coronavirus Crisis 2020). Within PPP, 600 loans totaling $96 million went to companies ineligible to receive funding; 10,850 more loans totaling $1 billion went to firms that received multiple loans despite regulatory prohibition of this; another 353 loans totaling $195 million went to government contractors who should have been disqualified because of "performance or integrity issues"; and $3 billion of additional loans were issued to what were considered "suspicious" borrowers.

Though discouraging, these figures of inequitable distribution across both the bad (firm losses) and the good (loan proceeds) are unfortunately not surprising. Similar to past responses to federal crises, it is clear that race matters and that it will have far-reaching and long-term implications. For example, most of the loans to black firms were to sole proprietorships, making them ineligible for forgiveness and requiring repayment, while billions of dollars to white firms that constitute the majority of employee-based firms will convert to grants (making them, in essence, free money). The combination of the disproportionate overrepresentation of black firm loss, likely as a result of the disproportionate underrepresentation of federal aid and other historic gaps, along with the forgivable nature of the PPP loan, will exacerbate the already extraordinary US racial wealth gap.

These data support the classic axiom that when the white community gets the flu, the black community catches pneumonia—and while the former community gets full medical treatment, the latter community gets no treatment or a placebo. It raises the question: When the white community gets coronavirus, what does the black community get, and what can and should be done about it? The goal of this chapter is to answer those critical questions and more—most notably, to comprehend the ultimate impact of COVID-19 on the American black business ecosystem. These inquiries are perhaps most importantly contextualized more broadly speaking within one definitive question: What does the future of the black economic landscape look like in America?

The Racial Business Ecosystem, Pre-COVID-19

Historically, communities have developed group-focused entrepreneurial ecosystems, with an eye toward either maintaining competitive advantage or combating or circumnavigating institutional barriers to entrepreneurial success (McKoy and Johnson 2018). These ecosystems are made up of trusted, mutually reinforcing, multisectoral, group-specific relationships, which are designed to facilitate, support, and advance entrepreneurship as an economic development strategy. These ecosystems allow for the resiliency and survival of the communities during structural changes to the economy, allowing them to grow and expand during good times, and ensuring they do not suffer irrecoverably during bad times. The current-day pandemic did not create the racial economic and entrepreneurial inequities we are now witnessing. Instead it has further exposed, exacerbated, and accelerated what was already, and has long been, present (McKoy 2020).

In an August 1897 *Atlantic* article, "Strivings of the Negro People," eminent scholar W. E. B. Du Bois decried that "to be a poor man is hard, but to be a poor race in a land of dollars is the very bottom of hardship" (Du Bois 1897). Nearly 125 years later, blacks remain a poor race in an extremely wealthy country and world, and they continue to bear the burden of what Du Bois called "the negro problem"—or the feeling of poverty: cent-less, home-less, land-less, tool-less and savings-less, yet having to continuously enter into competition with "rich landed, skilled neighbors." This phenomenon is predominantly evident when analyzing the racial entrepreneurial landscape. Blacks remain a poor race and business class in America, during both economic expansions and contractions, even after more than a century and a half of striving.

In recent decades, as blacks have increased their share of the overall American demographic, a corresponding rise in their entrepreneurial share has followed. At first glance, this pattern would appear to be a positive trend, since rises in entrepreneurship lead to rises in business growth and, presumably, increases in wealth. Instead, collective black wealth has steadily dropped, with estimated projections—based on trend data—of a decline to a median of $0 by 2053 (Collins et al. 2017). That prediction was made prior to COVID-19's arrival, and it is assured to be accelerated as a result of the pandemic's current impact on black America. A key factor in this counterintuitive trend of increased entrepreneurship and decreased wealth can be attributed, at least partly, to the types of businesses that dominant the black business landscape: sole proprietorships.

A typical business ecosystem includes both well-established and new entrepreneurial ventures (McKoy and Johnson 2018). These networks of interacting firms evolve over a long process, defining relationships among industry players, with entrepreneurial insights interacting with strategic thinking to create, shape, navigate, and exploit business ecosystems. In the process, these business ecosystems, as they grow, connect to communities via wealth creation, human capital investment, experiential capital investment, and job creation (Zahra and Nambisan 2012). However, even as blacks experienced a steady rise in business ownership during the years prior to COVID-19, it is important to look more closely at the data. While, in recent years, the popular press was replete with stories that highlighted the growing status of historically underutilized businesses, particularly black-owned firms, a more scholarly and expansive analysis uncovers a less rosy picture of modern trends. A critical aspect of measuring the relative economic status, strength, and resiliency of a community is to look at their entrepreneurial landscape—or more specifically, their relative position within the broader entrepreneurial ecosystem.

During America's last recession (2008–2012) blacks experienced the second-highest entrepreneurial growth of any population, at 34.5 percent, trailing only Hispanics at 46.3 percent, but significantly above Asians (23.8 percent) and American Indians (15.1 percent) (US Census Bureau 2012a). This minority business expansion stood in contrast to white firms, which experienced an overall business decline of nearly 5 percent. Black firms were seemingly making up ground on their white counterparts, moving 33.55 percent closer to being numerically and proportionately equitable based on population share relative to white firms between 2007 and 2012—the largest relative jump of any racial group (McKoy and Johnson 2018).

Yet, using an alternate quantitative vantage point provides a useful perspective when thinking about entrepreneurial equity. During that same time period, when measuring only for firms with paid employees—as opposed to all firms (those both with and without paid employees)—instead of losing ground, white firms actually grew overall by 2.2 percent during the Great Recession (US Census Bureau 2012a). In contrast to the previously reported aggregate overall firm growth of more than one-third, black firms with paid employees actually collectively declined 2.4 percent relative to their white counterparts—they were the only racial minority group in America to experience negative growth in this regard. As a result, prior to the COVID-19 pandemic black firms—when measured for parity—had just 13 percent of the firms with paid employees that they should have had when compared to white firms (McKoy and Johnson 2018).

Furthermore, black firms with paid employees were underrepresented when compared to all other racial groups as well. Blacks only had 10 percent, 21 percent, and 53 percent of firms when compared to Asians, American Indians, and Hispanics, respectively, to be considered equitable relative to those populations.[2] In short, black firms were being started at unprecedented levels in modern times prior to COVID-19, but unlike their counterparts of other races/ethnicities, they have not been, and are not, growing beyond a single worker-owner. In fact, black-owned firms with paid employees were, and are, declining rapidly (even prior to COVID-19) relative to their peer groups.

To illustrate why such continued decline is so troublesome, table 6.2 presents pre-COVID-19 data on racial business shares within leading US industries based on firms with paid employees. This snapshot paints a portrait of the disparate, perpetually underrepresented existence of black-owned firms. White firms control 80 to 90 percent of every major American industry with regard to firms with paid employees, providing their owners a basis for the continued formation of the key components of a thriving, robust, and growing entrepreneurial landscape; specifically, an ecosystem that can provide entrepreneurial capital (i.e., financial capital, experiential capital, human capital, and social capital) that intrinsically benefits their broader and race-specific community economic ecosystems, even if not distinctively aiming to.

When entrepreneurs launch firms, they eventually hire new employees, and most often those employees match the demographic of the founder or founders—in terms of both race and gender (Boston and Boston 2007). Typically, businesses with paid employees are the most viable and thus the most financially successful (Austin 2016). Businesses with paid employees outearn those without paid employees by a significant factor. In 2012, firms with paid employees generated 97 percent of the $33.5 trillion generated in sales, receipts, or values of shipments. Firms without paid employees produced the remaining 3 percent (just under $1 trillion) (McKoy and Johnson 2018). Employer businesses create the most wealth for their owners, employees, and associated communities. Consequently, if whites are significantly overrepresented in ownership of firms with paid employees, and if those firms routinely hire from their associated racial populations, then the ensuing outcomes will be evident in the broader community landscapes. In other words, the relative advantages and disadvantages will be distributed inequitably in visible ways.

Moving from the pre-COVID-19 industry perspective, to the aggregate viewpoint and employing six quantitative measurements, table 6.3 provides insights

TABLE 6.2. Selected industry breakdown share by percentage of race, pre-COVID

North American Industry Classification System (NAICS) code	US industry population	White 60.1% (%)	Black 13.4% (%)	American Indian 1.3% (%)	Asian 5.9% (%)	Hispanic 18.5% (%)
Business total	5,489,351	4,472,938	109,503	26,270	482,050	288,280
	100%	83.2	2.0	0.5	9.0	5.4
23	Construction	90.7	1.1	0.7	1.6	5.8
31–33	Manufacturing	90.0	0.5	0.5	4.9	4.2
42	Wholesale trade	82.4	0.8	0.3	11.0	5.5
44–45	Retail trade	79.1	1.3	0.4	14.2	5.0
48–49	Transportation and warehousing	82.9	3.8	0.5	3.9	8.9
51	Information	89.3	1.5	0.5	5.0	3.6
52	Finance and insurance	90.2	2.0	0.6	3.5	3.9
53	Real estate and rental leasing	90.1	1.1	0.3	4.6	3.8

Source: Author's analysis based on American Community Survey data (2010) and Survey of Business Owners data (2012) from US Census Bureau data estimates.

into both positive and negative economic distributions as they already were before the current pandemic. Both firm and revenue shares indicate which demographic populations are achieving representative success in their economic strivings. Since firm owners, as they grow, hire primarily those from their representative networks, poverty share is included in this analysis as a quantitative proxy indicator of how well the benefits of representative ownership are accruing from the entrepreneurial and business ecosystems to the broader community economic ecosystem.

As table 6.3 illustrates, and which was also evident from the previous eight sector industry-level analysis in table 6.2, when all economic sectors are accounted for, white firms already maintained a commanding aggregate economic presence prior to the COVID-19 pandemic: they were overrepresented in the positive metrics of community firm ownership and community revenue generation and underrepresented in the negative metric of community poverty share. Black firms and their community, in contrast, collectively held a much different position before COVID-19's arrival. These representative US entrepreneurial landscape data might be helpful in understanding why the "universal" nature of the PPP structure—especially in round one—likely worsened relative inequity among firms across race/ethnicity in America instead of improving it (SBA 2020a).

	Overall population (%)	All firms (%)	Firms with paid employees (%)	All firms revenue (%)	Paid-employee firm revenue (%)	Poverty (%)
White	60.1	72.7	82.8	88.9	89.8	45.7
Black	13.4	8.7	2.2	1.2	0.9	22.7
American Indian	1.3	0.9	0.6	0.3	0.3	1.6
Asian	5.9	6.5	9.0	5.7	5.6	4.1
Hispanic	18.5	11.2	5.6	3.9	3.4	27.5

Source: Author's analysis based on American Community Survey data (2010) and Survey of Business Owners data (2012) from US Census Bureau data estimates. Category overlap means columns may sum to more than 100%.

Among the simplest ways to racially categorize the (in)equity of America's business landscape prior to COVID-19, while juxtaposing that against the federal response, is to imagine that the millions of people, firms, and PPP loans in the United States were reduced to just factors of one hundred: one hundred people, one hundred companies, one-hundred dollars in business revenue, one-hundred dollars in entrepreneurial capital leverage, and one hundred PPP loans distributed.[3] Table 6.4 presents this data on relative entrepreneurial ownership and entrepreneurial wealth by race/ethnicity pre-COVID-19. An additional column, with data pulled from table 6.1, is added to reflect the corresponding figures related to the PPP loan distribution for supplementary analysis of the program's (in)equity.

Table 6.4 is consistent with previous data and studies that show both white and Asian firms—relative to their overall community population share—as routinely overrepresented in economic equity measurements, whereas black, American Indian, and Hispanic firms are consistently underrepresented (McKoy and Johnson 2018). In measurements related to number of companies (nine) and entrepreneurial wealth strength ($8), Asian firms are above equity, while at equity ($6) in terms of economic revenue (i.e., cash). White firms are significantly above equitable levels in all three categories: companies (eighty-three), cash ($90), and strength (ninety-two). Thus, in an America measured out of hundreds, the sixty white Americans own eighty-three of the one hundred firms, possess $90 of the $100 in cash, and control 92 percent of the national capital markets. Conversely, the thirteen black Americans own just two firms among themselves, survive on just $1 in cash shared between them, and collectively have $48 in *negative* financial leverage and equity. As of this writing,

TABLE 6.4. Pre-COVID-19 US racial entrepreneurial ownership, wealth, and PPP received (out of 100)[1]

Race/ethnicity	100 people	100 companies[2]	$100 firm cash ($)	Entrepreneurial wealth strength ($)	100 PPP loans received
White	60	83	90	92	83
Black	13	2	1	−48	2
American Indian	1	0.5	0.30	−2	0.6
Asian American	6	9	6	8	8
Hispanic	19	6	3	−54	7

Source: Author's analysis based on American Community Survey data (2010) and Survey of Business Owners data (2012) from the US Census Bureau data estimates, and Small Business Association (2020).

1. Figures are rounded, thus may not add to 100.

2. Paid-employee firms only.

following over a year of the federal PPP's operations, those two shared firms would have declined to one, and that shared $1 would be nearing $0 for black Americans.

In the earlier analysis represented in table 6.1, the significant inequity among firms of different races—based on the amount of PPP loans received relative to their overall population share—was the central focus. Conversely, using table 6.4 as a reference, one might be compelled to argue that if the percentage of firms with paid employees was used as the baseline demographic for the PPP loans, as opposed to the overall racial population share, then the program would prove appreciably more equitable in its distribution of loans. The firm shares and PPP shares are nearly identical. This analysis, however, ignores the two columns that sit between those data. There should be a convincing argument that when all of these pre-COVID-19 business characteristics are taken into consideration, that the PPP was distributed even more inequitably than even first posed.

If, as stated in the CARES Act, the purpose of the PPP was to help small businesses "survive the coronavirus crisis" and to "[reach] small businesses truly in need," then the program might have been better organized as one that was means-tested, instead of universal in nature (Select Subcommittee on the Coronavirus Crisis 2020). Kanye West's multibillion dollar apparel business was not the only one that rushed to the front of the PPP line. The companies approved for the larger loans—those above $150,000 that have been presented in this chapter—captured around 75 percent of the program's total funding, though they represent a relatively small percentage of the 4.1 million borrowers. Large, well-resourced companies, such as Soho House or Gores Vitac Holdings—both controlled by billionaire proprietors—as well as Ruth's Chris Steakhouse and Shake Shack, were among those who initially garnered PPP loans. Following mass public outcry, Ruth's Chris Steakhouse and Shake Shack hurriedly returned their funds, proving the dollars were not vital for their immediate survival to begin with. By contrast, in May 2020, nearly half of the remaining black business owners surveyed (following the first wave of closings when nearly half of black businesses shuttered in the United States) said they anticipated closing within six months (by November 2020) as only one in ten received the PPP funding they requested (Global Strategy Group for Color of Change and UnidosUS 2020). Based on their relative economic position to other races/ethnicities prior to the pandemic, with little capital at their disposal and an inability to leverage the strength of their entrepreneurial wealth, black-owned firms in the United States should have immediately been ushered to the front of the PPP line for federal assistance.

The "COVID-19 Health (i.e., outbreak) curve" has become the prevailing, but simple, hallmark visual representation of society's current collective health condition, with efforts to "flatten the curve" as the paramount indicator of success against the coronavirus spread—including infections, hospitalizations, and deaths. A comparable visual curve, and one also in need of flattening, is the racial entrepreneurial equity curve (see figure 6.1).[4] This plotted figure offers an equally simple quantitative representation of the collective health condition of America's entrepreneurs.

When utilizing data from table 6.3—population share, firm share, revenue share, and poverty share—to calculate a quantitative measurement of overrepresentation and underrepresentation of American racial ecosystems, a relative equity score categorized by race/ethnicity can be computed, indexed, and charted to produce a curve. A perfectly flat curve would represent a perfectly equitable business and entrepreneurial ecosystem, with each population receiving its equitable share of economic benefits and economic ills. For the associated racial business ecosystems to have benefitted similarly from the PPP, this curve would have needed to be flat (i.e., perfect equity) prior to loan disbursements, which would have been representative of an overall equitable economic distribution system. Instead, blacks and Hispanics were grossly and negatively inequitable relative to their other US racial counterparts, who were at, near, or well-above equitable economic levels, pre-COVID-19 (figure 6.1).

White firms, in aggregate—especially the largest ones—entered the pandemic with firm control over the US entrepreneurial and business economic ecosystems, finding themselves well positioned for opportunistic activity (i.e., mergers, acquisitions, etc.) and possessing the absorptive capacity for any negative

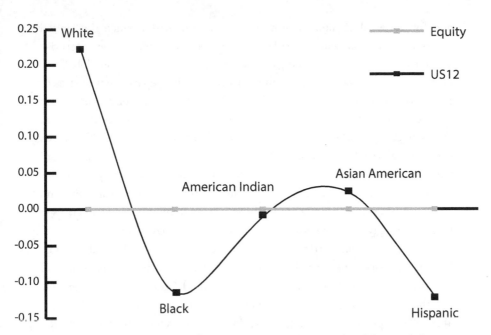

FIGURE 6.1. US Entrepreneurial Ecosystem Equity Curve indexed by race/ethnicity (prior to COVID 19). Plotted figures of entrepreneurial economic/wealth strength by race: whites (91.77); blacks (-47.67); American Indians (-2.00); Asian Americans (7.70); Hispanic (-54.21). Author's analysis of data from the American Community Survey (ACS) and Survey of Business Owners (SBO), 2010, 2012.

shocks. In contrast, black-owned firms in aggregate—with diminutive market ownership, miniscule revenue share, and negative capital leverage capacity—were (and continue to be) fighting for their collective survival: a perilous and precarious position they know, and have known, all too well throughout their history. This black American entrepreneurial journey, connected in its pathos to the global black diaspora but still distinct from other black parts of the world, must be both fully understood and reckoned with if black-owned firms in the United States hold any chance of surviving both the disproportionately negative impacts of the COVID-19 crisis on business and the subsequently inadequate policy responses.

How We Got Here

The notion that black entrepreneurship might altogether disappear from the American landscape, and black entrepreneurs from the economic ecosystem, as a result of COVID-19 might seem farcical. Blacks have been a constant, essential, and fundamental element of American entrepreneurship since the United States was a British colony. The black slave body was literally the enterprise around which capitalism was organized, instituted, expanded, and globalized, even before those same bodies could legally organize separate enterprises of their own (Beckert and Rockman 2016, 1–5). However, black entrepreneurship and business ownership—as a practice—existed even prior to the end of slavery in 1865, and even in the South. The total value of all free black-owned establishments and personal wealth in the United States in 1860 was at least $50 million—half of which was based in the slave South (Marable 1983, 141). Consequently, in the four hundred years since blacks have been in America, this entrepreneurial spirit and resilience has survived abundant intrinsic and existential threats and crises—many seemingly more trying and encompassing than COVID-19.

Despite numerous barriers and trials, black-owned firms have always historically outpaced the overall business market in new firm starts. The total number of black-owned businesses in the United States was approximately two thousand in 1863, four thousand in 1873, and ten thousand in 1883 (Marable 1983, 143). Growth rates for black businesses declined abruptly between 1883 and 1903, a result of the initial loss of whites patronizing black businesses following the end of Reconstruction and subsequent racial segregation (Marable 1983, 143–144). However, by 1914, the number of black businesses had increased to forty thousand (Marable 1983, 144). By 1929, the number of black firms was greater than seventy thousand—bolstered rather than hampered by legal racial segregation. This decade (1919–1929) that buttressed the Great Depression ended what some refer to as the "golden years of black business" (Marable 1983, 146). Thousands of black businesses went bankrupt during the Great Depression, with pre-Depression growth not resuming until after World War II (Marable 1983, 148–50). As a result of the Civil Rights Era, beginning in the 1950s and lasting through the 1960s, black firms grew at a brisk pace as politicians and corporate leaders sought to improve their relationship with the broader black community.

In 1972, the number of black businesses in America had grown to 187,602. A half-decade later, a more than 23 percent growth rate had increased that number to 231,203 (Stuart 1981). Still, as a percentage of the overall US economic ecosystem, black firms remained miniscule relative to the marketplace—2.4 percent in 1972 and 3.3 percent in 1977, during a time in which blacks composed roughly 12 percent of the overall population. Even with the 23 percent growth in firm count, in 1977, these black-owned firms accounted for just two-tenths of 1 percent of the total business revenue. At the time, 94 percent of black-owned businesses were sole proprietorships, 2 percent were corporations, and

4 percent were partnerships (Stuart 1981). Like now, black ownership figures in 1977 skewed smaller than the broader landscape, in which 77 percent of businesses were sole proprietorships, 15 percent were corporations, and 8 percent were partnerships.

Returning to 1972 as the year for comparison and focusing on three metrics (the count of all black firms, the collective revenue of all black firms, and the average revenue per firm), insights emerge as to the pathway to the precarious condition of the current black entrepreneurial ecosystem.

Table 6.5 (visually represented by figure 6.2) shows that despite constant increases in firm counts and steady revenue growth across the last half century, black firms—or perhaps more accurately, contemporary black entrepreneurs—are getting poorer on average. With the exception of 1977 to 1982, during which average firm revenue declined by over 16 percent—likely as a result of the inflationary pressures, oil crisis, and ensuing recession of the late 1970s—black businesses saw positive average revenue growth during the last three decades of the twentieth century. Contrast that to the twenty-first century (see figure 6.2), during which black firms have never experienced positive average revenue growth, averaging instead a per annum decline of more than 2 percent—a pattern that has persisted whether the economy was contracting or expanding. In short, black businesses are getting poorer with each passing year and have lost one-third of their total average revenue since the beginning of the 2000s.

A broad examination of black-owned business in America over the last four-to-five decades exposes many compelling and encouraging data points—points

TABLE 6.5. US black firms forty-year numerical change, revenue change, and average revenue change, 1972–2012

Year	All black firms	Change (%)	All black firm revenue ($)	Change (%)	Average revenue per firm ($)	Change (%)
1972	187,602	—	5.5B	—	29,317.38	—
1977	231,203	23.2	8.6B	56.4	37,196.75	26.9
1982	308,260	33.3	9.6B	11.6	31,142.54	−16.3
1987	424,165	37.6	19.8B	106.3	46,679.95	49.9
1992	620,912	46.4	32.2B	62.6	51,859.20	11.1
1997	823,500	32.6	71.2B	121.1	86,460.23	66.7
2002	1.2M	45.7	89.0B	25.0	74,166.67	−14.2
2007	1.9M	58.3	137.5B	54.5	72,368.42	−2.4
2012	2.6M	36.8	150.0B	9.1	57,692.31	−20.3

Source: Author's analysis of US Census Survey of Business Owner data (1972–2012).

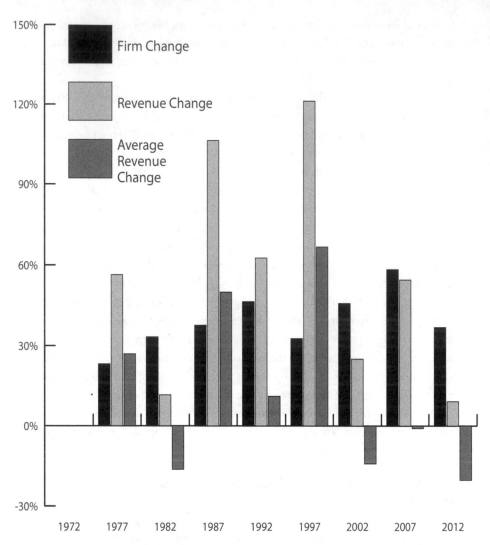

FIGURE 6.2. US black firm forty-year numerical change, average change, and average revenue change, 1972–2012. See table 6.5.

that are sometimes contradictory and seemingly inconsistent with the overall picture. From 1972 to 2012, the aggregate number of black-owned firms grew 1,286 percent, and aggregate black-firm revenue grew 2,627 percent: forty years of average annual growth at 32 percent and 66 percent, respectively. Black firms with at least $1 million in revenue grew more than twenty-fold—from around 715 in the mid-1970s to around 14,500 by the mid-2000s (Stuart 1981; US Census Bureau 2007). During that same period, aggregate black consumer buying power rose from an estimated $70 billion in 1973 (up from $30 billion in 1960) to nearly $910 billion in 2009; it is currently estimated at more than $1.3 trillion—an eighteen-fold increase (Marable 1983, 158; Nielsen Corporation 2019). Yet, in forty years, this development has only resulted in 97 percent total average revenue per firm growth for black entrepreneurs. During these four decades, average revenue per black firm increased by only 2 percent annually, preventing it even from doubling during that period.

To identify each economic impact—good or bad—that has left an impression on the trajectory of African American businesses would be impossible. However, characterizing the relationship between black entrepreneurship and business and the broader American (and global) ecosystem might be a useful analysis. These characterizations are divided into stages here and in table 6.6.

Deep-seated, entrenched, and systematic racism and discrimination have been the standard across all of these stages of black entrepreneurship in America. As a result, over time, the overall community economic ecosystem of black America has become increasingly fragile, weak, and hollowed.

The benefits that accompanied the emancipated black slave as a skilled and expert craftsman were countered by the two-thirds black illiteracy rate, a lack of business acumen resulting from centuries of bondage, and "black codes" (stage II) (Du Bois 1903). The benefits that accompanied segregation—forced black group economics—were countered by the serious violence that destroyed life and wealth in nearly fifty black communities across America between 1919 and 1923 alone, including in Tulsa, Oklahoma; Rosewood, Florida; and dozens of less well-known instances (stage III). Hundreds of black economic centers and business ecosystems would be destroyed in the decades ahead through federally funded urban renewal and highway projects. The "Silver Rights" benefits that accompanied the "Civil Rights Era" and the rise of black political influence, such as increased government contracting and opportunity, were countered by the unreciprocated and massive movement of consumer dollars from the black economic ecosystem to the white one (stage IV). The benefits that accompanied the recognition of the strength of the black consumer market by white

TABLE 6.6. Stages of black-owned firms in the United States, 1619–present

Stage	Time period	Key drivers	Characteristic outcomes
I—Slavery	1619–1865 (246 years)	Enslaved blacks were at the heart of enterprises as private property and means of production. Some free blacks in the North and South owned firms.	Enslaved blacks were denied the wealth they created. Free blacks were harassed, had businesses destroyed, or were killed in the North and South. Forced to rebuild from scratch.
II—Artisan entrepreneurs	1865–1883 (18 years)	Former slaves provided an array of services to primarily white patrons.	Black codes ("vagrancy codes") were instituted to deny blacks ability to be entrepreneurs. Illiteracy and lack of business education hampered efforts.
III—Segregation entrepreneurs	1883–1963 (80 years)	Growth of numerous black-owned businesses in array of industries including banks, insurance, media, press, retail, and hospitality. Rise of community anchoring black firms and organizations.	"Golden Years I" of black entrepreneurship bolstered by segregation. Series of US race massacres used to destroy black wealth, followed by black wealth destruction through urban renewal.
IV—Civil rights entrepreneurs	1963–1988 (25 years)	Black firms grew as politicians instituted affirmative action government business programs. This corresponded with growth of black political influence. Followed by decline of historic anchoring community institutions.	Social and economic integration went one way—black dollars into white communities, weakening and hollowing black economic base. Public sector promises to support black capitalism not kept. Number of federally protected business populations grew without growth of programs and resources.
V—Intermediary entrepreneurs	1988–2008 (20 years)	New black firms grew as white corporate elite sought to attract growing black consumer dollar, using black intermediary firms (media, advertising, etc.) to market. This (briefly) bolstered broader black entrepreneurial economic ecosystem.	Truncated "Golden Years II." Educated blacks entered white corporations at an increasing rate. White corporations began creating black focused divisions and talent recruitment. Black firms continually faced racial discrimination in public and private sectors.

(Continued)

TABLE 6.6. (*continued*)

Stage	Time period	Key drivers	Characteristic outcomes
VI—Hustle entrepreneurs	2008–present (12 years +)	Black firms see significant growth, but primarily in service industries, with more sole proprietorships, and with less average revenue. Black sports and entertainment entrepreneurs become the primary black entrepreneurial role models for society.	Black workers and black firms are continually displaced by globalization and automation. Black anchor institutions, such as banks, increasingly disappear from the black community economic ecosystem. Black firms are disconnected from the financial marketplace.

corporate elites were countered when those same corporations moved from procurement using black-owned intermediary firms to attract black dollars to transitioning that work in-house (stage V). This development led to a black business decline that was even quicker than the associated rise in black-owned businesses, as talent, along with opportunity, evaporated from black firms al most immediately. The benefits that have accompanied the rise of the black entrepreneurial startup in the twenty-first century, leading to nearly 2.6 million firms by the end of 2012, have been countered by the ongoing institutional racism and bias—specifically in banking and investment finance—that keeps them from growing beyond the founding entrepreneur (stage VI).

It is not the single contemporary effect of COVID-19 that threatens the survival of the black business ecosystem, but the uniqueness of the crisis coupled with the cumulative effects of past economic stressors and shocks. Black America as an entrepreneurial ecosystem is economically hollow—limited in absorptive capacity of both good and bad outcomes. Furthermore, the PPP is not the first program introduced under the guise of universality to address a major economic crisis that eventually exacerbated already present racial economic inequities. From the New Deal to the GI Bill to relief for distressed farmers and everything in between, blacks have absorbed the actual impact of most negative economic disruption in America's history with little to no cushion.

Each disruption, large and small, from the beginning of the seventeenth century until now, has tested the collective resilience and resolve of the black community and the associated black business ecosystem. Though black business has recovered from each blow, they have, collectively, rebounded more weakly following each aftershock. Stages II–VI were hampered and harshened by the re-

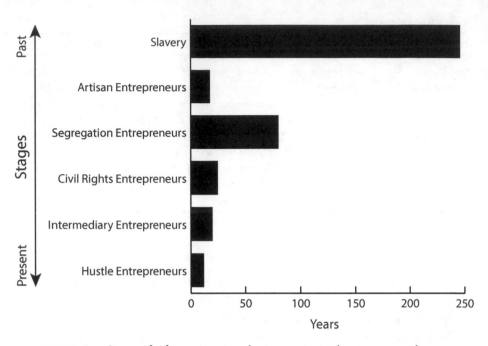

FIGURE 6.3. Stages of African American businesses in total entrepreneurial years. See table 6.6.

sidual impacts of stage I—by far the longest of all the stages (see figure 6.3)—the denial of two and a half centuries of enterprising wealth creation. Consequently, as a result of COVID-19's economic impacts, outcomes will continue to get worse for black business and entrepreneurship before they (maybe) get better.

Expected Postpandemic Outcomes for America's Black Business Ecosystem

Thus far, all data previously discussed have centered on the prepandemic racial business landscape, homing in on black-owned firms relative to their racial/ethnic counterparts as well as to the distinct stages that black entrepreneurship in the United States has followed. Attention will now be turned from the past and present toward the future and the expected outcomes from COVID-19's impact, specifically for the black-owned economy. What will the black entrepreneurial landscape look like after the storm has subsided? Until the health effects of the COVID-19 pandemic are addressed so that the American economy and the global economy can fully reopen, we can expect to see some version of the same types of negative economic impacts witnessed so far. Unfortunately, the black community and their associated businesses will likely bear the greatest brunt of the negative impacts. Even when the COVID-19 crisis no longer affects our daily lives, there will be at least four residual impacts that alter the US economic and entrepreneurial landscape.

INCREASE IN US OVERALL BLACK ENTREPRENEURSHIP

This first identified post-COVID-19 impact might appear inconsistent with previous statements, which suggests that the pandemic is threatening the very existence of black-owned business in America. However, what is in jeopardy is not the existence of black entrepreneurship in the rawest sense but instead a particular type of black entrepreneurship. Following COVID-19 there will be more black-owned businesses than prior to the pandemic, driven by new sole proprietorships that exist at even higher relative levels than in previous periods.

Analyses of US census data over time show that rises in self-employment—or entrepreneurship—follow and coincide with economic recessions. As people are displaced from paid labor, both in the short term and long term, they seek ways to replace and create incomes. These efforts to supplant and generate salaries, which all racial populations experience, often include leveraging human, social, experiential, and financial capital gained from past employment, education, and networks to launch businesses.

Black individuals are no different, and they are likely more prone to this path to entrepreneurship due to broader societal impetuses. The old adage suggesting blacks are the last racial group hired and the first one fired turns out to be true. This phenomenon is often most evident in and around economic recessions and subsequent recoveries. In economic recessions, across the board, unemployment increases for all demographics. However, the numbers are often most dramatic for black workers. During normal times, black unemployment is roughly twice that of white America. When companies begin shedding jobs, this ratio often remains consistent.

In the middle of the Great Recession, in July 2010, the official black unemployment rate stood at 15.6 percent—surprisingly not the highest for blacks during that period (US Bureau of Labor Statistics 2021). The white unemployment rate was 8.6 percent. Black US unemployment remained above 10 percent for nearly seven consecutive years during the Great Recession (July 2008–May 2015) with 2.5 consecutive years at or above 15 percent (July 2009–January 2012) (US Bureau of Labor Statistics 2021). The parallel and phenomenal above-average growth rate of black entrepreneurship during this same period is not coincidental. Similar patterns can be found in previous economic recessions.

Since during recessions a higher proportion of blacks lose their jobs than any other racial group, it stands that a higher proportion of blacks would launch businesses as an alternative to wage employment. This pattern is driven by the (un)availability of both short-term and long-term paid employment options, which historically differ by demographics. As recoveries occur, especially U-shaped ones (or recoveries taking several years), many employers start hiring or rehiring slowly, and they often rehire or hire white workers before others (Couch and Fairlie 2010). In addition, many firms do not return to prerecession employment numbers because of new operational efficiencies or automation—discovered or gained during the downturn—allowing them to utilize fewer workers while increasing productivity. These jobless recoveries often leave black wage earners out.

During the current health pandemic, even as blacks and other nonwhite groups are seeing higher shares of COVID-19 infections, hospitalizations, and deaths as a result of being classified as essential workers in many frontline jobs, the black community has simultaneously experienced the highest levels of continuous unemployment (CDC 2020).

All racial groups experienced a significant pandemic-induced year-over-year increase in unemployment (table 6.7). Despite the brief period in May 2020 when Hispanic unemployment eclipsed black unemployment, normal patterns reemerged upon a partial nationwide reopening of the economy in early summer. As reopenings lowered the unemployed US population from 49.8 million (May 2020) to 40.4 million (June 2020) to 31.3 million (July 2020), blacks resumed their status as the most unemployed group. This COVID-19-created recession and accompanying black unemployment should spark similarly aligned entrepreneurial-launch patterns of the past—especially postpandemic.

Entrepreneurship across all races will grow dramatically in the post-COVID-19 short term, but this pattern will be most dramatic for black Americans. Furthermore, even as the economy fully rebounds in the long term, many of those black entrepreneurs will remain self-employed. Some will remain self-employed

TABLE 6.7. US unemployment rates pre-COVID-19 and during COVID-19 by race/ethnicity

	May 2019 (%)	May 2020 (%)	August 2020 (%)	May 2021 (%)
White	3.3	12.4	7.3	5.1
Black	6.2	16.8	13.0	9.1
Asian	2.5	15.0	10.7	5.5
Hispanic	4.2	17.6	10.5	7.3

Source: US Bureau of Labor Statistics.

because they will enjoy it and have found success; many others will continue because they will not have viable options for returning to wage labor. Nevertheless, the overwhelming majority of these new black firms will be nonemployer firms—and will remain so in the long term.

INCREASE IN RACIAL INEQUITY (POVERTEERING)

Typically, a higher-than-average increase in black entrepreneurship relative to other groups would be coupled with corresponding anticipatory expectations of job growth, wealth creation, and the potential narrowing of the racial wealth gap. However, there is a considerable probability that the increase in entrepreneurship in the black community as a result of the COVID-19 recession will not only fail to narrow the racial wealth gap and corresponding racial inequity but will also increase it.

The forthcoming increase in black sole proprietorships will likely continue this current century's trajectory of falling average revenue per black-owned firm. As a result of this downward trend, coupled with the opportunistic movements of other entrepreneurial demographic populations and the disproportionate fraying of connective paths to wage employment for many blacks, inequality after the COVID-19 pandemic will grow across—and within—races.

In recent years, a group-level examination of black American demographic data trends yields a surprising discovery of a counterintuitive economic phenomenon: even as black Americans, with each subsequent year, continue to increase their proportionate demographic share of the overall American population as well as their proportionate share of the American business landscape, they are in aggregate holding a decreasing share of American wealth (US Census Bureau 2021a; US Census Bureau 2012b; Collins et al. 2017). I call this conflicting phenomenon *poverteering* (McKoy and Banks 2019).

Poverteering occurs when a distinct group or population simultaneously increases their societal population share and business share (through active entrepreneurship), while concurrently losing societal wealth share (presumably, while also increasing their overall societal buying power from their increase in population share). Blacks expanded their US population numbers by nearly 5 percent from 2007 to 2012 to an overall share of roughly 12.3 percent; that estimated share has now increased to 13.4 percent. Prior to the COVID-19 pandemic, the number of black businesses in the American economy (all firms) had increased by 34.5 percent during the last official US government Survey of Business Owners in 2012 and increased the group's overall share from 6.7 percent to 8.7 percent (McKoy Jr. and Johnson Jr. 2018). Black Americans also experienced increases in collective buying power from $845 billion in 2007 to \$1.1 trillion in 2012 (up from \$318 billion in 1990) (Humphreys 2008). However, trends showed that black median wealth was concurrently declining, with an expected decline to \$0 by 2053 (Collins et al. 2017). Presumably, white America is experiencing the opposite phenomenon—*inverse poverteering*, or the loss of population and business share while gaining wealth—seeing overall population shares decrease from 65.8 percent (2007) to 62.8 percent (2012) to 60.1 percent (2020) and business share from 79.1 percent (2007) to 72.7 percent (2012) (McKoy and Johnson 2018). In addition, though much larger in aggregate, white buying power is growing more slowly (124 percent) than black buying power (166 percent), though both trail Hispanic (307 percent) and Asian growth (294 percent) (Humphreys 2008).

Even prior to the COVID-19 pandemic, this racial inequity was anticipated to grow faster than previously estimated. This "road to zero wealth" in 2053 for black America (and Latinos in 2073) was estimated in September 2017, prior to the massive US Tax Cut and Jobs Act passed in December 2017. This legislation has largely benefitted wealthy, white Americans and has widened racial inequity, especially between white and black populations. COVID-19 will further accelerate and exacerbate these racial inequities across all populations, specifically as more black Americans begin poverteering.

RELATIVE AND ABSOLUTE DECREASE IN BLACK FIRMS WITH PAID EMPLOYEES

As previously stated, overall positive entrepreneurial growth among all populations will be a result of the COVID-19 economic crisis. The majority of that growth will be single-person, no employee firms—especially among African Americans. Moreover, during all major recessions, the number of firms with paid employees is expected to immediately decline as more will close down their operations from payroll strains than will create new employer firms. However, depending on the strength and speed of the subsequent economic recovery, employer firms would expect to eventually return to and surpass prerecession numbers. Within five years of the Great Recession, every racial and gender group (save black males) had surpassed their prerecession employer-firm absolute total (Austin 2016). Black males were net losers of employer firms (−2.2 percent), and the resulting positive overall growth within the black community was due only to the strong showing of black, female-owned employer firms that grew by 20.2 percent.

While percentage change offers some insight into how a racial entrepreneurial ecosystem is faring both relative to its own past performance and relative to that of other groups, there are also insights reflected in absolute numerical change as well. During the first five years of the previous recovery (table 6.8),

TABLE 6.8. Employer-firm absolute/percentage growth and changes 2007–2012 by race/ethnicity

Race/ethnicity	Five-year absolute numerical change	Five-year numerical percentage change (%)	Average numerical change per year (%)	Five-year average annual sales change (%)
Asian Americans	86,626	26.8	17,325	1.6
Whites	80,983	2.2	16,197	−2.7
Hispanics	44,717	21.2	8,943	2.0
Blacks	5,060	5.4	1,012	−9.6
American Indians	2,932	13.1	586	−13.9

Source: Author's analysis of data from the Survey of Business Owners (2007, 2012).

Asians and whites each increased their employer-firm totals by over eighty thousand, respectively. Hispanics added nearly forty-five thousand. These figures represented seventeen, sixteen, and nine times the rate of black employer firms added during the same period. Only American Indians trailed blacks in the average annual numerical growth, but American Indians far outpaced blacks per capita. As noted in previous studies, relative to employer firms, black Americans are losing ground to every other racial population, and they are the only group not making up ground on white firms when their population share is controlled for in the calculations (McKoy and Johnson 2018).

It is likely that black-owned employer firms will not only drop below prepandemic figures but also stay at that level for longer than their counterparts. Based on the most recent trends, employer firms owned by black males are likely to suffer the greatest setbacks. In addition, even as the recovery takes shape, black firms are likely to lose further economic ground to their counterparts via probable below-average sales figures—even as they are closing the gap in firm count on the strength of their above-average growth in sole proprietorships. As these black firms open or reopen, based on past trends, they may experience a significant drop in average annual sales revenue, meaning they may end up operating smaller employer firms, losing talent wars, suffering declining market prospects, and missing out on economic opportunities because of a lack of resources. Black women employer firms are the likeliest to suffer from these revenue declines and resource shortcomings.

Based on the small percentage of black-owned employer firms that received PPP proceeds—or other federal provisions—coupled with their lack of access to traditional broader private capital market as well as their lack of access to personal, familial, and community wealth to survive the extended closed economy, the time after the COVID-19 pandemic will see a dramatically shrunken black employer-firm ecosystem. Whereas many white firms with paid employees that closed during this pandemic will merge with or be acquired by other firms, as in past recessions, black firms with employees are not likely to see such activity. Instead, they will simply lay off their workforce and close their doors permanently.

DECREASE IN BLACK WEALTH (AND AN ACCELERATED ROAD TO ZERO WEALTH)

The fourth impact from the COVID-19 pandemic, and an attendant result of the three preceding impacts, will be a decreased level of collective black American wealth: an escalator on which blacks were already descending, now sped up by the pandemic.

Wealth is an economic measure of one's assets minus one's liabilities. If the determinants of wealth creation were to be categorized into five associated key drivers—income rate, savings rate, investment rate, inheritance rate, and business ownership rate—as well as the scale of those factors, it is possible to chart the likely post-COVID-19 aftereffects on black wealth, specifically those linked to and associated with racial business ownership rates and success. For all racial demographics of individuals, each of those key wealth drivers will contract, or altogether evaporate, in the current environment; these trends will occur in the black community at an augmented pace. The precise degrees of change across America's different demographic populations—positive and negative—will serve as the determinant of how much wider America's current racial wealth gap will expand post COVID-19. But make no mistake, it *will* be wider.

As the pandemic persists and more blacks lose wage employment, some permanently, maintaining current assets such as homes, investment securities, properties, savings, retirement accounts, and businesses may prove arduous, if not impossible. Blacks who lose businesses, with or without paid employees, will see their wealth diminished. Owners of employer firms will likely see greater losses, since those companies traditionally capture significantly more revenue than sole proprietorships. For those who successfully (re)start new businesses, they can expect to share in the pattern of declining average revenues for black firms mentioned earlier, as they vie for the same withering pools of minority-designated dollars, even as the minority business population grows. This will likely result in the increased chasm in America's racial wealth share generated by business ownership.

One example illustrates the scope of the racial wealth gap relative to US business ownership and operation. The *Forbes* list of American billionaires, released in September 2020, detailed a group of America's richest individuals who have all created their wealth through the founding and growth of business enterprises—or who are descendants of those who have done so. Despite the COVID-19 pandemic, where millions of Americans have experienced near fatal economic decline, America's 400 wealthiest individuals added more than $240 billion to their aggregate net worth during the twelve months from August 2019 to August 2020, for a combined $3.2 trillion in wealth (Rogers 2020). Globally, the world's twenty-five richest billionaires gained nearly $255 billion in the immediate two months following the US stock market's early pandemic low on March 23 (Ponciano 2020). These particular economic gains bypassed black America altogether. There are no black Americans among the world's twenty-five wealthiest individuals; only one investor—Robert Smith at 330—is among the 400 richest Americans (Dolan, Peterson-Withorn, and Wang 2020). Moreover, he is the rare billionaire who has lost wealth in the last year since the pandemic's start.

Even when expanding the pool of America's wealthiest to all billionaires, only seven of the estimated 615 total billionaires in America are black (Dolan, Peterson-Withorn, and Wang 2020). Hence, blacks comprise just 1.1 percent of American business billionaires, though constituting more than 13 percent of the overall populace. Of those seven, five—or 71 percent—are representative of sports or entertainment, one is a technologist, and one is an investor. The richest black business "moguls" in the United States represent just pennies on the dollar compared to the richest whites. The collective wealth of these seven African Americans is $16.1 billion: Robert Smith ($5.0B); David Stewart ($3.7B); Oprah Winfrey ($2.5B); Michael Jordan ($1.6B); Kanye West ($1.3B); Sean "Jay-Z" Carter ($1B); and Tyler Perry ($1B) (Dolan, Peterson-Withorn, and Wang 2020). Using Smith's status as the sole member of the *Forbes 400*, the black business proportionate wealth of the four hundred richest Americans is just $5 billion of $3.2 trillion, or 0.16 percent.

A more startling exemplification of the racial wealth gap, specifically black business disparities, might be to compare one of America's—and the world's—wealthiest entrepreneurs and business owners, Jeff Bezos of Amazon, to the roughly three-million firm black business ecosystem in America.[5] From 2007 to 2012, black-owned businesses expanded from 1.9 million to 2.6 million, with accompanying revenue growth of 9.1 percent from $137.5 billion to $150.0 billion (US Census Bureau 2021a). Assuming a similar annual revenue growth rate for black firms for the subsequent eight years, the aggregate total would have grown by about 14.6 percent to nearly $172 billion by 2020. An additional point of commercial optimism might postulate that as a result of the prepandemic bullish market, black business revenue more than doubled its growth rate from the previous 2012–2020 estimate of 14.6 percent to 30 percent, resulting instead in $195 billion in collective sales and receipts by 2020.

Even with such a sanguine (and doubtful) scenario of 30 percent growth over these eight years, these nearly three million black businesses collectively would still fail to match Bezos's sole personal wealth, which has expanded by 57 percent in the last year since the pandemic began (Rogers 2020). Bezos's wealth reached $205 billion on August 26, 2020, the first individual to ascend to that $200 billion milestone (Ponciano 2020). In July 2020, mid-pandemic, his personal worth increased by a record $13 billion in a single day—nearly as much wealth (81 percent) as all the black American billionaires have collectively earned over their lifetimes and careers in business (Pitcher 2020). Moreover, this increase was even after the divorce settlement that resulted in Bezos's ex-wife, Mackenzie Scott, receiving 25 percent of his Amazon stock—resulting in her becoming the thirteenth richest person in the world, with a net worth of $64 billion (Dolan, Peterson-Withorn, and Wang 2020). Furthermore, though his net worth has dropped slightly below $200 billion since its August 2020 peak, it still singly exceeds black American business' collective annual sales and revenue. Elon Musk, founder of Tesla and Space X, saw his wealth surpass $300 billion in November 2021, representing over 150 percent of the entire black business ecosystem (Haverstock 2021). Of course, these one-to-many comparisons do not even come close to representing the white business to black business wealth gap, which is exponentially greater.

For some, economic recessions are opportunities to expand wealth by acquiring assets at lower costs, inclusive of business acquisitions. This option does not exist for the majority of African Americans. The continuing deterioration of black American wealth, both absolute and relative to other US racial groups, will recycle itself through the reduction of future wealth generation prospects via business ownership—and consequently, for future opportunities to enhance overall community well-being—even after the COVID-19 pandemic is over. The loss of wealth will make it harder for African Americans to start and grow businesses. It will make it harder for them to pass down pecuniary endowments or make transfers to children that might result in business formation. It will make it harder for them to attain educational credentials, expand social networks, gain experiential opportunities, or otherwise develop foundations for successful entrepreneurship and business pursuits postpandemic.

The goal of this chapter is not to be fatalistic in regard to the ultimate survival of the black business ecosystem as a result of COVID-19. Instead, it offers key insights into why a thorough understanding of the prepandemic positioning of black-owned firms in the United States, their unique historic trajectory, and probable immediate postpandemic status, is critical to determining the best and most effective intervention: not only to save this racial classification of businesses but also to foster a sturdier, more durable, and more robust version of this ecosystem than before.

There are certainly urgent actions that are warranted to prevent the immediate extinction of the black entrepreneurial ecosystem in this present moment. Those actions should be pursued without delay, as stopping the black business hemorrhaging and preserving economic life is a necessity. However, as with any devastating storm that ravages the landscape, once survival is assured and the storm has passed, the true work begins in assessing what must be done to return or rebuild the topography.

Still, it is problematic to respond to what needs to be done on behalf of US black-owned businesses as a result of the COVID-19 crisis without concurrently speaking on what needs to be done on behalf of those black-owned businesses in general. Numerous policies should have been implemented prior to the pandemic to address black business degeneration in America. While the overall diversity of the business ecosystem has been changing rapidly for decades, the business success ecosystem has not been diversifying as fast, if at all (McKoy and Johnson 2018). Black businesses have been left behind.

It is necessary that any remedy aimed at addressing the specific effects of the COVID-19 pandemic on black-owned businesses in the United States must be simultaneously coupled with ecosystem-level cures for what ailed those businesses prior to the virus' arrival. There must be sequences of responses addressing the short-, medium-, and long-term horizons of black business survival for the remainder and immediate aftermath of COVID-19. Next, there must be a more comprehensive, but targeted, scheme to generate the broader conditions that support the inherent advancement of successful African American–owned businesses. Finally, specific and measurable goals must be established in order to track progress to entrepreneurial and business equity. This tripartite approach needs to be executed concomitantly and in parallel to be successful.

Short-Term, Medium-Term, and Long-Term Interventions

SHORT TERM: IMMEDIATE CASH INFUSIONS

In the short term and immediate term, it is most important to assist black businesses—as many as possible—to survive the crisis, even as economies continue to reopen. This should not be a controversial statement since saving as many American businesses as possible was the expressed impetus of the CARES Act, and specifically the PPP. However, the PPP, especially the first round, failed to adequately reach the most vulnerable and neediest businesses—which included the majority of black-owned firms in America. The second round, and subsequent attempts, did not fare much better even with such targeting language. Figure 6.4 presents a framework of tiered responses that could better support the short-term, medium-term, and long-term survival of US-based black businesses.

Cash is king, and it is important to be prudent while also finding the most direct way to get cash to black business owners. Thus far, with the PPP, the primary vehicles for cash distributions have been traditional banks. As of May 2021, of the 5,242 PPP lenders who participated since the program's inception, nearly all are categorized as traditional banks (4,217, or 80 percent) or credit unions (859, or 16 percent) (SBA 2021). Financing has always been problematic for black businesses. While 77 percent of US adults rely on traditional banks or credit unions, 14 percent of blacks are unbanked and 35 percent are underbanked, rates higher than those of Hispanics (11 percent and 23 percent) and whites (4 percent and 11 percent), respectively (Board of Governors of the Federal Reserve System 2019). Furthermore, across all income levels, blacks are more

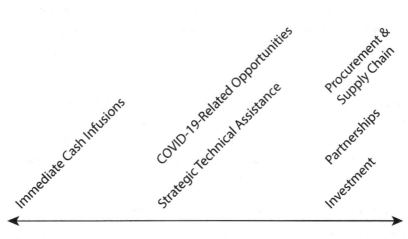

FIGURE 6.4. Tiers and timeline of needed COVID-19 responses for US black-owned businesses.

likely to be denied credit compared to their counterparts. As recently as 2017, nearly half (45 percent) of black loan applicants, compared to only 18 percent of white loan applicants, reported being denied for bank credit. Even at income levels above $100,000, blacks were still more than 2.5 times more likely than whites to be denied credit (21 percent vs. 8 percent) (Board of Governors of the Federal Reserve System 2019). These statistics indicate how traditional banking is ineffective in reaching many black business owners.

Instead, Congress should allocate and target a significant amount of funding specifically to black-owned businesses through different and more targeted financial vehicles and intermediaries. Instead of the SBA being designated to work on such a targeted program, that task should fall to the Minority Business Development Agency (MBDA), which was established in March 1969 and has long been dedicated exclusively to minority business enterprise (Minority Business Development Agency 2021). The MBDA has a more direct history supporting minority businesses than the SBA, which has been questioned in recent years on its commitment to black business lending as SBA-backed loans have declined for African American business owners, even as the agency's overall lending has increased to other business populations—with little other explanation beyond racial bias (Bates and Robb 2020).

These targeted funds should be delivered through means most likely to reach those firms. For example, Self-Help Credit Union, a white-founded-and-led community development financial institution (CDFI) based in Durham, North Carolina, with a sizable minority clientele, managed $183 million of PPP loans, totaling 1,758 loans with 59 percent of the loans received by businesses led by people of color (Gentry 2021). To target the funding even more precisely, supplementary capital could be allocated specifically to a coalition of CDFIs led by African Americans—who have customer bases of predominantly black-owned businesses.[6] Moreover, these loans could be provided to both sole proprietorships and employer firms and be fully forgivable (with no tax penalty) to both groups.

A targeted allocation of federal capital could also explore other vehicles for swift deployment to eligible black firms. In addition to providing forgivable lending capital through African American–led CDFIs, Congress could create a substantial black business block grant program, modeled after current federal block grant projects like the Community Development Block Grant (CDBG) program, in existence since 1974.[7] CDBG is the annual US Housing and Urban Development agency's program that allocates capital to state governments and local municipalities of a certain size to address housing and poverty issues. This funding formula is based on a series of quantitative factors such as population, age and condition of housing stock, and area poverty rates as determined by census tract data, with the greatest pro rata allocation going to the neediest areas. A new block allocation could be designated specifically for African American–owned businesses and distributed to state and local governments for rapid deployment, with the most pro rata funds going to the neediest areas and businesses.

Both state and local governments have struggled throughout the pandemic to figure out how to get capital to minority businesses, specifically black-owned firms, without running afoul of discriminatory laws. As a result, some governments have partnered with statewide or local anchor institutions—including nonprofits, foundations, and universities—who possess better track records or more relevant missions in reaching those target populations (Goad 2020). However, these programs have also proven largely ineffective and unsuccessful, with some black business owners complaining that these state or localized capital programs were stricter and more onerous than the federal ones.[8] As a result, even among some of the most broadly crafted local and state business funds, the capital distribution rates seemed to parallel the bleak federal distribution levels. In addition, even among those local or state programs that were more successful in reaching black firms, the grant or loan size was so small, because of the fund's diminutive scale, that it was largely inconsequential.[9] Moreover, for some businesses, these funds were too little and too late anyway, since many relied on CARES Act funding to create these programs.

Thus, a block grant program dedicated to African American business owners could include some of the same capital-matching components of CDBG but also offer state and local governments the flexibility to partner with other resourced institutions to get funding onto the street more broadly and quickly. Finally, an additional aspect of the program could allow for retroactive grant making to black-owned firms that shuttered their doors as a consequence of inadequate and inequitable distribution of original PPP funding. In other words, if a black business owner can prove they had a business prior to COVID-19 and were denied an adequate opportunity to save their business, they would be able to get a retroactive loan or grant to restart their firm.

These represent two short-term and immediate actions that the federal government could implement to provide capital to black-owned businesses across the United States, addressing a critical need that PPP has failed to satisfy. Deploying capital through both African American–led CDFIs and through a special purpose state and local government block grant program would ensure that a significant number of the remaining black businesses will survive the pandemic or be resurrected.

MEDIUM TERM: MARKET-BASED STRATEGIC TECHNICAL ASSISTANCE AND CONNECTIVE OPPORTUNITIES

Though immediate capital distribution allows for short-term survival of African American businesses in the midst of the ongoing pandemic and tepid reopening of the economy, it fails to adequately address the future positioning of those businesses in the broader marketplace. As expressed previously, to some extent the majority of black businesses, even prepandemic, were merely—and barely—surviving. The goal should be to advance a greater share of those firms from a state of surviving to thriving. To achieve this, black firms will need to both adjust to the modified and truncated pandemic-induced marketplace as well as position themselves more strongly for the postpandemic return to a fully opened economy.

Strategic Technical Assistance (STA)

To support adjustments to a modified marketplace, black firms must be supported in this transition to ensure that as markets are reopened they can take advantage of their new knowledge. As the marketplace has shifted, so have the parameters for operating within it. Some black-owned businesses, because of limited capital resources in the past or just outdated operational strategies, have been unable to evolve prior to and during the COVID-19 pandemic. For instance, most restaurants were required to shut down during the height of COVID-19's spread and were only allowed to seat a reduced number of patrons as reopenings started. Black-owned restaurants that have operated as cash-and-carry businesses might need assistance moving to operations that include accepting payments via debit and credit cards, utilizing online and cellphone application-based ordering for curbside pickup, and employing delivery services such as Uber Eats, GrubHub, and DoorDash. This type of strategic technical assistance (STA) would have both immediate and long-term positive impacts on businesses, allowing them to remain operational during truncated marketplace conditions as well as better positioning them for after those conditions have stabilized.

Restaurants are not the only business sector that could benefit from market-based strategic technical assistance in this new era. Such strategic assistance could range from traditional areas such as legal and accounting advice to ensure that the organization is on solid footing, to less traditional advisory assistance.

Black business owners could receive consultation on how to protect their brands, copyrights, patents, or other intellectual property. Technical assistance could also be provided to firms that would benefit from gaining federal, state, and local certifications and designations important to qualifying for government contracting opportunities, such as Historically Underutilized Businesses (HUB), Small Business Enterprises (SBE), Minority Business Enterprises (MBE), the SBA 8(a) Business Development Program, and others. Though these skills and designations were equally important prior to the pandemic, they might allow black firms to better position themselves for postpandemic opportunities. Technical assistance should be strategic to the firm's competitive positioning, as opposed to focusing on arbitrarily chosen topics. Black-owned firms should be able to procure these services from any provider in the marketplace, and not rely on having to go through government-specific programs.

To support this range of strategic technical assistance activities, which could occur simultaneously to short-term cash infusions, surplus funding could be included in the previously outlined immediate cash provisions. To procure these services, African American business owners would access these medium-term strategic technical assistance funds directly through either the CDFIS or block grant funds. Small businesses that request supplementary resources for STA would have those funds fully forgiven if they provided proof of procuring the strategic assistance. There are some state governments already leveraging CARES Act dollars to support entrepreneurial technical assistance.[10] However, these programs do not allow entrepreneurs to engage in broader training activities that would also support firm advancement, such as educational workshops or higher education courses, nor do they provide the funds directly to entrepreneurs. In addition, technical assistance programs are customarily limited to the business owners as opposed to all employees. Yet, for those black firms that have paid employees, those employees should also be able to engage in STA trainings relevant to their work duties since many of these duties also have been permanently altered by the pandemic. Each of these added allowances would expand the impact of these STA efforts supported by federal funding.

Connections

Given that the results of some strategic technical assistance might take time, the direct federal cash infusions could provide a bridge for firms that are reskilling and retooling their leaders and workers for the ongoing economic reopening and post-COVID-19 economy. However, this approach might not be adequate for all firms within the black entrepreneurial ecosystem. Some black firms are already properly equipped and simply need to be pulled into the COVID-19-related business opportunities that have emerged in the marketplace. This is a medium-term strategy that some, but not enough, US communities have used during the COVID-19 pandemic to assist black-owned businesses in an attempt to offset lost revenue.

The closure of school districts across the United States in mid-March 2020 as a result of the pandemic simultaneously created several community quandaries. Nationally, school districts were faced with having to figure out how to deliver educational content to students at home who might be without adequate learning resources and environments. A supplementary challenge was that a significant portion of those same students also lost access to at least two of the meals they generally ate at school each day: breakfast and lunch. While many school districts are familiar with this during summer vacation months, they were unprepared for this problem in early spring. As a response, some communities, through public funds and/or funds raised from charitable sources, moved to provide daily meals for those adversely affected students and families.

A key strategy in some geographies was the intentional procurement of those school meals from black-owned restaurateurs and caterers. In some places, this process was also inclusive of broader supply chains—such as procuring fresh fruits and vegetables from black-owned farms or other associated supplies from black business owners. This opportunity for double-positive impact allowed children and families to be fed and, simultaneously, for some black-owned firms to generate revenue: helping cash-starved businesses while filling an immediate, real, and pressing community need.

State and local governments can utilize similar creative strategies by surveying the landscape to identify real and immediate, as well as ongoing, COVID-19-related opportunities that can be subsequently connected to and procured by qualified black firms. Though such efforts might not replace all revenue loss, they can offer needed lifelines, concurrently allowing some firms to survive while maintaining—and on occasion expanding—payrolls that keep community members working.

These medium-term strategies would provide black-owned firms with more sustainable and supplemental means of survival than the one-time cash loans or grants. The ultimate goal would be to help these firms survive, reposition, and strengthen themselves in the short term and medium term, allowing them to thrive in the long term.

LONG TERM: SCALED-UP PUBLIC AND
PRIVATE INVESTMENT AND OPPORTUNITY

It is unclear what the future of business will look like including when, and if, the economy returns to its full, pre-COVID-19 pandemic form. Still, now is an ideal time and opportunity for the public and private sectors, who have both publicly pledged commitments to invest more in the economic growth of the black community and to reevaluate and alter their actual practices. Once the economy returns to its normal operations, there is a strong likelihood that things will return to business as usual. The same inequities, general and race specific, that existed prior to and during the COVID-19 pandemic will exist following it.

Though many municipal and corporate leaders have recently made public proclamations, pronouncements, and even capital investments in response to increased attention paid to America's racial inequities and injustices—particularly relating to the black community—it is unclear how sustainable and durable these commitments are. Furthermore, the majority of these investments have centered around support for historic social justice organizations, as opposed to providing conduits for the bolstering of the US black business ecosystem.

It will matter very little if short-term strategies of cash infusions, and medium-term strategies of strategic technical assistance and COVID-related opportunities, position black American firms for a future of wider prospects that never materializes. Prior to the full reopening of the economy, all levels of government and major corporations should undergo intensive evaluations of their internal cultures and policies related to supporting black businesses across their respective footprints. These are endeavors that must be commenced by white-led institutions that control the majority of the economic landscape and accompanying resources, in order to fashion a less hostile and more welcoming environment for black firms attempting to do business in the full, unabridged economy.

Any allied efforts, if they aim to produce lasting transformation of a system that has been designed to be exclusionary since its founding, must go beyond perfunctory tactics, strategies, campaigns, and gestures, such as instituting new diversity, equity, and inclusion policies; commissions; or token positions that are little more than symbolic. As the old axiom professes, "Culture trumps policies every time." Though inclusionary policy is important, as are devoted and enthusiastic diversity champions, if measurable impact toward equity is the goal, societal institutions must change enduring cultural practices that have become organizational features.

Procurement

Both public and private entities should reevaluate their procurement portfolios, supply chains, policies, and practices—as well as the cultures that drive them. When the first government and corporate procurement programs were instituted in the early 1970s, black Americans were the primary if not exclusive focus of minority business programs. Black Americans then constituted roughly 11 percent of the US population. Therefore, the subsequent 10 percent target goal set as a general standard for minority participation and procurement made relative sense. In the half-century since those original policies, the definition and pool of populations classified as minority has expanded (as has the overall minority population of the United States) to recognize and include many more racial identities, gender categorizations, sexual orientations, and veteran statuses. Yet, many procurement programs continue to utilize the 10 percent goal—not only as a guidepost but also as a ceiling for this collection of protected classes. Even as whites constitute a smaller share of the overall US populace, their businesses continue to control 90 percent of most industries and sectors—with every other group competing for the same remaining 10 percent. Consequently, a first step toward economic equity is for public and private sector players to reconstitute their procurement goals to be more reflective of America's changing demographic landscape.

Sliding racial procurement goals should be adopted based on the demography of the geographic landscape where they operate, combined with their customer or resident composition. Doing so would increase the probability that tax payments or consumer dollars paid and spent by the black community would recycle back through the black community economic ecosystem, with similar effects for other groups. Though this change would shift around the current revenue shares within the business landscape, every demographic would benefit as collective well-being increases.

President Joseph Biden, speaking on June 1, 2021 in Tulsa, Oklahoma, to commemorate the one-hundredth anniversary of the Greenwood race massacre, announced his intention to increase federal procurement and contracting dollars under his control from 10 to 15 percent for disadvantaged businesses. To ensure the desired impact on the long-term viability of the black business ecosystem, President Biden should not only direct his proposed procurement increase to go specifically to black entrepreneurs but also take the lead from some other local governments and create stretch goals such as 30 to 35 percent of federal procurement. Only then will there be adequate progress toward equity in the American procurement system.

Partnership

Public and private institutions should also examine their partnership portfolios. All levels of government engage in some degree of public-private partnerships to spur job creation and economic development. More public resources should be leveraged specifically with and on black-owned businesses. At the federal level, this practice might mean creating more trade agreements and activities with predominantly black countries or providing federal tax policy favorable to black-owned business expansion across the United States. At the state and local levels, it would entail creating dedicated pools of corporate recruitment incentives, programs, and policies, specifically to support black businesses.

White-owned firms are constantly offered recruitment incentive packages that include billions of dollars in tax credits, workforce development investments, and property/site development subsidies, leveraged at both the state and local levels. Black-owned firms rarely, if ever, receive access to such subsidies, which further widens the associated business inequity and wealth gaps. The public sector should prepare for a postpandemic landscape that supports black business growth and expansion through leveraging dedicated efforts and resources to black-focused public-private partnerships.

Major corporations also have portfolios of strategic partnerships, joint ventures, and similar alignments with other businesses for mutual benefit. These organizations should identify opportunities to partner with black-owned firms to pursue new marketplace prospects, not merely for the purpose of increasing scores on government contract bids or checking a diversity or inclusion box. Since many start-up firms emerge as a result of employee churn from larger corporations, if larger firms alter their partnership portfolio to include black firms, the area most affected could be the future start-up economy. Pairing more early stage black firms with other groups in emerging markets and spaces could dramatically alter business-associated wealth opportunities for black-founded firms. A post-COVID-19 environment that is welcoming to such business-to-business strategic partnerships would create greater opportunities for black firms and entrepreneurs. Whether in the public or private sector, these partnerships have to be racially equitable in their structures to maximize impact and see measurable change.

Investment

Public and private sectors should also reevaluate and overhaul how they currently invest into the black business marketplace and ecosystem. Expanding procurement and supply chain dollars to reach more black firms, as well as more partnerships, would have significant long-term impact on racial entrepreneurial equity; however, cash investment, a predecessor to organizational capacity, is just as critical.

Though state and local governments have continued to face COVID-19-related revenue uncertainty throughout the pandemic, and will continue to do so as the economy ramps back up, they should still consider organizing special purpose capital funds for black-owned business support in the long term. The American Rescue Plan of 2021 was signed into law on March 11, 2021, with $350 billion of the $1.9 trillion total designated for local and state government control (White House 2021). Local and state government leaders should petition the federal government to allow a portion of federal rescue act dollars to form evergreen investment funds for black-owned firms. These local and state government rescue funds, which under federal statute must be spent by December 31, 2024, have a set of allowed uses, including aid to small businesses. A special clause could and should be adopted by Congress allowing the previously proposed "special purpose capital fund" to be an eligible activity under the act. In addition, any unspent funds after 2024 should be permitted to remain at the state or municipal levels if they are dedicated to providing equity capital for black business investment. These funds would move beyond current "minority loan pool" debt models popular with governments, which generally come with higher interest rates, to capital pools that can be distributed in equity or equity-like forms.

Moreover, investments in the entrepreneurial landscape—if they pan out—turn businesses into potential acquisition targets, or strategic partners, in the future. Major corporations should carve out designated capital to invest in funds dedicated to black firms in their industry (or supporting the entry of such firms) as a method of diversifying the entrepreneurial marketplace. As the demographic landscape has diversified, corporations for several decades have poached black talent to enter into new markets or have acquired black-owned firms. These strategies can remain, but they ought to be supplemented with investment dollars that build the capacity of future independent partner firms instead.

A Transformation of National Culture

Though institutional culture is critical to any substantial change, societal culture is paramount to any broader and permanent systemic shift in racial equity. Interest in business-related societal inclusion and diversity comes in periodic waves and cycles. The usual pattern finds these societal inclusive impulses most

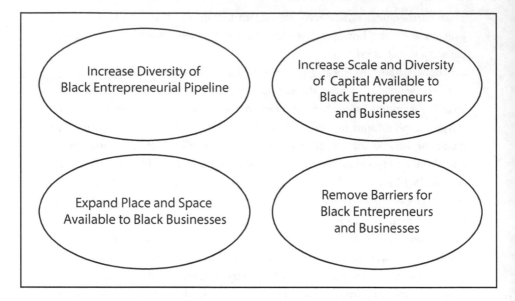

FIGURE 6.5. Four key strategies for permanent transformation of US black business competitive ecosystem.

pronounced when economic growth is at its peak and least evident during economic downturns. Presumably at the apex of growth, as some racial groups have been left out, there are pressures, inclinations, and aspirations to pull those populations into the economic tent. Alternatively, when markets are constrained and in duress, the prevailing attitude is often that racial equity must take a backseat to overall economic growth.

Figure 6.5 provides an approach beyond inclusionary and exclusionary cycles keyed on four strategies for permanent transformation of the US competitive black business ecosystem. The pattern of "peak growth/peak inclusion" and "slow growth/slow inclusion" in the business ecosystem runs inverse to business and market readiness for many black firms. This asymmetric pattern persists ironically for the same reason that drives the dynamic growth of black entrepreneurship during recessionary periods. In down markets, black-owned firms are among the last to be called upon for opportunities, as all business demographics scramble for contracting prospects. As the economy begins initial expansion following a recession, white-owned firms are among the first to be called back into action—partly because of their industry networks and partly because their resource base often allows them to withstand the downturn, unlike many black-owned firms—and maintain their capacity in the process.

Conversely, when black firms are sidelined for years without opportunities for revenue, those entrepreneurs choose, or are forced to find, alternative means for survival. Moreover, those black entrepreneurs who decide to stay the course often do so as sole proprietors, without access to adequate capital resources to build capacity. Consequently, as the economy approaches an apex, and well-meaning people begin looking for diverse firms to work with across an array of industries, there are few, if any, black-owned firms of scale remaining in the market.

As these inclusive opportunities arrive in the marketplace that is without an adequate supply of diverse firms—especially black-owned ones—an array of programs arise attempting to fulfill the demand. In these programs and during these periods, black entrepreneurs learn skills, launch firms, and gain industry and government certifications and designations, with the intention of taking advantage of these presumptive market opportunities. However, two timing-related factors undermine these opportunistic plans.

First, market opportunities are not everlasting. When those offering the opportunities are unable to find the diverse supply of contractors to fulfill their immediate demands, they assume there are none available in the marketplace, shrug their shoulders, rejoice in offering their best effort, and move forward with the standard industry players. Second, this preliminary outreach usually occurs at or near the peak of the associated economic growth cycle. By the time black firms have achieved readiness to take advantage of these inclusive opportunities, these advantages have been extended to others and recessionary pressures are shrinking the overall marketplace, beginning a descent into an economic trough. Thus, there exists a supply of ready black firms in the midst of an economic recession, where they will once again be the first to lose out on opportunities and contracts and the last to gain them. This asymmetric cycle continues perpetually. Eventually, black entrepreneurs grow weary and concentrate on smaller scale, service-based endeavors that can be operated as sole proprietorships, can be more easily attained, have lower barriers and costs to entry, and can be undertaken in both bull and bear markets—or simply focus on wage employment, if it is available to them.

If America is to permanently break these asymmetric cycles and remove the entrepreneurial disincentives that suppress black business wealth creation, and thus provide a post-COVID-19 ecosystem for black-owned firms stronger than the one that existed prepandemic, it must focus on four concurrent strategies in relation to the black entrepreneur: pipeline, place and space, capital, and barriers. The United States government, the only entity with enough resources and wherewithal to invest and respond at an appropriate and adequate postpandemic scale to foster a new national culture of equity for black-owned businesses, should advance substantial federal dollars in each of these efforts over a sustained period of time, and it should consider previous and current pandemic response funding as only a beginning.

PIPELINE

First, the black entrepreneurship pipeline must be broadened, strengthened, and diversified across all sectors and industries. Black entrepreneurs are often pigeonholed into narrow constructs within key industries, expected to only engage in entrepreneurial efforts related to their race/ethnicity, or aggregated into low-margin and low-wealth service sectors. Lifestyle businesses such as barbershops, beauty salons, lawn-care businesses, janitorial services, and handy services are fine undertakings, but they cannot be the sole or primary players in a business ecosystem that expects to thrive and create wealth for the broader community. The implementation of this strategy must focus on increasing the representative pipeline of black-owned firms with paid employees and those that operate nationally and globally. In addition, attention must be paid to increasing the scalable business success pipeline beyond black athletes and black entertainers to the "everyday" black entrepreneur. Each of these various pipelines—industry, size, and type—will regenerate itself once it is adequately built. At that point, successful mentor entrepreneurs and businesses from the black community will support the next generation of black individuals and firms by providing inspiration, experiential opportunities, social networks, familial networks, employment, and financial support (i.e., entrepreneurial capital), ensuring a pipeline of skilled black entrepreneurs and more racially equitable business outcomes in perpetuity.

PLACE AND SPACE

Black-owned businesses should not be resigned to exist only in low-income and high-poverty census tracts, nor exclusively in racially monolithic ones. Commercial and retail gentrification in many major markets quickly follows or occurs in parallel to residential gentrification. As a consequence of economic integration following the Civil Rights Era only consisting of black dollars integrating into white businesses and communities, the black geographic economic ecosystem has been left barren and depleted. Furthermore, historic racial migration patterns, such as white flight from city centers to the suburbs—and then back again—often displace black firms that cannot absorb the accompanying rent or property tax hikes. Consequently, black firms get pushed into the most economically desolate zip codes, until those zip codes themselves begin to gentrify—at which time, those same increasingly nomadic black firms get pushed into ever poorer areas (if they exist), or they shuttered altogether.

In 2020, fifty-two former black McDonald's franchisees filed a federal lawsuit against the corporation alleging the organization "engaged in blatant and implicit racial discrimination" against them (*Triangle Business Journal* 2020b). These plaintiffs, who collectively operated more than two hundred stores, alleged they each lost between four and five million dollars because they were assigned undesirable locations, complaints that predated the pandemic-induced decline in the hospitality sector. This pattern of assigning black franchisees the worst locations might correlate with the dramatic decline of black-owned McDonald's, which has decreased from 2.5 percent of total franchises in 1998 to less than half a percent currently.

Black businesses should be given strategic resources and help in positioning themselves within valuable real-estate areas. In addition, these firms should be given the opportunity to lead and anchor those efforts when revitalization is happening along historically black corridors. Financial resources or government-owned property should be made available, specifically at the municipal level, to support real-estate positioning to ensure that black firms are not left out of high trafficked and high growth, nonminority areas of the city. Such expanded geographic positioning will allow black firms to capture more diverse dollars.

CAPITAL

The scale and diversity of capital available to black-owned firms and the entrepreneurs who create them is crucial to any strategy to broaden the business success landscape. Lack of adequate access to capital stymies not only the types of industries and sectors that an entrepreneur can enter but also what types of entrepreneurs will even attempt to enter the market. Industries with high capital barriers to entry are often those with the potential to generate the greatest wealth. In contrast, black entrepreneurs, because of ongoing struggles to access all kinds of capital—from friends and family to bank debt to venture and equity funds—are forced to enter into low-cost, low-margin, and low-wealth industries. Furthermore, the black prospective entrepreneurs most qualified, experienced, and likely to succeed might choose to remain in corporate America—often with a white-owned firm—if the prospects of taking the entrepreneurial leap is too risky for them or their familial networks because of discriminatory capital options and lower wealth creation prospects.

In addition, geographic positioning in the highest potential markets also requires access to substantial, patient capital. Capital currently available to black businesses is both limited and restrictive. Half of black-owned businesses have expressed difficulty with the availability of credit; nearly one-third indicated that they had difficulty purchasing inventory or supplies to fulfill contracts (US Federal Reserve Bank 2017). Additionally, 37 percent expressed difficulty making their debt payments. These challenges existed prior to the COVID-19 pandemic and were unsurprisingly higher than for any other racial group. Unquestionably, black entrepreneurs and businesses need access to more equitable bank credit, but they need access to more diverse kinds of capital as well. Most critically, they need access to venture, equity, and more flexible forms of capital at significantly greater and equitable scales. Equity capital allows firms to grow faster and create more wealth than debt does. If the black business ecosystem is to ever equitably compete and compare to their demographic counterparts, they will have to surpass the less than 1 percent share of equity investments that they now garner annually. Even when overt racism is not a direct exclusionary factor in business and entrepreneurship, capital access can be.

BARRIERS

Finally, black-owned businesses have not suffered because of one or two racist policies or practices: they have had their success suppressed by the sheer magnitude and voracity of the barriers—entrepreneurial, business, and economic death by a thousand paper cuts. Truthful conversations should be conducted with black entrepreneurs and firm owners to capture information on the myriad of barriers that they face on a routine basis, which cause individual and collective harm to the entrepreneurs, businesses, and overall black business ecosystem. Each and every one of these barriers should be categorized as either internal or systematic and addressed and remediated to the fullest extent possible. Frequent, persistent, and unremitting barriers are inherent and expected elements of the entrepreneurial vocation, but they should not be specifically attached to any particular racial demographic.

Undertaken collectively, cooperatively, and consistently, these four complementary strategies have the potential to provide the groundwork for an entrepreneurial and business ecosystem evolution that prevents black-owned firms in America from becoming extinct. The most important aspect is to normalize both black business inclusion and success and expand its relevance beyond diversity and inclusion cycles into the national culture of America. A sustained and significant congressional commitment to invest in these strategies after the COVID-19 pandemic would begin this important effort. The composition of the current inequitable landscape did not happen overnight; it culminated from more than four centuries of social and economic oppression, exclusion, and suppression. As a consequence, racial equity and systemic cultural change and practice across the business landscape will not come immediately. However, the most effective pathway toward permanent transformation is to identify key metrics that will serve as the foundation of this aspirational and ambitious national cultural change—and to intently and diligently track them.

Monitoring Specifics

Any meaningful effort without definitive metrics to track progression toward success is one that is doomed to fail.[11] This effort should become as naturalized and normalized as standard economic and business development is for white entrepreneurs. Nevertheless, in order to track and measure progress, at least

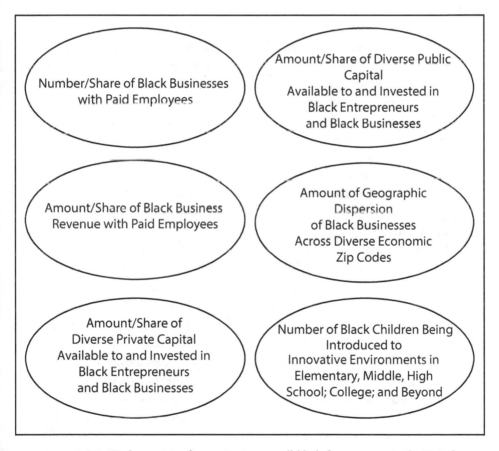

FIGURE 6.6. Six key metrics for monitoring overall black firm progress in the United States.

six key metrics (see figure 6.6) should be monitored at routine intervals to determine whether the four-pronged broader ecosystem strategies outlined in the previous section are working or if strategic adjustments are warranted.

PAID BUSINESS SHARE

While the number and share of black-owned businesses in the United States should be tracked relative to other demographic populations, specific focus should be allotted to firms with paid employees. Increasing the black relative share of this measurement should provide some indication of prospective well-being of the broader community economic ecosystem, since those firms would presumably benefit the black population through job creation and employment, retirement accounts, experiential learning, income, and wealth generation.

PAID REVENUE SHARE

Along with monitoring the share of black employer businesses, there should exist an accompanying tracking and measurement of those firms' relative share of business revenues. Specifically, monitoring average firm revenue and overall share—to see if these metrics are rising over time, or at least in conjunction with overall market conditions—would be key to understanding the potential of those firms to leverage such revenues into further entrepreneurial opportunities such as expansion into new markets, nationally and globally. Such a development would impact the same wealth and well-being factors previously mentioned, but more directly than simply increasing the numerical share of paid-employee firms.

PUBLIC AND PRIVATE INVESTMENT

The third and fourth metrics are both associated with access to capital. Though public and private capital sources are frequently conjoined and often allied, they are distinct-sourced pools. Public capital can be inclusive of tools such as actual cash, tax breaks, incentives, workforce resources, building and site resources, and others. Private capital is more often associated with various pools of debt and equity investment. In either case, black firms get miniscule amounts of it relative to their economic contribution into the pools that provide the capital and their relative population share. Capital is the lifeblood of the economy, meaning that black entrepreneurs and businesses must see a dramatic increase in their share of the economy's overall capital to be competitive and successful relative to their peers. Access to capital may be the most important of any of these factors; tracking the black share of public and private capital investment is imperative to tracking overall community well-being and success.

DIVERSE ZIP CODES

This metric will help to address the asymmetric outcomes of the one-way consumer capital flow, from the black community to the white community, following the civil rights movement. The expectation of social integration by African Americans was that economic integration would follow. Rising consumer buying power for the black diaspora in America, and even the world, has not resulted in a boom to black firm growth. Very few dollars of *any* demographic enter into the black business ecosystem, including *black* dollars. For black businesses, one of the challenges in capturing diverse dollars is that they are often relegated to segregated and low-wealth areas. As economic development takes place in cities across the United States, very few African American–owned businesses are included in those rising geographies. A major step in the right direction would be to track and monitor the geographic location and positioning of black businesses (including virtual/online positioning) to ensure they have adequate placing and opportunities to capture more diverse dollars, including, but not exclusively, those of the black community.

YOUTH INNOVATION EXPOSURE

The final metric, crucial to understanding the future strength of the black business ecosystem, is the amount of innovative exposure gained by the youth of the black business ecosystem. Findings suggest that gaps in adult innovation may be driven by differences in childhood environment, including role model or network effects, rather than varying abilities to innovate or differing quality of schools (Bell et al. 2019). Though children from high-income (top 1 percent) families are ten times as likely to become inventors as those from below median-income families, evidence suggests minorities and children from low-income families would likewise have had highly impactful inventions had they been exposed to innovation in childhood. Inventions and innovations such as patents, copyrights, and other intellectual property are the basis of the majority of business-created wealth in society. Increasing the exposure of black youth to innovation at earlier ages, in formal educational environments and outside of them, will be the foundation and connective tissue of the previous five metrics, as doing so would ensure a hearty and abundant black entrepreneurial ecosystem for generations to come.

BENCHMARK = EQUITY

What are the desired numerical and calculable goals—how many black firms are enough, how much revenue is enough, how much capital investment is enough—to declare equity (or for blacks to *feel* equitable)? As an anchoring benchmark, US demographic population share should be used as a reflective and suitable guide of equity and distributive outcomes in business and entrepreneurship statistics. That is to say, as populations that have historically been classified as majority and minority attain smaller/larger respective shares of the overall population, including black Americans, so presumably would their proportional representative business share. Though this relative target is not hard and fast, it offers a guidepost to benchmarking success in the pursuit of full equity across all US demographic populations.

As affirmed recurrently throughout this chapter, the existing statistics for black America related to these six identified metrics are vastly inequitable compared to every other US racial population, and they will be even more so following the COVID-19 pandemic. However, this time the burden of existential survival cannot be placed solely on the shoulders on black Americans. Instead, historic action must be coupled with considerable and unprecedented economic resources—and scaled and sustained to match the unparalleled nature of the problem. The future of black America is dependent on how the nation moves forward to address these now *more* exacerbated postpandemic gross inequities.

Conclusion

African American businesses have traveled through six distinctive stages relative to the broader US economic ecosystem. Since the centuries where black bodies, backs, and hands served literally as the primary capital base of American capitalism, to their golden years as segregated entrepreneurs from 1919 to 1929, to their current status as hustle entrepreneurs, black firms have nakedly absorbed every substantial blow that has accompanied four centuries of economic calamities. The COVID-19 pandemic is itself a once-in-a-lifetime-type catastrophe requiring an equally rare type of response. Moments like these, because of their uniqueness, often have the potential to shift the wider landscape.

One of those factors during the COVID-19 pandemic was the ability of the global populace to watch an inconceivable series of oppressive—actually deadly—actions taken against an array of black Americans in real time (i.e., Ahmaud Arbery, George Floyd, Breonna Taylor, among others). These acts, as horrendous as they were, were inconceivable only to a large portion of white America and the white world—they were unsurprising to the black populace. Nevertheless, these extraordinary images of modern, overt, and deadly racism toward black America and the resulting outcry led to unprecedented protests, marches, and demands for change to systematic racism directed at black Americans. Consequently, in a rare synchronous moment, extending beyond usual considerations of narrow social justice levers (i.e., legal, educational), the world collectively pointed to gross economic imbalances that black Americans face as an effort worth paying specific attention to—after the peaceful protests and demonstrations gave way to a secondary faction of looters and rioters that destroyed many white-owned businesses in downtowns across America. As a result, increasing the success of black-owned businesses became the central focus of a national movement in the United States—at least for an initial period.

My Black Receipt was an initiative started with an "aim to make buying from black-owned businesses more than a trend" (Bond 2020). In 2020, from the symbolic Juneteenth (June 19) to the equally symbolic Independence Day (July 4), in the midst of the pandemic, consumers were encouraged to buy from black-owned businesses with a goal of customers spending and posting at least five million dollars in receipts by the end of the 2020 campaign. Blackout Day 2020 similarly called for all black Americans—as well as for other people of color—to refrain from spending any money on Tuesday, July 7, in a show of solidarity against the killing of unarmed black citizens by law enforcement (Brooks 2020). For any consumer planning to spend money on that date anyhow, the organizers called for them to patronize black-owned businesses only. Though Juneteenth 2021 was historic, becoming the eleventh designated federal holiday in the United States and the first since Martin Luther King Jr. Day nearly forty years prior, there was no continuation of the previous Juneteenth and Independence Day "buy black business" campaigns.

Throughout the months following 2020's so-called "racial reckoning," some historically black institutions (such as banks and universities) also received significant depository and donation increases, as did many other black-led organizations (*Triangle Business Journal* 2020a). Furthermore, organizations such as Google and Yelp created technology tools to make it easier for consumers to identify black-owned businesses in their searches (Bond 2020). Nevertheless, these consumer-, philanthropy-, and corporate-driven initiatives—even as well meaning as they are and might have been—represent only a tiny portion of what needs to be done to support the infrastructure of African American–owned businesses in this country; moreover, they fail to adequately address the historical institutional impediments that remain barriers to success.

Historically, especially in an election year, there might have been an expectation from the federal government of at least a token effort aimed at the voting portion of the forty-four million black Americans—undertaken to stoke greater turnout in November for whichever party made the latest and greatest economic effort on their behalf (US Census Bureau 2021b). However, these were not conventional times.

On September 4, 2020, less than sixty days from the US presidential election, Donald Trump directed the leadership of all federal agencies and executive departments, via a memo from the White House Office of Management and Budget (OMB) to "list all contracts related to training sessions involving 'white privilege' or 'critical race theory,' and do everything possible within the law to cancel those contracts" (Dawsey and Stein 2020). According to the OMB memo, then President Trump deemed any belief that whites in America "benefited from racism" as "divisive, anti-American (and un-American) propaganda."

Despite this denial that racism exists in America, and therefore declaring that efforts to address it have "no place in the federal government," the memo ended by stating that "the president has a proven track record of standing for those whose voices have long been ignored and who have failed to benefit from all our country has to offer"—seemingly contradicting the memo's notion of a nation that has always been fair to all people (Vought 2020). Not only does four hundred years of recorded American history serve as a counter to former President Trump's assertion of a completely equitable country, but the broad array of inequitable racial responses to the COVID-19 crisis currently means the representation of that inequity is only a daily newsfeed away. This attempted retreat from federal programmatic responses to proven historic, and contemporary, racial inequities must be countered with both dramatic counteracting words as well as with bold reparative actions on behalf of the black business ecosystem in the United States. More challenging is that such efforts must occur in an environment that has quickly returned hostile toward *racial acknowledgement* and *racial remedy* by some political actors following a divisive election; the January 6, 2021, riot on the US Capitol; and rising aggression to not only critical race theory but also factual history related to black American oppression.

The activities and recommendations proposed throughout this chapter offer such bold proceedings. Throughout the history of this country the federal government has intervened with dramatic financial responses following crises that have threatened the nation's survival, specifically those economically related— including massive capital investments in other countries: the New Deal, in the 1930s; the Marshall Plan (1940s); the GI Bill (1950s); the American Recovery and Reinvestment Act (2010s); and now the pandemic-related CARES (2020) and American Rescue Plan (2021) Acts. However, each time, those responses have been racially inequitable, with particular benefits aimed at white America's survival while black America was left to fend for itself. The black business ecosystem in America has always been in a state of perpetual crisis—and in need of devoted attention and intervention. Its depleted, fast-declining status now threatens the nation's survival. The survival of all America is tied to the survival of black America, and the survival of black America, in turn, is tied to the survival of black American businesses.

The US black business ecosystem has been hollowed out from centuries of fiscal exclusion and economic discrimination, and the CARES Act has been no differently structured. However, this time, if left unattended, this economic exclusion could have a fatal impact on the future of black America—and America as a whole. America is becoming blacker and browner, on its way to becoming a majority-minority country. If the majority of a country has low, no, or negative wealth, then it is a problem not just for that population but for the entire country. If black businesses in the United States become functionally extinct and no longer play a significant role in the functioning of the overall American ecosystem, then there will be grave and negative consequences for the entire country. The unrest during the COVID-19 summer of 2020 might prove a mild preview of what is to come, if these swelling and intensifying economic disparities are unaddressed and further deteriorate.

The American Rescue Plan Act of 2021 seems to make an attempt at using federal capital in targeted ways to address historic racial inequities. Though the act is not specific to black America, President Biden has indicated that monies from the legislation should seek to address historic racial gaps. The $1.9 trillion Rescue Act, a part of what Biden calls his plan to Build (America) Back Better, is the third COVID-19 focused economic legislation passed since March 2020—following the $2 trillion CARES Act and $910 billion Consolidated Appropriations Act of 2021. These are touted as once-in-a-generation investments, as they are among the largest economic rescue plans in American history. Still, these investments should include more funds targeted toward black America's economic development. It is impossible to build America back better unless it builds black American business back better. Targeted investments by the Biden administration to black entrepreneurship are a good start, but they are not sufficient for the scope of the current disparities.

Thus, as part of this ongoing pandemic relief, Congress should not only provide substantial supplementary capital to address the immediate and short-term needs of black-owned American firms but also allocate additional distinct funding aimed at addressing historic inequities in the black business landscape. Congress should authorize the creation of a permanently funded US black business development block grant program for both the short term and the long term, which would thereafter garner a significant annual appropriation.

The immediate dollars would cover much-needed cash infusions to black firms and strategic technical assistance. Though the short-term cash allocation would disappear in future appropriation bills, the STA funds would become a permanent component of the block grant program. Additional annual funding as part of the block grant would go to support the creation and operation of a new AmeriCorps-type service program called *Equity Corps*. Equity Corps would fund the training and intensive service of a group of young and diverse postcollegiate Americans to spend two years working with municipalities and states around the country on creating more equitable local entrepreneurial, business, and economic ecosystems—aimed at transforming the national inclusive culture. The largest proportion of the block program would be dedicated to the distribution of block grants to local and state governments on an annual formulaic basis, in order to fund all associated efforts in creating a racially equitable business environment.

Perhaps a first step toward more ambitious and sustainable federal support for minority businesses arrived with the passage of the Minority Business Development Act of 2021. The bill's passage codified the Minority Business Development Agency (MBDA) as a permanent agency under the guidance of a newly created undersecretary role; expanded its geographic scope to include regional offices and rural business centers; and increased its ability to collaborate with both public- and private-sector partners to support the development of minority business enterprises (Bienasz 2021). The more than $1 trillion Infrastructure Investment and Jobs Act, passed in November 2021, provided $110 million annually through 2025 for the MBDA, up from $48 million allocated by Congress in 2021. Though this allocation is miniscule when considering the problem and degree of need—it is not enough to support the current black business ecosystem let alone the nine million minority businesses across the United States it aims to—the legislation may be a starting point. It *must* be seen as merely that. If black America, and America as a whole, are to achieve social and economic equity, the black business ecosystem alone must start seeing its own $1 trillion-plus in annual allocations and investments.

The weakened state of the black economy before the COVID-19 pandemic did not arise by chance, and it will not be changed by chance. In fact, the United States government played the central role in the African American business ecosystem arriving at such a depleted status, a situation that has been further hampered by the ongoing crisis and insufficient responses related to black American businesses. Consequently, the United States government must play an equally important role in building it up following the COVID-19 pandemic. Thus, there is substantial and significant ground in America to make up if there is any hope of ever curing the other deadly disease that has been ravaging the country since its founding: systemic racism.

NOTES

1. These loan count figures by race/ethnicity are estimates based on data extrapolated from SBA figures of the 94,501 applicants who filled out demographic information for the 661,218 actual total loans distributed that were above $150,000.

2. Author's analysis based on American Community Survey (ACS) data (2010) and Survey of Business Owners (SBO) data (2012) from US Census Bureau data estimates.

3. Entrepreneurial Capital Leverage (ECL) is the access to additional capital through means such as capital markets, banks, investors, and the such.

4. For more context on this curve, also called the Hygioeconomic Parity Index (HEPI), see McKoy and Banks (2019).

5. Three million is a modest estimate by the author of all black firms, with and without employees in 2020, based on prior growth trends. Estimated at 15.4 percent increase from 2012 to 2020—pre-COVID-19.

6. For more context, see African American Alliance of CDFI CEOs (2021).

7. For more context, see HUD (2021).

8. Based on information collected by the author in Durham, NC, July–August 2020.

9. Based on information collected by the author in Durham, NC, July–August 2020.

10. Based on the author's marketplace knowledge, 2020.

11. The word *effort* is utilized versus opposing language such as *initiative* or *project*, which belies some bounded start and end times.

REFERENCES

Abramson, Alana. 2020. "How Black-Owned Businesses Were Shut Out of Coronavirus Aid." *Time*. June 5. https://time.com/5848557/black-owned-business-coronavirus-aid/.

African American Alliance of CDFI CEOs. 2021. Accessed November 1, 2021. https://aaacdfi.org.

Austin, Algernon. 2016. *The Color of Entrepreneurship: Why the Racial Gap among Firms Costs the US Billions*. Center for Global Policy Solutions. http://globalpolicysolutions.org/report/color-entrepreneurship-racial-gap-among-firms-costs-u-s-billions/.

Bates, Tim, and Alicia Robb. 2020. "Decline in SBA Loans to Blacks Raises Questions about Obama Administration's Commitment." National Black Chamber of Commerce. Accessed September 18. https://www.nationalbcc.org/news/latest-news/1752-decline-in-sba-loans-to-blacks-raises-questions-about-obama-administrations-commitment.

Beckert, Sven, and Seth Rockman, eds. 2016. *Slavery's Capitalism: A New History of American Economic Development*. Philadelphia: University of Pennsylvania Press.

Bell, Alexander, Raj Chetty, Xavier Jaravel, Neviana Petkova, and John Van Reenen. 2019. "Who Becomes an Inventor in America? The Importance of Exposure to Innovation." *Quarterly Journal of Economics* 134, no. 2 (May): 647–713.

Bienasz, Gabrielle. 2021. "A Key Piece of the Infrastructure Bill Aims to Help Minority-Owned Businesses." *Inc.* November 8. https://www.inc.com/gabrielle-bienasz /infrastructure-bill-minority-business-development-agency-house-codified.html.

Board of Governors of the Federal Reserve System. 2019. *Report on the Economic Well-Being of US Households in 2018.* https://www.federalreserve.gov/publications/files/2018 -report-economic-well-being-us-households-201905.pdf.

Bond, Casey. 2020. "'My Black Receipt' Aims to Make Buying from Black-Owned Businesses More Than a Trend." *HuffPost.* July 17. https://www.huffpost.com/entry/my -black-receipt-buying-from-black-owned-businesses_l_5eeb97dac5b60f114ac54354.

Boston, Thomas D., and Linje R. Boston. 2007. "Secrets of Gazelles: The Differences between High-Growth and Low-Growth Business Owned by African American Entrepreneurs." *Annals of the American Academy of Political and Social Science* 613, no. 1 (September): 108–30. https://doi.org/10.1177/0002716207303581.

Brooks, Khristopher J. 2020. "Blackout Day Draws National Attention to Black Spending Power." *CBS News.* July 8. https://www.cbsnews.com/news/blackout-day-2020-black -owned-businesses/.

CDC (Centers for Disease Control and Prevention). 2020. "Risk for COVID-19 Infection, Hospitalization, and Death by Race/Ethnicity." Accessed September 18. https://www .cdc.gov/coronavirus/2019-ncov/covid-data/investigations-discovery/hospitalization -death-by-race-ethnicity.html.

Collins, Chuck, Dedrick Asante-Muhammad, Josh Hoxie, and Emanuel Nieves. 2017. "Report: The Road to Zero Wealth." *Institute for Policy Studies.* November 7. https:// www.ips-dc.org/report-the-road-to-zero-wealth/.

Couch, Kenneth A., and Robert Fairlie. 2010. "Last Hired, First Fired? Black-White Unemployment and the Business Cycle." *Demography* 47, no. 1 (February): 227–47. https://doi.org/10.1353/dem.0.0086.

Dawsey, Josh, and Jeff Stein. 2020. "White House Directs Federal Agencies to Cancel Race-Related Training Sessions It Calls 'Un-American Propaganda." *Washington Post.* September 5. https://www.washingtonpost.com/politics/2020/09/04/white-house -racial-sensitivity-training/.

Dolan, Kerry A., Chase Peterson-Withorn, and Jennifer Wang, eds. 2020. "The Forbes 400 2020: The Richest People in America." *Forbes.* September. https://www.forbes .com/forbes-400/.

Du Bois, W. E. B. 1897. "Strivings of the Negro People." *Atlantic.* June 24. https://www .theatlantic.com/magazine/archive/1897/08/strivings-of-the-negro-people/305446/.

Du Bois, W. E. B. 1903. *The Souls of Black Folk.* Chicago: A. C. McClurg and Co.

Duffy, Clare. 2020. "How Kanye West Embodies the Payroll Protection Program's Big Problems." *CNN.* July 9. https://www.cnn.com/2020/07/09/economy/yeezy-ppp -coronavirus-relief/index.html.

Fairlie, Robert. 2020. "The Impact of COVID-19 on Small Business Owners: Evidence of Early-Stage Losses from the April 2020 Current Population Survey." Working Paper w27309, National Bureau of Economic Research, Cambridge, MA. https://doi.org/10 .3386/w27309.

Flitter, Emily. 2020. "Black Business Owners Had a Harder Time Getting Federal Aid, a Study Finds." *New York Times*. July 15. https://www.nytimes.com/2020/07/15/business /paycheck-protection-program-bias.html.

Gentry, Connie. 2021. "Helping Provide the Foundation: How CDFIs Are Supporting the Small Businesses That Help the Triangle Attract Big-Name Firms." *Triangle Business Journal*. June 3. https://www.bizjournals.com/triangle/news/2021/06/03/how-cdfis -support-many-essential-businesses.html.

Global Strategy Group for Color of Change and UnidosUS. 2020. "Federal Stimulus Survey Findings." *The Black Response*. May 13. https://theblackresponse.org/wp-content /uploads/2020/05/COC-UnidosUS-Abbreviated-Deck-F05.13.20.pdf.

Goad, Matt. 2020. "How Duke University Is Helping the Durham Community during the Coronavirus Pandemic." *News and Observer*. June 30. https://www.newsobserver.com /news/local/counties/durham-county/article243899477.html.

Haverstock, Eliza. 2021. "Elon Musk Is the First Person Worth More Than $300 Billion." *Forbes*. November 2. https://www.forbes.com/sites/elizahaverstock/2021/11/02 /elon-musk-is-the-first-person-worth-more-than-300-billion-but-hertz-uncertainty -threatens-tesla-stock-tear/?sh=2c15528221f4.

HUD (US Department of Housing and Urban Development). 2021. "Overview, Community Development Block Grant Program." https://hud.gov/program_offices/comm _planning/cdbg.

Humphreys, Jeffrey. 2008. "The African-American Market." *Georgia Trend Magazine*. July 1. https://www.georgiatrend.com/2008/07/01/the-african-american-market/.

Kranhold, Kathryn, and Chris Zubak-Sees. 2020. "Small Business Loan Data Includes Little about Race." Center for Public Integrity. July 6. https://publicintegrity.org/health /coronavirus-and-inequality/small-business-loan-data-includes-little-on-owners-race -paycheck-protection-program/.

Lederer, Anneliese, Sara Oros, Sterling Bone, Glenn Christensen, and Jerome Williams. 2020. "Lending Discrimination within the Paycheck Protection Program." National Community Reinvestment Coalition. https://ncrc.org/lending-discrimination-within -the-paycheck-protection-program/.

Marable, Manning. 1983. *How Capitalism Underdeveloped Black America*. Boston: South End Press.

McKoy, Henry C., Jr. 2020. "Column: Averting Economic Crisis Needs Intentional Disruption." *Triangle Business Journal*. August 6. https://www.bizjournals.com/triangle /news/2020/08/06/averting-economic-crisis-needs-intentional-disrupt.html.

McKoy, Henry C., Jr., and LaChaun J. Banks. 2019. *City Economic Equity Rankings: Analysis of 21 US Cities—Inclusive Economic Development November 2019*. Ash Center for Democratic Governance and Innovation, Harvard Kennedy School. https:// socialequity.duke.edu/wp-content/uploads/2019/11/PMI-CITY-ECONOMIC-EQUITY -INDEX-HARVARD-NOV-2019.pdf.

McKoy, Henry Clay, Jr., and James H. Johnson Jr. 2018. "Do Business Ecosystems See Color?" *International Journal of Social Ecology and Sustainable Development* 9, no. 3: 80–91. https://doi.org/10.4018/ijsesd.2018070106.

Nielsen Corporation. 2019. "African American Spending Power Demands That Marketers Show More Love and Support for Black Culture." September 12. https://www.nielsen.com/us/en/pressreleases/2019/african-american-spending-power-demands-that-marketers-show-more-love-and-support-forblack-culture/.

Pitcher, Jack. 2020. "Jeff Bezos Adds Record $13 Billion in Single Day to Fortune." *Bloomberg*. July 20. https://www.bloomberg.com/news/articles/2020-07-20/jeff-bezos-adds-record-13-billion-in-single-day-to-his-fortune.

Ponciano, Jonathan. 2020. "The World's 25 Richest Billionaires Have Gained Nearly $255 Billion in Just Two Months." *Forbes*. May 24. https://www.forbes.com/sites/jonathanponciano/2020/05/22/billionaires-zuckerberg-bezos/#2f152f257ed6.

Rogers, Taylor Nicole. 2020. "America's 400 Wealthiest People Added $240 Billion to Their Net Worths in the Past 12 Months despite the Pandemic." *Business Insider*. September 8. https://www.businessinsider.in/thelife/news/americas-400-wealthiest-people-added-240-billion-to-their-net-worths-in-the-past-12-months-despite-the-pandemic/articleshow/78002046.cms.

Select Subcommittee on the Coronavirus Crisis. 2020. *Preliminary Analysis of Paycheck Protection Program Data*. https://coronavirus.house.gov/sites/democrats.coronavirus.house.gov/files/2020-09-01.PPP%20Interim%20Report.pdf.

Stuart, Reginald. 1981. "Businesses Owned by Blacks Still Fighting an Uphill Battle." *New York Times*. July 26. https://www.nytimes.com/1981/07/26/us/businesses-owned-by-blacks-still-fighting-an-uphill-battle.html.

Triangle Business Journal. 2020a. "M and F Bank Sees Uptick from Social Justice Campaigns." August 28.

Triangle Business Journal. 2020b. "11 Area Stores Included in McDonald's Suit." September 11.

US Bureau of Labor Statistics. 2020. https://www.bls.gov.

US Bureau of Labor Statistics. 2021. https://www.bls.gov.

US Census Bureau. 2007. Survey of Business Owners 2007. https://www.census.gov/library/publications/2007/econ/2007-sbo-business-owners.html.

US Census Bureau. 2012a. Survey of Business Owners 2007–2012. https://www.census.gov.

US Census Bureau. 2012b. Survey of Business Owners 2012. https://www.census.gov/library/publications/2012/econ/2012-sbo.html.

US Census Bureau. 2021a. "American Community Survey (ACS)." https://www.census.gov/programs-surveys/acs/.

US Census Bureau. 2021b. "QuickFacts United States." https://www.census.gov/quickfacts/fact/table/US/PST045219.

US Department of Commerce, Minority Business Development Agency. 2021. Accessed November 1, 2021. https://www.mbda.gov/.

US Department of the Treasury. 2020. "Assistance for Small Businesses." https://home.treasury.gov/policy-issues/cares/assistance-for-small-businesses.

US Federal Reserve Bank. 2017. Small Business Credit Survey.

US Small Business Administration (SBA). 2020a. "Flash Report: Small Business Administration's Implementation of the Paycheck Protection Program Requirements." May 8. https://www.oversight.gov/sites/default/files/oig-reports/SBA_OIG_Report_20-14_508.pdf.

US Small Business Administration (SBA). 2020b. "Paycheck Protection Program: An SBA Loan That Helps Businesses Keep Their Workforce Employed during the Coronavirus (COVID-19) Crisis." https://www.sba.gov/funding-programs/loans/coronavirus-relief -options/paycheck-protection-program.

US Small Business Administration (SBA) Office of Capital Access. 2020. "SBA Paycheck Protection Program Loan Level Data." https://data.sba.gov/dataset/ppp-foia.

US Small Business Administration (SBA). 2021. "PPP Data." https://www.sba.gov/funding -programs/loans/covid-19-relief-options/paycheck-protection-program/ppp-data.

Vought, Russell. 2020. "Training in the Federal Government." Office of Management and Budget. https://www.whitehouse.gov/wp-content/uploads/2020/09/M-20-34.pdf.

White House. 2021. "Fact Sheet: The American Families Plan." April 28. https://www .whitehouse.gov/briefing-room/statements-releases/2021/04/28/fact-sheet-the -american-families-plan/.

Zahra, Shaker A., and Satish Nambisan. 2012. "Entrepreneurship and Strategic Thinking in Business Ecosystems." *Business Horizons* 55, no. 3 (May–June): 219–29. https://doi .org/10.1016/j.bushor.2011.12.004.

7. COVID-19 Effects on Black Business-Owner Households

CHRIS WHEAT, FIONA GREIG, AND DAMON JONES

The COVID-19 pandemic and its aftermath will likely have disparate impacts on black business-owning households relative to their white counterparts for a number of reasons: the concentration of essential workers in specific neighborhoods, differential access to healthcare, and wealth inequality, among others. Given what we know about overall black-white wealth gaps, we might expect black households to generally be more vulnerable to the various shocks brought upon by the global health crisis. In particular, the financial resilience of households that generate wealth and income through small business ownership may be especially correlated with race during this period. In this chapter, we explore the potential implications of these baseline disparities for the financial health of black business-owning households during the pandemic, and the likelihood of success of the businesses they own as the economy begins to emerge from the public-health-induced recession.

Long-standing gaps in income and wealth between white families and black and Latino families have been well documented and grew following the Great Recession (Bayer and Charles 2018; Chetty et al. 2019; McKernan, Ratcliffe, Steuerle, and Zhang 2014; Thompson and Suarez 2019). Many factors have systematically contributed to wealth building of many white families while impeding wealth building among black and Latino families, including intergenerational wealth transfers (e.g., Meschede et al. 2017; Chiteji and Hamilton 2002; McKernan, Ratcliffe, Simms, and Zhang 2014); neighborhood conditions such as poverty rates, racial bias, and home values (e.g., Chetty et al. 2019; Perry, Rothwell, and Harshbarger 2018); geographic and financial barriers to human capital accumulation (e.g., Dobbie and Fryer 2011; Jackson and Reynolds 2013; Addo, Houle, and Simon 2016); racial segregation and discrimination in the labor market (e.g., Grodsky and Pager 2001; Bertrand and Mullainathan 2004); and racial biases in the policies and practices of government, institutions, and the private sector (e.g., Oliver and Shapiro 2013; Katznelson 2005; Robles et al. 2006; Bayer, Ferreira, and Ross 2014; Asante-Muhammad et al. 2017; Bartlett et al. 2019). These forces, most of which have substantial if underexamined structural components (Emmons and Ricketts 2017; Aspen Institute 2004; Kijakazi, Smith, and Runes 2019), not only have a direct effect on wealth and wealth accumulation at a given point in time but also may create racial differences in the key determinants of wealth over time and across generations.

While business ownership is often cited as a mechanism that might close this wealth gap (Bradford 2014; Herring and Henderson 2016), some researchers have suggested that this may not in fact be true, as the large number of exits among black business owners might actually lead to losses in overall household wealth (Shapiro 2019). Even in a growing economy, black-owned businesses tend to have lower revenues, lower profit margins, and less cash liquidity than those of white owners (Farrell, Wheat, and Mac 2020a). Although small business ownership is therefore not a likely channel through which the racial wealth gaps can be completely eliminated (Darity et al. 2018), tracking the health and solvency of small businesses can still provide insights into the financial well-being of households. Prior research suggests that household wealth, housing wealth, and small business outcomes are closely linked, even if the causal mechanism of these linkages are unclear (Hurst and Lusardi 2004; Fairlie and Krashinsky 2012). Substantial differences in household wealth and housing wealth by race (Darity et al. 2018), viewed alongside depressed cash liquidity among small businesses in neighborhoods with lower housing values and higher shares of black residents (Farrell, Wheat, and Grandet 2019), as well as racial differences in small business financial outcomes (Farrell, Wheat, and Mac 2020a), suggest that this link may be particularly strong among black business-owning households.

The COVID-19 pandemic is laying bare many of the structural forces at play, threatening to exacerbate racial gaps in income and wealth, and small-business outcomes for these households is likely to be an important part of the story. Specifically, the COVID-19 pandemic is likely to impact the economic well-being of black business-owning households. This chapter provides preliminary evidence to suggest the ways in which this might happen.

Our analysis draws on a novel data set we constructed using administrative bank data on households and small businesses, combined with publicly available voter registration records from Florida, Georgia, and Louisiana that collect information on race.[1] This pairing allows us to construct highly granular data on household and small business finances, cash flows, and liquidity, while also identifying family and business-owner race. We leverage these data, along with recent data about the impact of COVID-19 on household and small-business financial well-being, to outline the likely evolution of these phenomena during the current crisis.

We begin with an analysis of the relative financial health of black and white households. We highlight racial gaps in overall wealth and in liquid assets, in particular. We then summarize the differential sensitivity of consumption to income shocks for black households relative to their white counterparts. Using what we know about differential impacts on employment across racial groups during the COVID-19 pandemic, we speculate on the relative impact on households by race.

We then present analyses of racial disparities in scale, cash flow, and credit access for small-business owners. These differences feed directly into the likelihood of small-business survival during relatively stable economic times. Combined with the aforementioned discussion of more pronounced negative income shocks for black families during the COVID-19 crisis, we then delineate the expected effects on exits for black-owned businesses. These business outcomes will then feed back into household wealth and balance sheets, further leaving black households even more exposed to income shocks in general and positioned to fall even farther behind in wealth accumulation relative to white households. We conclude with potential policy interventions that may be useful given these considerations.

Data and Methodology

The analyses in this chapter are based on two data sets leveraging de-identified data from a sample of JPMorgan Chase (JPMC) customers who are registered to vote in and live in Florida, Georgia, and Louisiana. The first of these captures financial outcomes for 1.8 million families associated with personal deposit accounts whose primary account holders meet these criteria, and the second captures financial outcomes for 150,000 small businesses associated with business deposit accounts with owners who meet these criteria. In both cases, we determine self-identified race by matching account data with voter registration files from Florida, Georgia, and Louisiana. Both data assets cover account activity from 2012 through 2021.

Our family sample differs from the nation in a few noteworthy respects, but it gives us a reliable window into racial gaps in financial outcomes compared to benchmarks. More specifically, our sample is not fully representative of the general population in that it excludes the unbanked and anyone who is ineligible or not registered to vote. It overrepresents black and Latino households, families in urban areas, and younger primary account holders. That said, our sample frame offers an income distribution that is broadly representative of the respective income distributions of black, Latino, and white families. In addition, we find that racial gaps in median checking account balances and take-home income as observed in JPMC accounts are of the same order of magnitude as benchmarks from the nation and among banked, registered voters.

We use this sample to measure racial gaps in family take-home income and liquid assets and to study the consumption response to fluctuations in income. Take-home income reflects a family's purchasing power on a cash-flow basis and includes income deposited into one's checking account such as labor income after taxes and other payroll deductions, unemployment insurance (UI) and other government benefits, tax refunds, capital and retirement income, ATM deposits, check deposits, and other electronic deposits. We define liquid assets as the sum of balances in one's checking, prepaid debit, savings, money market, and certificates of deposit accounts.

The small-business sample has a higher share of black- and Latino-owned businesses as compared to the overall US population of small businesses, but a broadly comparable share of black- and Latino-owned businesses as compared to the population of small businesses in Florida, Georgia, and Louisiana. Notably, the sample is larger and covers a much more recent time period than the 2003 Survey of Small Business Finances—the most recent publicly available source of data on small-business cash flows and balances by race. Accordingly, the sample provides a unique lens into differences in small-business outcomes by owner race in recent years.

We use this sample to study differences in small-business financial and survival outcomes, and in particular how financial circumstances shape survival outcomes. Specifically, we identify revenues and expenses as inflows and outflows out of business deposit accounts less identified financial cash flows; we identify cash balances as the sum of cash across all accounts associated with a firm at a given point in time; and we identify firm exit as indicated by the closure of all business deposit accounts.[2]

Pandemic Effects on Black Household Finances

When assessing racial disparities in financial outcomes, it is important to distinguish between income and wealth. Income is earned from year to year, while wealth is accumulated over time and often passed down to the next generation. Liquid assets, a small piece of the wealth picture, play a central role as a first line of defense in a crisis; they serve as a form of private insurance in helping families and businesses weather volatility. Our data show that for every dollar of income earned by white families, black families earn roughly 72 cents. These gaps actually widen for the highest earning families—for every dollar earned by the ninetieth percentile white family, the ninetieth percentile black family earns just 60 cents, raising the question as to whether black and Latino families face the greatest barriers in accessing the highest income-generating opportunities.

The wealth gap between black and white households is much larger than the gap in income. Figure 7.1 shows liquid assets for black, Latino, and white households at the median as well as the tenth and ninetieth percentiles. In 2018, the typical white family had $3,247 in liquid assets, while the typical black family had just $1,029. Put differently, for every dollar the typical white family held in liquid assets, the typical black family held only 32 cents. These differences did not shrink meaningfully among families with relatively more wealth—at the ninetieth percentile, for every dollar in liquid assets held by the typical white family, the typical black family held 34 cents and the typical Latino family held 52 cents. Moreover, these differences do not go away when we account for racial gaps in income. Take two families with the same levels of income, and the black families will have roughly half the liquid assets of the white family (Farrell, Greig, Wheat et al. 2020).

When we consider net worth, reflecting the full balance sheet of a household in terms of the excess of a family's assets over its debts, the racial gaps are even larger. According to the 2019 Survey of Consumer Finances, the median black family has just $0.13 of net worth for every dollar of net wealth of the median white family.

The black-white gap in wealth has important consequences for families when they experience income volatility. For example, we show that under normal circumstances prior to the COVID-19 pandemic, among families who receive unemployment insurance, a $1.00 decline in income due to involuntary job loss (after accounting for unemployment insurance benefits received) is associated with a fall in nondurable spending of $0.46 among black families, $0.43 among Latino families, and $0.28 among white families (figure 7.2). Thus, while all families tend to reduce spending on necessary goods upon job loss, black and Latino families do so to a larger extent. These numbers imply

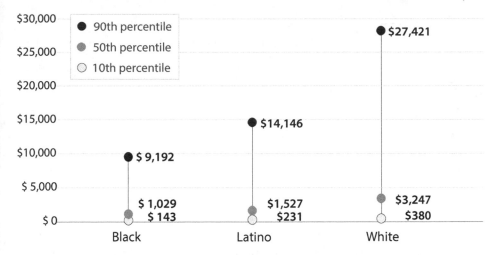

FIGURE 7.1. Distribution of liquid assets (2018) by race. Sourced from the JPMorgan Chase Institute (Farrell, Greig, Wheat, et al. 2020). We define liquid assets as the sum of balances in one's checking, prepaid debt, savings, money market, and certificates of deposit accounts.

that when families experience a $500 decline in monthly income as a result of job loss, black families reduce their monthly spending by $90 more than white families, resulting in perhaps one less trip to the grocery store per month.

We see a similar disparity in consumption changes among individuals who face moderate income losses—for instance, among workers who are not laid off but whose hours are cut. We examine the path of families' spending when their employer raises or lowers pay for all employees (Ganong et al. 2020). Even in the face of these smaller employer-driven income changes, black families alter consumption by 50 percent more than white families, and Latino families by 20 percent more than white families. For example, a one-month decline in labor income of $500 leads to a one-month decline in consumption of $146 for black families compared to $100 for white families.

Importantly, we find that, in a statistical sense, racial differences in liquid assets almost entirely account for differences in consumption sensitivity. When we control for racial disparities in liquid assets (specifically measured as liquid asset buffer, or how many months' worth of spending one has in liquid assets), racial gaps in the spending response to income fluctuations largely disappear. Thus, among black, Latino, and white families with similar levels of liquid assets, we might expect to see almost no racial differences in their spending response to involuntary job loss or payroll fluctuations.

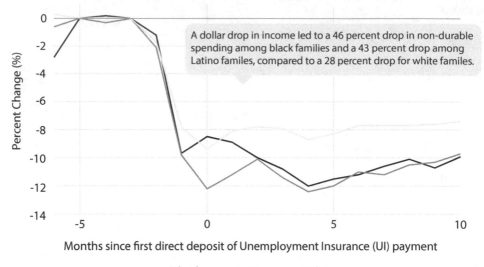

FIGURE 7.2. Change in nondurable spending from five months prior to first unemployment insurance (UI) receipt between 2013 and 2018. Sourced from the JPMorgan Chase Institute (Farrell, Greig, Wheat, et al. 2020). Unemployment Insurance refers to UI payments direct deposited in the checking account; labor income only includes inflows to the checking account identifiable as labor income; and nondurable spending refers to expenditures on nondurable goods from the checking account and using Chase credit cards. The ratio is relative to month −5 (five months before first UI payment).

How did household income, spending, and liquid asset patterns evolve during the COVID-19 pandemic? First, financial need was not evenly distributed by race. Public survey and administrative data sources show that job losses were concentrated among black workers. The unemployment rate soared in April 2020 to 16.7 percent for black workers compared to 14.2 for white workers and has since then fallen more slowly to 9.1 percent as of May 2021 for black workers compared to 4.8 percent for white workers (US Bureau of Labor Statistics 2020, 2021). Even as small businesses start to open back up, they have been slower to recall their black employees compared to white employees (Bartik et al. 2020).

We would expect these more pervasive and sustained employment shocks for black households to exact a disproportionately larger toll on the welfare of black families given their thinner cash reserves and greater sensitivity of consumption to income shocks (Farrell, Greig, Wheat, et al. 2020; Ganong et al. 2020). Importantly, the CARES Act expanded unemployment insurance (UI) eligibility and provided a $600 federal supplement to the level of UI benefit payments through July 2020. Subsequent rounds of legislation delivered $300 weekly UI supplements and two more rounds of stimulus in January and March of 2021.

As a result, checking-account inflows, inclusive of both labor income and generous government income supports, actually increased during the COVID-19 pandemic, especially for black families (figure 7.3). Checking-account outflows, which include everyday spending, debt payments, and transfers, mirrored this pattern, recovering more quickly for black families after the initial drop in March 2020 and spiking concurrently with the second and third rounds of stimulus (figure 7.4). These results remain when we focus on more narrow measures of income and spending and when we look exclusively at low-income families (Greig and Deadman 2021).

Similarly, we find that families who received UI also increased their spending relative to baseline, a phenomenon that was particularly true among lower-income workers for whom the $600 supplement represented a larger (percentage) benefit increase. The fact that jobless workers receiving UI increased their consumption is surprising given the fact that under normal times, jobless workers decrease their spending (figure 7.2), and during the pandemic, spending had initially declined in general (figure 7.4).

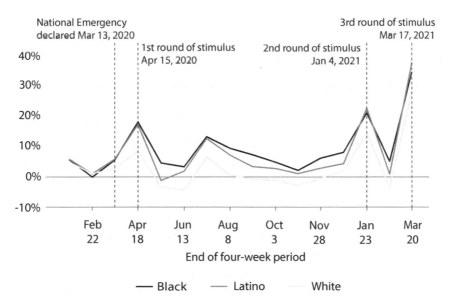

FIGURE 7.3. Year-over-year percent change in median account inflows (four-week periods). Sourced from the JPMorgan Chase Institute (Greig and Deadman 2021).

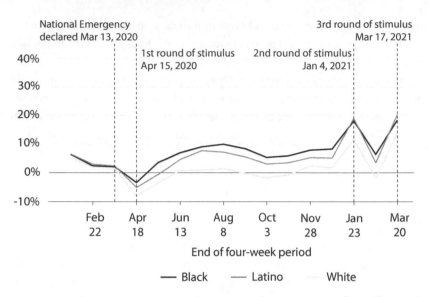

FIGURE 7.4. Year-over-year percent change in median account outflows (four-week periods). Sourced from the JPMorgan Chase Institute (Greig and Deadman 2021).

Turning to checking-account balances, we observe large increases in cash balances following the arrival of each round of stimulus (figures 7.5 and 7.6). On a percentage basis, these increases were greater for black families because of their lower baseline levels prior to the pandemic. In other words, pandemic-related government supports were progressive in that they delivered cash to low-liquidity families, disproportionately boosting the cash balances of black families.

Also evident in figures 7.5 and 7.6, however, is that black and Latino families' balances were depleted faster than white families' after the arrival of stimulus payments, signaling the criticality, but also temporality, of those supports. While median cash balances were still elevated at the end of 2020, black and Latino families maintained a smaller proportion of their initial balance boost than white families. The fact that black and Latino families depleted their cash balances faster than white families after each round of stimulus may indicate that these families faced circumstances that made it more difficult to maintain a cash buffer. It underscores the relative precarity of their financial position should they experience more prolonged unemployment.

In short, government income support played a critical role in boosting the spending and saving of black and Latino workers. These programs both insured households against the hardships of job loss, allowing them to maintain their everyday spending, and stimulated aggregate demand in the overall economy.

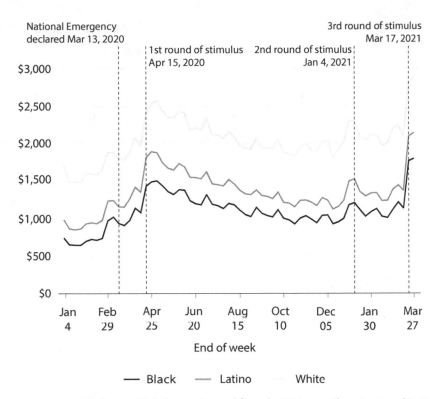

FIGURE 7.5. Median weekly balances. Sourced from the JPMorgan Chase Institute (Greig and Deadman 2021).

In fact, we know that families cut their spending by an additional 2 percent for each additional week of delay they face in receiving UI benefits (Farrell, Ganong, Greig, et al. 2020) and by an additional 12 percent at the expiration of UI benefits (Ganong and Noel 2019). As workers lose their UI benefits, we might expect consumption drops, particularly among households who face slower re-employment or who have lower cash reserves, of whom black households constitute a disproportionate share.

What do these household dynamics mean for black business-owning families? First, under normal circumstances to the extent that black business owners generally have more wealth than black families who do not own businesses, they still are likely to have substantially less liquidity than white business owners. Thus, without the extraordinary stimulus efforts, we might worry that, in the face of an economic disruption, black business-owning families would be less likely to be able to support their businesses. Recognizing that the economic impacts of the COVID-19 pandemic are likely to outlast the existing

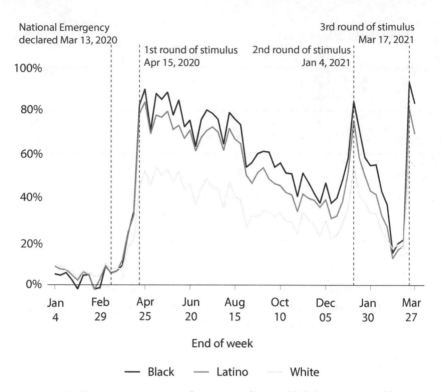

FIGURE 7.6. Year-over-year percent change in median weekly balances. Sourced from the JPMorgan Chase Institute (Greig and Deadman 2021).

stimulus efforts, without renewal, black families are at risk of more dramatic welfare losses in the form of larger spending cuts. Black families who own small businesses—which tend to be disproportionately located in majority-black neighborhoods—may see meaningful declines in cash inflows over time.

Pandemic Effects on Black-Owned Businesses

The effect of a pandemic on black families who own small businesses may be especially severe, even as compared to the effect of an economic disruption on black families overall. Business ownership is often cited as an important mechanism in generating wealth and closing the black-white wealth gap. While business owners stand to create wealth through starting and growing successful businesses, such gains are modest over the first few years of operations of those businesses that survive and show little evidence of closing liquid wealth gaps (Wheat, Mac, and Tremper 2021). Moreover, small businesses may face substantial losses in household wealth upon firm exit.[3] Notably, exit rates were higher among black-owned businesses in the early months of the pandemic (Fairlie 2020a, 2020b) suggesting that black families with a substantial share of assets in a business may be particularly exposed to wealth losses. As key drivers of the sustainability of businesses with owners of any race, cash liquidity and revenue levels are both likely to fall through the course of the pandemic, with downstream impacts on the financial well-being of black families who own them.

As a first observation, even in a growing economy, black-owned businesses have substantially lower revenues than white-owned businesses and have meaningfully less cash liquidity (Farrell, Wheat, and Mac 2020a). Figures 7.7 and 7.8 illustrate these gaps among a cohort of young black-, Latino-, and white-owned businesses founded in 2012 and 2013. Figure 7.7 shows median revenue for surviving firms aged one to five with black, Latino, and white owners. At less than $39,000, the median revenue of a black-owned business in its first year is less than 42 percent of the median revenue of a first-year white-owned

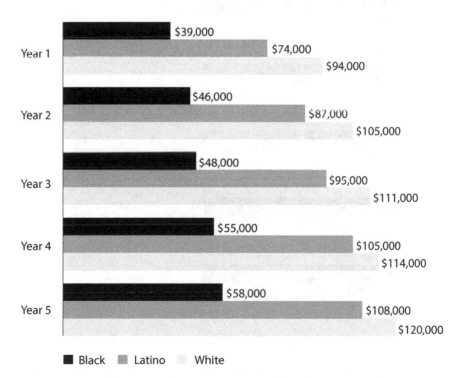

FIGURE 7.7. Median revenue by owner race. Sourced from the JPMorgan Chase Institute (Farrell, Wheat, and Mac 2020a). Sample includes firms founded in 2013 and 2014.

business. While median annual revenues are higher for firms that survive until their fifth year among all businesses, the revenue gap stays large, with black-owned firms generating only $0.48 of revenue for every dollar generated by white-owned firms. Notably, these gaps in revenue are substantially larger than black-white household income gaps among non-business-owning families.

Figure 7.8 shows a measure of the cash liquidity of the typical black-, Latino-, and white-owned firm from its first year through its fifth. Specifically, the chart shows the median number of cash buffer days in each group, computed as the number of days a firm could continue to support its typical level of cash outflows given its typical cash balance. Cash buffers are small for most small businesses, with the typical white-owned business only carrying eighteen or nineteen cash buffer days over its first five years. However, cash buffers for black-owned businesses are especially small, with the typical business carrying twelve cash buffer days in its first year and only eleven in its second through fifth year.

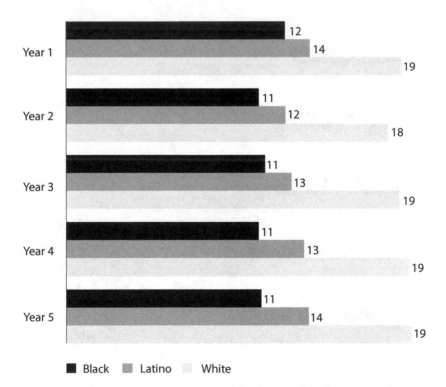

FIGURE 7.8. Median cash buffer days by owner race. Sourced from the JPMorgan Chase Institute (Farrell, Wheat, and Mac 2020a). Sample includes firms founded in 2013 and 2014. Estimated values control for industry, metro area, owner age, and gender.

Lower revenues among black-owned businesses suggest that these businesses are likely generating lower levels of income for the families who own them. Lower levels of cash liquidity suggest that these businesses are using less capital, consistent with other research that has shown the difficulties black business owners have attaining credit (Bates and Robb 2015a, 2015b; Fairlie, Robb, and Robinson 2016; Robb, de Zeeuw, and Barkley 2018; Lederer et al. 2020). While these differences are critically important during times of economic growth for the ability of a small business to survive, revenue gaps and differential access to cash liquidity are likely even more so during a pandemic in which revenues have declined and long-term access to cash has not been guaranteed.

Figures 7.9 and 7.10 illustrate the relationship between cash liquidity, revenue levels, and survival by showing observed exit rates among three-year-old businesses by the race of their owners and contrasting that to predicted exit rates from a counterfactual model in which businesses have the same revenue and cash liquidity levels. Figure 7.9 shows that 11.2 percent of three-year-old black-owned businesses exit before reaching their fourth year, as compared to only 9.1 percent of three-year-old white-owned businesses.

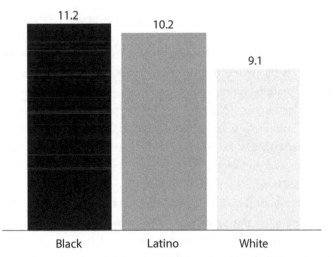

FIGURE 7.9. Observed share of firms that exit in year 3. Sourced from the JPMorgan Chase Institute (Farrell, Wheat, and Mac 2020a). Sample includes firms founded in 2013 and 2014. Estimated exit rates control for industry, metro area, owner age, and gender. Counterfactual exit rates assumed that all firms have the median revenues and cash buffer days.

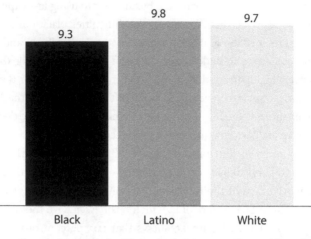

Counterfactual (%)

9.8

9.3

9.7

Black   Latino   White

FIGURE 7.10. Counterfactual share of firms that exit in year 3. Sourced from the JPMorgan Chase Institute (Farrell, Wheat, and Mac 2020a). Sample includes firms founded in 2013 and 2014. Estimated exit rates control for industry, metro area, owner age, and gender. Counterfactual exit rates assumed that all firms have the median revenues and cash buffer days.

Given the strong relationship between small-business survival, revenue, and cash liquidity, policymakers might be especially concerned about the impact of a pandemic on families that own small businesses—and black small-business owning families in particular. In fact, most small businesses saw large revenue and cash liquidity declines at the onset of the COVID-19 pandemic (Farrell, Wheat, and Mac 2020b). Moreover, the cash liquidity declines experienced by black-owned businesses were especially sharp. Figure 7.11 shows annualized declines in cash balances for white-, Asian-, Latino-, and black-owned firms in March and April 2020. Notably, cash balances were already down substantially for black-owned businesses in early March 2020 and were down 26 percent by the end of that month. This fall suggests that the already thin cash buffers black-owned businesses had during recent years of economic growth were especially strained during the beginning of the pandemic.

The recovery in balances toward the end of April 2020 depicted in figure 7.11 may well have been a response to programs and policies rather than the ability of business owners to cut revenues in excess of expenses. Overall, typical small-business revenues fell faster than expenses through the end of March, and expenses fell somewhat slower than revenues throughout April 2020 (Farrell,

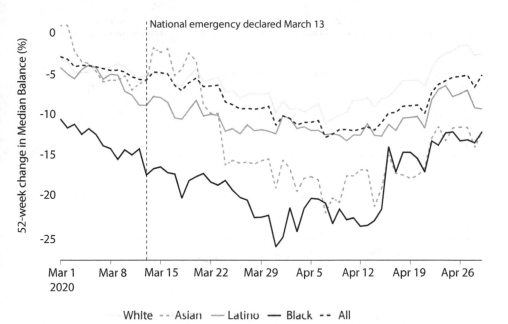

FIGURE 7.11. Change in median cash balance by owner race. Sourced from the JPMorgan Chase Institute (Farrell, Wheat, and Mac 2020b). Sample includes firms operated in the period shown as well as the same period fifty-two weeks earlier.

Wheat, and Mac 2020b). However, the differences may not have been large enough to drive the uptick in balances observed in figure 7.11.

In particular, there were some segments in which the typical small business saw material balance increases that aligned with the timing of CARES Act programs. As shown in figure 7.12, cash balances of white-owned restaurants doubled in early May 2020, while cash balances of black-owned restaurants increased, but only by 38 percent (Farrell, Wheat, and Mac 2020c). This timing is at least consistent with the resumption of Paycheck Protection Program applications on April 27, 2020. Figure 7.13 shows that black-owned personal service firms also saw large increases in cash balances starting in mid-April 2020, experiencing as high as a 62 percent increase in early May (Farrell, Wheat, and Mac 2020c). These cash balance increases began around the time that CARES Act stimulus payments began to arrive. While these payments were targeted at households rather than small businesses, they potentially provide an additional illustration of the close relationship between household and small-business finance, particularly among more minute small businesses, many of which are black owned.

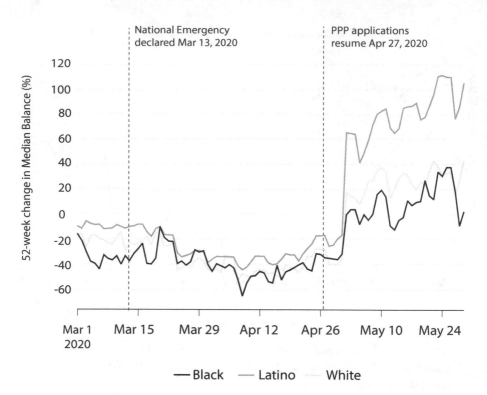

FIGURE 7.12. Changes in cash balances of small restaurants by owner race. Sourced from the JPMorgan Chase Institute (Farrell, Wheat, and Mac 2020c). Sample includes firms in Florida, Georgia, and Louisiana that were operating in the period shown as well as the same period fifty-two weeks earlier.

Overall, these results complement the view of the financial lives of black business-owning families presented in the earlier section by drawing attention to the importance of both household and business cash liquidity.

Conclusions and Implications

In summary, preexisting differences in financial well-being between white and black business-owning households suggest that black business-owning households will face substantial challenges during the COVID-19 pandemic and any subsequent recovery. Our results show the multiple channels through which such an event can affect the financial well-being of black business-owning families. These families are disproportionately subject to both labor-market income losses and business revenue losses. Moreover, to the extent that the businesses they own are located in majority-black neighborhoods, they may

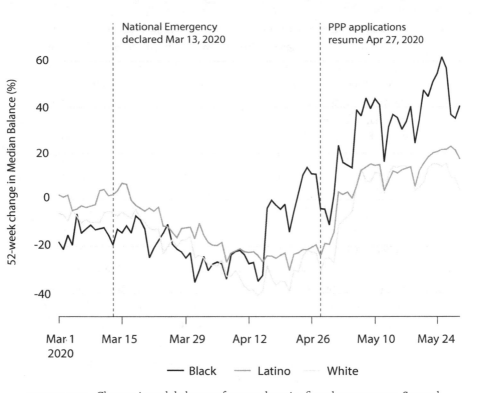

FIGURE 7.13. Changes in cash balances of personal service firms by owner race. Sourced from the JPMorgan Chase Institute (Farrell, Wheat, and Mac 2020c). Sample includes firms in Florida, Georgia, and Louisiana that were operating in the period shown as well as the same period fifty-two weeks earlier.

be subject to even sharper revenue losses. They may have neither the household nor the business liquidity to buffer either loss, potentially leading to family hardship and business exit. Indeed, empirical results during the COVID-19 pandemic illustrate the continued sensitivity of households in general to economic shocks—and specifically sharply decreased cash liquidity among black-owned businesses. These results suggest the following implications for policymakers interested in supporting these households, the businesses they own, and the communities in which they are located:

1. Limited cash liquidity among black business-owning families will continue to pose challenges for the survival of their businesses during an ongoing pandemic. Both black families and black-owned businesses have substantially less cash liquidity than white families and white-owned businesses. These differences in cash liquidity limit the ability

of black families to withstand economic shocks, and the ability of any businesses that they own to survive. Early data from the pandemic suggest that cash liquidity has dropped among these families and may have dropped even more so were it not for large-scale intervention from the public sector. Without continued intervention, liquidity is likely to materially fall among these families and the businesses they own.

2. Stimulus efforts and income supports targeted progressively at low-income families generate a larger spending response. Karger and Rajan (2020) estimate that had the CARES Act been delivered to families with the highest marginal propensity to consume, the aggregate effect on consumption could have been 45 percent higher. Notably, income levels are not the only way to target relief. Arguably, unemployment insurance is effective at targeting relief to families in the most need—*those who lost a job*—and we have documented a large increase in spending among UI recipients during the pandemic (Farrell, Ganong, Greig, et al. 2020). In addition, families with the *lowest liquid assets* exhibit the highest marginal propensity to consume out of tax refunds and UI, and, given large racial wealth gaps, black and Latino families disproportionately benefit from income supports (Farrell, Greig, and Hamoudi 2019; Ganong and Noel 2019; Farrell, Greig, Wheat, et al. 2020).

3. Programs and policies targeted at stimulating spending among black families may also increase survival rates among black-owned busi-nesses. Programs and policies that stimulate overall spending will likely be critical to supporting the small business sector as a whole, especially to the extent that many firms cease to have enough liquid-ity to absorb longer-term revenue losses. However, targeted pro-grams that focus on black families or places where black families live could support black-owned businesses in two ways. First, programs that seek to stimulate demand through cash transfers to families may transfer cash to families who own businesses, who in turn may invest some or all of the proceeds into the businesses they own. This would increase the ability of these businesses to withstand longer short-falls in revenue. Second, increased spending among black families may indirectly support black-owned businesses if these families, through preference or through local market structures, are differentially likely to spend at black-owned businesses. This additional spending could offset revenue declines and similarly extend the otherwise limited cash liquidity held by these businesses, substantially enhancing their survival prospects.

4. Policies that facilitate overall asset building among black families might improve the financial stability of black-owned businesses for a future pandemic or other large-scale economic shock. Notably, our results are consistent with empirical results from many other studies in showing black-white gaps across several asset classes, including but not limited to household liquid assets, housing wealth, business ownership assets, and liquid assets within the businesses they own. While identifying mechanisms that might cause these asset levels to move together was beyond the scope of the current study, our results suggest that unpacking these mechanisms might be a fruitful area for future research. To the extent that, for example, overall wealth drives both household consumption smoothing and survival rates for any owned businesses, policies that support housing wealth accumulation among black families might also increase survivorship rates among black-owned businesses. Accordingly, both researchers and policymakers might benefit from increased investigation into these linkages and the programs and policies that might leverage their potential.

NOTES

1. See Farrell, Greig, Wheat, et al. (2020) for a detailed description of the data asset.

2. Further details about the construction of the household data asset, its representativeness, and the construction of household financial outcome measures are reported by Farrell, Grieg, Cox, et al. (2020) and Farrell, Greig, Wheat, et al. (2020). Further details about the construction of the small business asset, its representativeness, and the construction small business financial outcome measures are reported by Farrell, Wheat, and Mac (2020a).

3. Data from the Panel Survey of Income Dynamics at least preliminarily shows that, among owners with businesses founded in 2005, those that exited by 2009 saw a median $65,826 decline in owner wealth (Shapiro 2019).

REFERENCES

Addo, Fenaba R., Jason N. Houle, and Daniel Simon. 2016. "Young, Black, and (Still) in the Red: Parental Wealth, Race, and Student Loan Debt." *Race and Social Problems* 8, no. 1: 64–76. https://doi.org/10.1007/s12552-016-9162-0.

Asante-Muhammad, Dedrick, Chuck Collins, Josh Hoxie, and Emanuel Nieves. 2017. *The Road to Zero Wealth: How the Racial Wealth Divide Is Hollowing Out America's Middle Class.* Washington, DC: Prosperity Now, Institute for Policy Studies.

Aspen Institute Roundtable on Community Change. 2004. *Structural Racism and Community Building.* Washington, DC: Aspen Institute. https://www.aspeninstitute.org/wp-content/uploads/files/content/docs/rcc/aspen_structural_racism2.pdf.

Bartik, Alexander, Marianne Bertrand, Zoe Cullen, Edward L. Glaeser, Michael Luca, and Christopher Stanton. 2020. "How Are Small Businesses Adjusting to COVID-19? Early Evidence from a Survey." Working Paper w26989, National Bureau of Economic Research, Cambridge, MA. https://doi.org/10.3386/w26989.

Bartlett, Robert P., Adair Morse, Richard H. Stanton, and Nancy E. Wallace. 2019. "Consumer Lending Discrimination in the FinTech Era." Public Law Research Paper, University of California, Berkeley. http://dx.doi.org/10.2139/ssrn.3063448.

Bates, Timothy, and Alicia Robb. 2015a. "Has the Community Reinvestment Act Increased Loan Availability among Small Businesses Operating in Minority Neighborhoods?" *Urban Studies* 52, no. 9: 1702–21.

Bates, Timothy, and Alicia Robb. 2015b. "Impacts of Owner Race and Geographic Context on Access to Small Business Financing." *Economic Development Quarterly* 30, no. 2: 159–70.

Bayer, Patrick, and Kerwin Kofi Charles. 2018. "Divergent Paths: A New Perspective on Earnings Differences between Black and White Men since 1940." *Quarterly Journal of Economics* 133, no. 3 (August): 1459–5101.

Bayer, Patrick, Fernando Ferreira, and Stephen L. Ross. 2014. "What Drives Racial and Ethnic Differences in High-Cost Mortgages? The Role of High-Risk Lenders." *Review of Financial Studies* 31, no. 1 (January): 175–205.

Bertrand, Marianne, and Sendhil Mullainathan. 2004. "Are Emily and Greg More Employable Than Lakisha and Jamal? A Field Experiment on Labor Market Discrimination." *American Economic Review* 94, no. 4 (September): 991–1013.

Bradford, William. 2014. "The 'Myth' That Black Entrepreneurship Can Reduce the Gap in Wealth between Black and White Families." *Economic Development Quarterly* 28, no. 3: 254–69. https://doi.org/10.1177/0891242414535468.

Chetty, Raj, Nathaniel Hendren, Maggie R. Jones, and Sonya R. Porter. 2019. "Race and Economic Opportunity in the United States: An Intergenerational Perspective." Working Paper w24441, National Bureau of Economic Research, Cambridge, MA. https://doi.org/10.3386/w24441.

Chiteji, N. S., and Darrick Hamilton. 2002. "Family Connections and the Black-White Wealth Gap among Middle-Class Families." *Review of Black Political Economy* 30, no. 1 (Summer): 9–28.

Darity, William, Jr., Darrick Hamilton, Mark Paul, Alan Aja, Anne Price, Antonio Moore, and Caterina Chiopris. 2018. "What We Get Wrong about Closing the Racial Wealth Gap." Durham, NC: Samuel DuBois Cook Center on Social Equity and Insight Center for Community Economic Development. https://socialequity.duke.edu/wp-content/uploads/2020/01/what-we-get-wrong.pdf.

Dobbie, Will, and Roland G. Fryer Jr. 2011. "Are High-Quality Schools Enough to Increase Achievement among the Poor? Evidence from the Harlem Children's Zone." *American Economic Journal: Applied Economics* 3, no. 3 (July): 158–87.

Emmons, William R., and Lowell Ricketts. 2017. "College is Not Enough: Higher Education Does not Eliminate Racial and Ethnic Wealth Gaps." *Review* (Federal Reserve Bank of St. Louis) 99, no. 1: 7–39.

Fairlie, Robert. 2020a. "The Impact of COVID-19 on Small Business Owners: Evidence of Early-Stage Losses from the April 2020 Current Population Survey." Working Paper

w27309, National Bureau of Economic Research, Cambridge, MA. https://doi.org/10
.3386/w27309.

Fairlie, Robert. 2020b. "The Impact of COVID-19 on Small Business Owners: The First
Three Months after Social-Distancing Restrictions." Working Paper w27462, National
Bureau of Economic Research, Cambridge, MA. https://doi.org/10.3386/w27462.

Fairlie, Robert, and Harry Krashinsky. 2012. "Liquidity Constraints, Household Wealth,
and Entrepreneurship Revisited." *Review of Income and Wealth* 58, no. 2 (June):
279–306. https://doi.org/10.1111/j.1475-4991.2011.00491.x.

Fairlie, Robert, Alicia Robb, and David Robinson. 2016. "Black and White: Access to
Capital among Minority-Owned Startups." Working Paper w28154, National Bureau of
Economic Research, Cambridge, MA. https://doi.org/10.3386/w28154.

Farrell, Diana, Peter Ganong, Fiona Greig, Max Liebeskind, Pascal Noel, and Joe Vavra. 2020.
"Consumption Effects of Unemployment Insurance during the COVID-19 Pandemic."
Research paper, JPMorgan Chase Institute, New York. https://www.jpmorganchase.com
/institute/research/labor-markets/unemployment-insurance-covid19-pandemic.

Farrell, Diana, Fiona Greig, Natalie Cox, Peter Ganong, and Pascal Noel. 2020. "The
Initial Household Spending Response to COVID-19: Evidence from Credit Card
Transactions." Research paper, JPMorgan Chase Institute, New York. https://www
.jpmorganchase.com/institute/research/household-income-spending/initial-household
-spending-response-to-covid-19-evidence-from-credit-card-transactions.

Farrell, Diana, Fiona Greig, and Amar Hamoudi. 2019. *Tax Time: How Families Manage Tax Refunds and Payments.* New York: JPMorgan Chase Institute. https://www
.jpmorganchase.com/content/dam/jpmc/jpmorgan-chase-and-co/institute/pdf
/institute-tax-time-report-full.pdf.

Farrell, Diana, Fiona Greig, Chris Wheat, Max Liebeskind, Peter Ganong, Damon Jones,
and Pascal Noel. 2020. *Racial Gaps in Financial Outcomes: Big Data Evidence.* New
York: JPMorgan Chase Institute. https://www.jpmorganchase.com/content/dam/jpmc
/jpmorgan-chase-and-co/institute/pdf/institute-race-report.pdf.

Farrell, Diana, Chris Wheat, and Carlos Grandet. 2019. *Place Matters: Small Business
Financial Health Urban Communities.* New York: JPMorgan Chase Institute. https://
www.jpmorganchase.com/content/dam/jpmc/jpmorgan-chase-and-co/institute/pdf
/institute-place-matters.pdf.

Farrell, Diana, Chris Wheat, and Chi Mac. 2020a. *Small Business Owner Race, Liquidity,
and Survival.* New York: JPMorgan Chase Institute. https://www.jpmorganchase.com
/content/dam/jpmc/jpmorgan-chase-and-co/institute/pdf/institute-small-business
-owner-race-report.pdf.

Farrell, Diana, Chris Wheat, and Chi Mac. 2020b. "Small Business Financial Outcomes
during the Onset of COVID-19." Research paper, JPMorgan Chase Institute, New York.
https://www.jpmorganchase.com/institute/research/small-business/small-business
-financial-outcomes-during-the-onset-of-covid-19.

Farrell, Diana, Chris Wheat, and Chi Mac. 2020c. "Small Business Financial Outcomes
during the COVID-19 Pandemic." Research paper, JPMorgan Chase Institute, New
York. https://www.jpmorganchase.com/institute/research/small-business/report-small
-business-financial-outcomes-during-the-covid-19-pandemic.

Ganong, Peter, Damon Jones, Pascal Noel, Diana Farrell, Fiona Greig, and Chris Wheat. 2020. "Wealth, Race, and Consumption Smoothing of Typical Income Shocks." Working Paper, Becker Friedman Institute for Economics, University of Chicago. https://doi .org/10.3386/w27552.

Ganong, Peter, and Pascal Noel. 2019. "Consumer Spending during Unemployment: Positive and Normative Implications." *American Economic Review* 109, no. 7 (July): 2383–2424. https://www.aeaweb.org/articles?id=10.1257/aer.20170537.

Greig, Fiona, and Erica Deadman. 2021. "Financial Outcomes by Race during COVID-19." Research paper, JPMorgan Chase Institute, New York. https://www.jpmorganchase .com/institute/research/household-income-spending/financial-outcomes-by-race -during-COVID-19.

Grodsky, Eric, and Devah Pager. 2001. "The Structure of Disadvantage: Individual and Occupational Determinants of the Black-White Wage Gap." *American Sociological Review* 66, no. 4 (August): 542–67.

Herring, Cedric, and Loren Henderson. 2016. "Wealth Inequality in Black and White: Cultural and Structural Sources of the Racial Wealth Gap." *Race and Social Problems* 8, no. 1: 4–17.

Hurst, Erik, and Annamaria Lusardi. 2004. "Liquidity Constraints, Household Wealth, and Entrepreneurship." *Journal of Political Economy* 112, no. 2 (April): 319–47.

Jackson, B. A., and J. R. Reynolds. 2013. "The Price of Opportunity: Race, Student Loan Debt, and College Achievement." *Sociological Inquiry* 83, no. 3 (August): 335–68.

Karger, Ezra, and Aastha Rajan. 2020. "Heterogeneity in the Marginal Propensity to Consume: Evidence from COVID-19 Stimulus Payments." Working Paper 2020-15, Federal Reserve Bank of Chicago. http://doi.org/10.2139/ssrn.3612828.

Katznelson, Ira. 2005. *When Affirmative Action Was White: An Untold History of Racial Inequality in Twentieth-Century America.* New York: W. W. Norton and Company.

Kijakazi, Kilolo, Karen Smith, and Charmaine Runes. 2019. "African American Economic Security and the Role of Social Security." Brief, Center of Labor, Human Services, and Population, Urban Institute, Washington, DC.

Lederer, Anneliese, Sara Oros, Sterling Bone, Glenn Christensen, and Jerome Williams. 2020. "Lending Discrimination within the Paycheck Protection Program." National Community Reinvestment Coalition. https://ncrc.org/lending-discrimination-within -the-paycheck-protection-program/.

McKernan, Signe-Mary, Caroline Ratcliffe, Eugene Steuerle, and Sisi Zhang. 2014. "Disparities in Wealth Accumulation and Loss from the Great Recession and Beyond." *American Economic Review* 104, no. 5: 240–44.

McKernan, Signe-Mary, Caroline Ratcliffe, Margaret Simms, and Sisi Zhang. 2014. "Do Racial Disparities in Private Transfers Help Explain the Racial Wealth Gap? New Evidence from Longitudinal Data." *Demography* 51, no. 3 (April): 949–74.

Meschede, Tatjana, Joanna Taylor, Alexis Mann, and Thomas M. Shapiro. 2017. "Family Achievements? How a College Degree Accumulates Wealth for Whites and Not for Blacks." *Review* (Federal Reserve Bank of St. Louis) 99, no. 1: 121–37.

Oliver, Melvin L., and Thomas M. Shapiro. 2013. *Black Wealth/White Wealth: A New Perspective on Racial Inequality.* New York: Routledge.

Perry, Andre M., Jonathan Rothwell, and David Harshbarger. 2018. *The Devaluation of Assets in Black Neighborhoods: The Case of Residential Property.* Washington, DC: Metropolitan Policy Program, Brookings Institution. https://www.brookings.edu/wp-content/uploads/2018/11/2018.11_Brookings-Metro_Devaluation-Assets-Black-Neighborhoods_final.pdf.

Robb, Alicia, Mels de Zeeuw, and Brett Barkley. 2018. "Mind the Gap: How Do Credit Market Experienes and Borrowing Patterns Differ for Minority-Owned Firms?" Discussion Paper 03-18, Community and Economic Development, Atlanta. https://www.atlantafed.org/-/media/documents/community-development/publications/discussion-papers/%202018/03-mind-the-gap-how-do-credit-market-experiences-and-borrowing-patterns-differ-for-minority-owned-firms-2018-09-14.pdf.

Robles, Barbara, Betsy Leondar-Write, Rose Brewer, and Rebecca Adamson. 2006. *The Color of Wealth: The Story behind the U.S. Racial Wealth Divide.* New York: New Press.

Shapiro, Thomas. 2019. "Wealth Inequality: Challenges and Opportunities for Entrepreneurs of Color." Panel presentation at Capital Matters: Race, Gender and Entrepreneurship, Durham, NC, October 23–25, 2019.

Thompson, Jeffrey P., and Gustavo A. Suarez. 2019. "Accounting for Racial Wealth Disparities in the United States." Research Department Working Paper 19-13, Federal Reserve Bank of Boston. https://www.bostonfed.org/publications/research-department-working-paper/2019/accounting-for-racial-wealth-disparities-in-the-united-states.aspx.

US Bureau of Labor Statistics. 2021. "The Employment Situation—May 2021." June 4. https://www.bls.gov/news.release/archives/empsit_06042021.htm.

US Bureau of Labor Statistics. 2020. "Unemployment Rate Rises to Record High 14.7 Percent in April 2020." May 13. https://www.bls.gov/opub/ted/2020/unemployment-rate-rises-to-record-high-14-point-7-percent-in-april-2020.htm.

Wheat, Chris, Chi Mac, and Nich Tremper. 2021. "Small Business Ownership and Liquid Wealth." Research paper, JPMorgan Chase Institute, New York. https://www.jpmorganchase.com/institute/research/small-business/small-business-ownership-and-liquid-wealth-report.

8. Closing Racial Economic Gaps during and after COVID-19

JANE DOKKO AND JUNG SAKONG

The severe and prolonged economic consequences of the COVID-19 pandemic have stressed the earnings of tens of millions of households. The pandemic has also elevated concerns about further widening the racial disparities in economic outcomes for black and Latino families (for example, see figure 8.1). The unemployment rate surged at the start of the pandemic, with black and Latino workers experiencing higher rates of unemployment. And while the unprecedented fiscal support over the course of the pandemic helped stave off large increases in the poverty rate, the timing of this support still left uncertainty for households' economic resources. Indeed, as figure 8.2 shows, the estimated poverty rate among black and Latino households fluctuated more during the pandemic, thanks to the outsized role of the social safety net and fiscal support for the adequacy of their economic resources relative to their needs. And on top of the many challenges with reduced or uncertain incomes, the pandemic has featured large racial disparities in health outcomes and access to education. Taken together, these shortfalls are likely to affect not just black and Latino households' immediate needs but also, as research suggests, their long-term economic prospects (Hendren and Sprung-Keyser 2020).

Policymakers, philanthropists, nonprofits, and business leaders may wish to contemplate interventions that jointly address the immediate economic distress and lay the groundwork to help close economic gaps for black and Latino households. Given the persistence of earnings shocks and the challenges of re-employment after extended unemployment, black and Latino households may

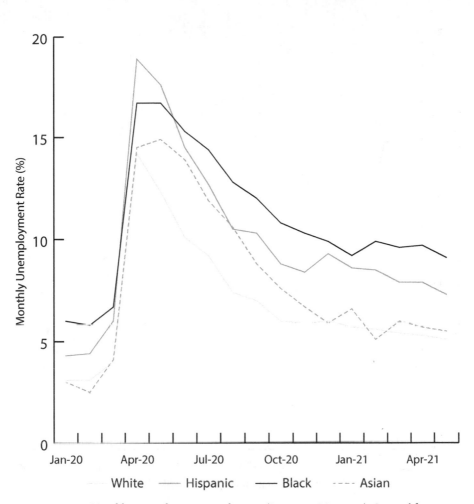

FIGURE 8.1. Monthly unemployment rate by race (Jan 2020–May 2021). Sourced from the US Bureau of Labor Statistics. Black and Hispanic workers experienced higher unemployment during the COVID-19 pandemic.

be at heightened risk of falling even farther behind white households as a result of this protracted public-health and economic crisis.

In this chapter, we highlight evidence-based approaches—approaches based on empirical research—to reducing racial disparities in economic opportunity, particularly in light of the COVID-19 pandemic and economic downturn. Focusing on interventions with high private and social net benefits (or returns) leads us to emphasize strategies in three areas: (1) those related to children's education and health; (2) those providing support for adults that typically have

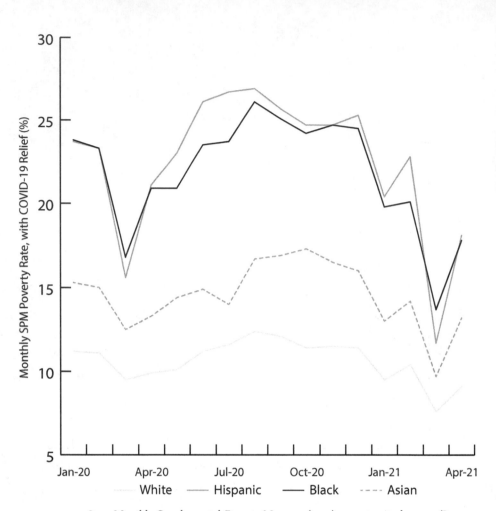

FIGURE 8.2. Monthly Supplemental Poverty Measure (SPM) poverty rate by race (Jan 2020–May 2021). See Parolin et al. 2020. Racial gaps in estimated poverty increased during the COVID-19 pandemic.

spillovers to children; and (3) those focused on juvenile and criminal justice. We also briefly discuss interventions that have been evaluated and demonstrate low returns and interventions that have yet to be evaluated, including those targeting gaps in homeownership and wealth accumulation.

There are many possible policy interventions, so we limit our discussion in three ways. First, we focus on interventions that have been sufficiently evaluated, but there may be some that have not been evaluated and are still high-return. There may also be new interventions in development. In both cases, greater scrutiny would help broaden our understanding of the high-return interventions that are available. Second, low-return interventions may be worth considering if they help achieve desirable noneconomic objectives, but this discussion is outside our scope. Third, often the purpose of interventions is to help people with immediate needs, and such strategies are worth pursuing without regard as to whether they lead to a large or permanent narrowing of opportunity gaps.

Even though the interventions we review are wide-ranging, those with high documented returns share some common characteristics. First, they tend to have benefits that extend over a number of years. Second, they tend to have benefits that spill over, such as to children or to the surrounding communities. Third, they tend to provide direct material benefit or reinforce noncognitive capabilities (soft skills) rather than giving beneficiaries complex information or incentives. Finally, they have been evaluated empirically for both immediate and long-term impacts.

High-Return Interventions

CHILDREN'S EDUCATION AND HEALTH

Absent intervention, economic disadvantage begins in utero and may compound over time. Extensive research in economics, neuroscience, and psychology points to large and durable economic impacts of early childhood programs that narrow achievement gaps in older grades, boost earnings and strengthen labor force attachment later in life, and reduce kids' exposure to the criminal justice system (Bartik, Gormley, and Adelstein 2012; Cascio and Schanzenbach 2013). The specific features of these programs can vary but they often involve addressing the following: in utero nutrition and environmental exposure to stress (Almond 2006; Royer 2009); work/life balance issues of parents/caregivers, as well as their education and training; availability of educational materials; parental habits and behaviors; lead abatement; and access to healthcare (Chay, Guryan, and Mazumder 2009). Still, public investments in young children tend to be lower than for older children, and parents of young kids tend to be at a stage in their careers when they are least able to invest in their children using their own income or savings.

The COVID-19 pandemic has disrupted investments in minority children in at least two ways. First, day-care and school closures have limited educational opportunities, and early evidence points to widening achievement gaps (Bacher-Hicks, Goodman, and Mulhern 2021; Dorn et al. 2020). Second, black and Latino parents have lost earnings and are experiencing additional stress and hardships, making the funding misalignment discussed in the previous paragraph more serious. Both of these factors generate a critical need for more support to black and Latino families with young children. Indeed, Ryan et al. (2020) document disruptions in parents' income stability, mental health, and support for children's learning, particularly among low-income families. Moreover, the risks of being unable to reenter the workforce loom larger for black and Latino workers and working minority mothers in particular (Alon et al. 2020; Couch, Fairlie, and Xu 2020).

Many studies also underscore the high returns from increasing high school graduation rates, improving college readiness, and boosting college completion rates. Greater per-pupil spending in K-12 education not only increases low-income students' educational attainment but also leads to higher wages and lower poverty for them when they grow up (Jackson, Johnson, and Persico 2016). High-performance charter schools also may have large effects on narrowing achievement gaps for low-income and minority students (Dobbie and Fryer 2011).[1]

At the college level, high-return interventions include steering low-income students to selective institutions; providing "last dollar" scholarships to bridge the gap between financial aid and the all-in costs of college; high-touch support services, like comprehensive advising, career services, and tutoring; and even low-touch programs, like personalized text messages reminding students to renew financial aid applications. Today's strained finances and uncertain job markets make student loans more burdensome, and college enrollment may even rise if high unemployment rates persist and typical recessionary patterns take hold. In the absence of job opportunities, more students may choose to continue their education until labor markets improve, often by financing college with student loan borrowing. Interventions to increase students' odds of college completion and to lower their risk of being financially burdened by student loan debt are particularly important for first-generation students, older students living independently from their parents, part-time students, and those attending nonselective institutions.[2]

SUPPORT FOR ADULTS

The private and social returns on interventions targeting adults tend to be substantially smaller than for children, on balance. Among other reasons, the benefits from investing in adults accrue over a shorter horizon. However, there are some notable exceptions: select job training programs; work subsidies to encourage work among low-skilled workers (including add-ons to the earned-income tax credit like Paycheck Plus) (Miller et al. 2018); and interventions with large spillovers to children, such as subsidized moves to low-poverty neighborhoods and health insurance for pregnant women (Miller and Wherry 2019). In these last two cases, the effects on children include higher educational attainment and earnings long after the interventions have taken place. The pandemic's sharp employment losses among black and Latino workers, especially among black women and Latinas, mean that income support for adults is a critical component of economic recovery. Subsidies for affordable and high-quality childcare and eldercare may also be needed to allow workers to reenter the labor market.

In addition, job losses in the pandemic have not been even across geographies, as low-wage retail and service sector workers have lost their jobs at a higher rate. As such, the geographical concentration of workers without jobs will likely require new interventions to target the racially segregated and occupationally segregated neighborhoods that characterize many cities. This is especially the case because high-return neighborhood job creation strategies have been difficult to develop, as we discuss below.

JUVENILE AND CRIMINAL JUSTICE

Disadvantaged youths are at high risk of becoming victims or perpetrators of crime. When juvenile and criminal justice interventions have high returns, two mechanisms are usually present: teens build human capital and become less likely to be exposed to the criminal justice system, expanding their future job opportunities, and safety and quality of life improve in disadvantaged neighborhoods where violent crimes disproportionately occur. As one example of a high-return intervention, the Becoming a Man (BAM) program prevents automatic escalation into violent crimes through cognitive behavioral therapy (CBT) group sessions that help youths reevaluate their automatic responses (Heller et al. 2017). Another set of interventions creates summer jobs and transitional employment for teens, which in turn lowers their risk of arrest for violent crime (Heller 2014). These latest interventions have been evaluated through randomized controlled trials and distinguish themselves from older interventions in that they require lower costs to implement. While research is ongoing to determine the exact mechanism, both interventions point to the role of soft-skill development, either in CBT sessions or on the job. This theme is consistent with the large and growing evidence on the importance of soft skills—autonomy, self-control, etc.—on market and nonmarket outcomes. The effects also persist beyond the program duration, pointing to a durable impact on the youths' human capital. At a time when COVID-19 has disproportionately challenged low-income neighborhoods and our society is reexamining the appropriate role of police, interventions to reduce teens' and young adults' exposure to the juvenile and criminal justice system can have important long-run payoffs for black and Latino youth.

SUMMARY

To date, the strongest evidence for high-return interventions apply to human capital formation. We believe this occurs for at least two reasons. First, market incompleteness may apply more to human capital investments than other areas, leaving considerable scope for policies to make a difference. Second, using the methods of causal identification, microeconomists have looked the hardest at human capital interventions.

Interventions with Less Evidence of High Returns

We now turn to important areas where interventions are necessary but where there is less evidence of their efficacy. Across these areas, some interventions have been evaluated and demonstrate low returns, while other interventions have yet to be evaluated. Considering the former, low-return interventions targeting opportunity gaps typically have some or all of the following distinguishing features: (1) the evidence suggests the economic gains are small or not widespread enough; (2) the intervention is not well targeted; (3) the intervention is very costly or resource intensive; and (4) unintended consequences undermine the intent of the intervention and may even lead to harm.

Closing racial gaps in nonhuman capital aspects of wealth requires targeting tangible and intangible aspects of household balance sheets. At the risk of oversimplifying, many existing interventions related to gaps in homeownership, financial wealth accumulation (by way of financial literacy programs and savings policies), and place-based economic opportunities possess some or all of these distinguishing features.

These interventions are partly motivated by the strong correlations that wealth displays with each component: high-wealth households are more likely to own their homes as well as own investment real estate; they have disproportionately more financial assets and invest them more in risky assets that earn premiums; they are more likely to be self-employed and own disproportionate shares of private business; and they live in neighborhoods that are characterized by better amenities, other high-wealth peers, and higher house prices.

However, the evidence we have on various interventions is not as robust and often shows mixed results. While it is difficult to generalize over such heterogeneous policies and aspects of household finance, it is possible to point out two likely causes. First, unlike in human capital, where market incompleteness is more likely to be a feature, there is greater scope for private-sector intermediaries to respond to market incompleteness. The ability to make and capture profit is higher when the assets are more tangible or if they can be traded or collateralized, neither of which applies to human capital. Second, while interventions targeting the household balance sheet have been researched considerably, less research employs the causal identification methods typically used by applied microeconomists, whose topics of study overlap the most with human capital.

To narrow racial disparities in areas beyond human capital, new interventions may be needed to achieve high returns. For each of these areas, we provide our interpretation of why the evidence may be more limited and point to new possibilities where there may be more scope to close racial opportunity and wealth gaps. We caution that such new interventions would need to be rigorously evaluated and compared against those that offer more certainty of high returns.

HOMEOWNERSHIP

Homeownership is often considered a pathway to wealth accumulation, possibly because of the robust correlation between homeownership and wealth or because of the long history of policy interventions to encourage it. Research evidence is limited, however, on whether homeownership itself actually causes faster wealth accumulation, suggesting that interventions to increase homeownership may not have the intended effect of increasing wealth unless other factors are also addressed.

One reason why homeownership may not increase wealth is that buying a home exposes households to a volatile and leveraged risky asset with high transaction costs. Financial gains through homeownership substantially depend on what happens to housing markets following the home purchase (Wainer and Zabel 2020). Weaker housing demand in minority neighborhoods, as well as lower provision of amenities and schools, may weigh down home price growth and housing returns. Moreover, if subsidies to homeownership are structured to subsidize greater leverage, this policy design can leave households exposed to more risk.

An important consideration is whether the nonfinancial benefits of homeownership can offset the aforementioned risk. There is a stronger evidence base that the nonfinancial benefits are positive, including tax exemptions on mortgage and imputed rent, access to neighborhoods with limited rental options, greater attachment to the community, and the automatic savings feature of amortized mortgage payments (Laibson 1997). However, research is lacking on whether these nonfinancial benefits and expected financial returns outweigh the aforementioned risk.

Economic research suggests there may be more scope for interventions that keep struggling homeowners from losing their homes, such as by providing loan relief during periods of falling or stagnant house prices. This is consistent with three evidence-based findings in the literature. First, there is robust evidence that the main drawback to homeownership is the downside risk. Second, liquidity is important for keeping homeowners in their homes. Third, liquidity-driven defaults negatively affect future wealth building. As such, an intervention that acts as an insurance scheme, rather than a price subsidy, may be more effective at helping homeowners build wealth. For example, mortgage products can mimic equity by making the repayment amount contingent on local house price indices (Mian and Sufi 2015). Another potential intervention might support new mortgage loan products that help homeowners build equity (liquidity) faster than the amortization schedule of a traditional thirty-year fixed-rate mortgage (Oliner, Peter, and Pinto 2020).

WEALTH ACCUMULATION PROCESS

To date, the most promising interventions on personal financial decisions have been along behavioral dimensions, including nudges and intelligent defaults. These interventions engage noncognitive aspects of behavior and can simplify choices without adding to the cognitive burdens of households (Madrian and Shea 2001; Thaler and Benartzi 2004). For example, default options into savings in retirement accounts have been successful in increasing 401(k) participation and allocations that include risky-asset exposure (Beshears et al. 2009). Such nudges have shown to be effective across various domains, including personal finance. Some evidence suggests that limited cognitive slack may be exacerbated for low-wealth households who face more tough choices throughout the day (Mani et al. 2013; Mullainathan and Shafir 2013). This explanation contrasts with the stereotypes that associate minorities with low savings and spendthrift behavior.

A shift of focus in interventions to effective yet safe nudges would be useful, aided by more evidence from field experiments. We believe this shift would entail less emphasis on interventions that aim to improve financial literacy, which have, on balance, produced nonrobust results (Hastings, Madrian, and Skimmyhorn 2013). This result may frustrate policymakers as higher-wealth households make decisions that contribute more to wealth accumulation over time, such as investing in risky assets with higher average returns and avoiding costly behavior (Campbell 2006). Moreover, in surveys, financial literacy—

measured as knowledge about financial concepts—is also greater for higher-wealth respondents (Lusardi and Mitchell 2014).

Across the range of wealth accumulation interventions, there are important risks to consider. Because it is difficult to affect how individuals make decisions consistently, successful nudges often change the environment or choice set in which decisions are made, for example, by changing the default options in 401(k) automatic enrollment or target-date fund selection. Inertia from households then makes them stick with these options instead of opting out. When nudges and defaults are designed well, they benefit households even without their paying too much attention, but the same inertia means that poorly designed nudges and defaults can have lasting welfare costs. Many behavioral interventions with robust evidence have been and are being adopted. Research in this area has been fruitful as field experiments have been easier to roll out with the collaboration of employers and benefit providers (Harrison and List 2004).

ENTREPRENEURSHIP AND SMALL-BUSINESS OWNERSHIP

Research suggests that interventions to create wealth through business ownership may be challenged. Despite the archetype of the successful innovator entrepreneur along the path to wealth, whether there are high-return interventions that yield this outcome remains an open question. Importantly, when comparing the same individuals before and after their transition into self employment, small-business owners earn less on average, and few report desires of expanding their businesses. Autonomy, flexibility, and leisure may be prevalent benefits of small businesses and may offset lower earnings to some extent (Hurst and Pugsley 2011). The vast majority do not hire more than one employee, leaving little room for employment spillovers to boost hiring. This is especially a concern among minority-owned small businesses and their scope to hire minority employees. Lastly, average productivity tends to be low, and given that, on average, higher-income individuals enter self-employment, subsidies may be regressive.

An emerging literature recognizing the heterogeneity in small businesses may one day support the development of high-return interventions. After all, business owners have higher incomes (Evans and Jovanovic 1989) and private-business equity takes up disproportionately large shares of balance sheets among high-wealth households (Campbell 2006). Small businesses are not a monolith, and recent research is beginning to understand which small businesses contribute to growth, employment, and wealth. For example, young businesses are on average faster growing, whereas older small businesses more likely provide leisure (Haltiwanger, Jarmin, and Miranda 2013). Research on venture capital and deterrents to access venture capital is also progressing.

A stronger safety net for business owners who want to transition out of self-employment may be a promising policy response. While older small firms do not grow and are not productive, the business owners themselves made fixed investments that make it difficult to transition out. Furthermore, successful ventures are risky, so stronger safety net protection in cases of failure can encourage risky innovation (Hombert et al. 2020).

PLACE-BASED ECONOMIC OPPORTUNITIES

Federal, state, and local governments spend about $95 billion per year on place-based policies that seek to strengthen and move the location of economic activity, thereby reducing inequality and opportunity gaps (Kline and Moretti 2014b). But recent research on place-based policies, such as state enterprise zones and federal empowerment zones, casts doubt on their effectiveness. Nevertheless, there may be a large need for such place-based policies (Austin, Glaeser, and Summers 2018). Most obviously there is a large geographical component to the wealth distribution, and places of residence are often segregated by wealth. In addition, place-based policies have several theoretical benefits, ranging from synergy among beneficiaries in geographically concentrated areas and localized market failures to improved public services (Bartik 2020).

Place-based policies may be challenged for several reasons. First, such policies may target too large a geography, as often the wealth distribution is still substantial within the targeted areas. Furthermore, place-based policies are often intermediated through employers or other suppliers, who also capture some of the benefit themselves.

Another fundamental issue is that of information. Neighborhoods and cities are constantly rising and falling in their economic prosperity. It is difficult for policymakers to gauge whether an area is temporarily distressed or whether a fundamental and secular decline is taking hold. While places are important, policies seek to improve outcomes for the people in those places, with improvements to the physical infrastructure of places providing an input to that process. In this light, place-based policies can also be contrasted against policies that support moves to growing areas or areas with more opportunities. While there have been fewer interventions of this kind, research evidence has demonstrated their effectiveness in improving economic outcomes of the targeted households (Ludwig et al. 2013; Chetty, Hendren, and Katz 2016; Bergman et al. 2019). Moving is costly, of course, not just in economic costs but also in lost social connections and the costs to rebuild them. A silver lining from the COVID-19 pandemic may be that many more Americans have become more familiar with online communications, which can help retain value from long-distance social connections and thus improve the net welfare gains from moves to pursue opportunities.

One final challenge with today's place-based policies may be their small scale. Massive Great Depression-era programs were effective, most notably the Tennessee Valley Authority (Kline and Moretti 2014a); select, large-scale interventions have also been effective, a primary example being the Rosenwald rural schools' initiative in the early twentieth century (Aaronson and Mazumder 2011).

Discussion

Taking an even broader view of the recent evidence on interventions to close racial opportunity gaps, we outline and discuss four overarching themes. Our perspective is that new policies to close economic opportunity gaps may achieve a more effective design, should policymakers take these themes into consideration.

Human capital development requires both economic and noneconomic inputs. The many randomized controlled trials and quasi-experimental studies in recent years point to the importance of both economic and noneconomic inputs for human capital development, including better outcomes for employment and earnings. Importantly, interventions that increase noneconomic resources, like reducing exposure to lead or improving women's access to health insurance during pregnancy, have large effects on human capital outcomes (education, earnings, and employment). Conversely, economic inputs, such as participation in summer youth employment programs, improve noneconomic outcomes (e.g., violent crime arrests). A more holistic view of human capital development emphasizes the vast range of policies that must work together to reduce racial opportunity gaps.

The intergenerational economic benefits of social safety net programs deserve greater emphasis in policy debates. As discussed above, in the last two decades, many studies have identified robust causal effects of social safety net policies for strengthening the long-run economic prospects of low-income and minority children. For example, social safety net programs providing supports like healthcare (Medicaid), food (Supplemental Nutrition Assistance Program and WIC), earnings (earned income tax credit), cash assistance (welfare), and education (Head Start) have causally improved many economic and health outcomes for low-income children (see Brown, Kowalski, and Lurie 2019; Ludwig and Miller 2007; Hoynes, Schanzenbach, and Almond 2016; Bailey et al. 2020). Policymakers would be well served to balance this evidence against complaints—which are often based on insufficient evidence—about the social safety net exacerbating cycles of economic dependency, idleness, and individuals' moral failings. The positive evidence also diverges from the negative and racially charged stereotypes that tend to accompany such gripes.

Focusing housing and financial wealth-building interventions on behavioral nudges and defaults can have larger effects over price subsidies or individual incentives, especially in the short run. The more limited evidence base for nonhuman capital interventions suggests there may be opportunities for new policies to help narrow racial disparities in wealth. Our earlier discussion emphasizes how behavioral nudges and defaults have large effects on retirement savings, college attendance, and health insurance plans (Chetty 2015). Research shows great promise for adding these new policy tools to existing efforts seeking to improve financial outcomes for low-wealth, minority households. Importantly, behavioral nudges and defaults are often cheaper to implement than price subsidies (Benartzi et al. 2017). The private sector can also play a role.

For closing large wealth gaps, deliberating about incremental policy changes with large important impacts and larger-scale policy changes will likely prove challenging. To date, the most convincing and policy-relevant research evidence stems from either actual randomized controlled trials in real-life settings (field experiments) or natural experiments. Such methods have been widely used across subfields and interventions, but still a large bulk of such evidence is limited to topics studied by applied microeconomists. The use of natural and field experiments has been spreading into macroeconomics and finance as well, and accumulating more convincing evidence will delineate the most effective interventions in those areas for reducing racial opportunity gaps.

However, in experimental settings, the majority of interventions or policy changes studied are incremental. Costs, ethical concerns, and disruptions to people's lives limit the applicability of large-scale field experiments to many important settings, while large changes threaten the validity of the study design in natural experiments. But theory suggests that even interventions that are effective in small doses will experience decreasing returns as they are scaled up, both in terms of returns for a given recipient as well as in terms of returns for the broader economy. While making educated assessments may be possible using models disciplined by empirical estimates from more incremental experiments, the research has less to say about larger-scale policy changes. This limitation could be ameliorated through more small-scale field experiments of larger-scale policy changes, as well as through policy experiments and data from around the world.

Conclusions

In this chapter, we reviewed three categories of high-return interventions that can help address the immediate needs of families and close economic opportunity gaps. These interventions include those related to children's health and education, income supports for adults that spill over onto children, and youth crime prevention. All of these interventions affect the human capital of young individuals, who have many years over which the benefits can accrue. Relative to adults, they may be more malleable and likely to be receptive to behavioral "nudges," as well as material support.

However, of the wide inequality in wealth and especially of the wealth gap between racial groups, only about half can be accounted for by differences in earnings, the main byproduct of human capital. This incomplete answer motivates researchers to understand better how those earnings accumulate into wealth, such as through homeownership and financial-market participation— and especially how that process varies across people. More work is needed to develop and validate interventions in this area; we highlight a few nonhuman capital interventions that seem to show promise, but these still need to be evaluated. Lastly, we must consider important trade-offs in dedicating limited resources to new interventions over proven ones; it is a topic that warrants robust debate.

NOTES

The views in this chapter are those of the authors and do not reflect those of the Federal Reserve Bank of Chicago, the Federal Reserve Board, or their staffs.

1. The evidence on the returns for inputs beyond traditional resource-based ones and community programs that are often bundled with charter schools suggests more muted effects.

2. A 2019 speech by Charles L. Evans, president of the Federal Reserve Bank of Chicago, provides a framework for thinking about the risks of attending and financing college, as well as risk-mitigating policy interventions. https://www.chicagofed.org /publications/speeches/2019/the-risks-of-attending-and-financing-college.

REFERENCES

Aaronson, Daniel, and Bhashkar Mazumder. 2011. "The Impact of Rosenwald Schools on Black Achievement." *Journal of Political Economy* 119, no. 5 (October): 821–88.

Almond, Douglas. 2006. "Is the 1918 Influenza Pandemic Over? Long-Term Effects of In-Utero Influenza Exposure in the Post-1940 US Population." *Journal of Political Economy* 114, no. 4 (August): 672–712.

Alon, Titan, Matthias Doepke, Jane Olmstead-Rumsey, and Michèle Tertilt. 2020. "The Impact of the Coronavirus Pandemic on Gender Equality." *COVID Economics Vetted and Real-Time Papers* 4: 62–85.

Austin, Benjamin, Edward Glaeser, and Lawrence Summers. 2018. "Jobs for the Heartland: Place-Based Policies in 21st Century America." *Brookings Papers on Economic Activity*, no. 1 (Spring): 151–255.

Bacher-Hicks, Andrew, Joshua Goodman, and Christine Mulhern. 2021. "Inequality in Household Adaptation to Schooling Shocks: COVID-Induced Online Learning Engagement in Real Time." *Journal of Public Economics* 193: 104345.

Bailey, Martha J., Hilary W. Hoynes, Maya Rossin-Slater, and Reed Walker. 2020. "Is the Social Safety Net a Long-Term Investment? Large-Scale Evidence from the Food Stamps Program." Working Paper w26942, National Bureau of Economic Research, Cambridge, MA. https://doi.org/10.3386/w26942.

Bartik, Timothy J. 2020. "Using Place-Based Jobs Policies to Help Distressed Communities." *Journal of Economic Perspectives* 34, no. 3 (Summer): 99–127.

Bartik, Timothy J., William Gormley, and Shirley Adelstein. 2012. "Earnings Benefits of Tulsa's Pre-K Program for Different Income Groups." *Economics of Education Review* 31, no. 6: 1143–61.

Benartzi, Shlomo, John Beshears, Katherine L. Milkman, Cass R. Sunstein, Richard H. Thaler, Maya Shankar, Will Tucker-Ray, William J. Congdon, and Steven Galing. 2017. "Should Governments Invest More in Nudging?" *Psychological Science* 28, no. 8: 1041–55.

Bergman, Peter, Raj Chetty, Stefanie DeLuca, Nathaniel Hendren, Lawrence F. Katz, and Christopher Palmer. 2019. "Creating Moves to Opportunity: Experimental Evidence on Barriers to Neighborhood Choice." Working Paper w26164, National Bureau of Economic Research, Cambridge, MA. https://doi.org/10.3386/w26164.

Beshears, John, James J. Choi, David Laibson, and Brigitte C. Madrian. 2009. "The Importance of Default Options for Retirement Saving Outcomes: Evidence from the United States." In *Social Security Policy in a Changing Environment*, edited by Jeffrey R. Brown, Jeffrey B. Liebman, and David A. Wise, 167–95. Chicago: University of Chicago Press.

Brown, David W., Amanda E. Kowalski, and Ithai Z. Lurie. 2019. "Long-Term Impacts of Childhood Medicaid Expansions on Outcomes in Adulthood." *Review of Economic Studies* 87, no. 2: 792–821.

Campbell, John Y. 2006. "Household Finance." *Journal of Finance* 61, no. 4 (August): 1553–1604.

Cascio, Elizabeth U., and Diane Whitmore Schanzenbach. 2013. "The Impacts of Expanding Access to High-Quality Preschool Education." *Brookings Papers on Economic Activity* (Fall): 127–78.

Chay, Kenneth Y., Jonathan Guryan, and Bhashkar Mazumder. 2009. "Birth Cohort and the Black-White Achievement Gap: The Roles of Access and Health Soon after Birth." Working Paper w15078, National Bureau of Economic Research, Cambridge, MA. https://doi.org/10.3386/w15078.

Chetty, Raj. 2015. "Behavioral Economics and Public Policy: A Pragmatic Perspective." *American Economic Review* 105, no. 5 (May): 1–33.

Chetty, Raj, Nathaniel Hendren, and Lawrence F. Katz. 2016. "The Effects of Exposure to Better Neighborhoods on Children: New Evidence from the Moving to Opportunity Experiment." *American Economic Review* 106, no. 4 (April): 855–902.

Couch, Kenneth A., Robert W. Fairlie, and Huanan Xu. 2020. "Early Evidence of the Impacts of COVID-19 on Minority Unemployment." *Journal of Public Economics* 192 (December): 104287.

Dobbie, Will, and Roland G. Fryer Jr. 2011. "Are High-Quality Schools Enough to Increase Achievement among the Poor? Evidence from the Harlem Children's Zone." *American Economic Journal: Applied Economics* 3, no. 3 (July): 158–87.

Dorn, Emma, Bryan Hancock, Jimmy Sarakatsannis, and Ellen Viruleg. 2020. "COVID-19 and Student Learning in the United States: The Hurt Could Last a Lifetime." McKinsey and Company, New York. https://www.mckinsey.com/industries/education/our-insights/covid-19-and-student-learning-in-the-united-states-the-hurt-could-last-a-lifetime.

Evans, David S., and Boyan Jovanovic. 1989. "An Estimated Model of Entrepreneurial Choice under Liquidity Constraints." *Journal of Political Economy* 97, no. 4 (August): 808–27.

Haltiwanger, John, Ron S. Jarmin, and Javier Miranda. 2013. "Who Creates Jobs? Small versus Large versus Young." *Review of Economics and Statistics* 95, no. 2 (May): 347–61.

Harrison, Glenn W., and John A. List. 2004. "Field Experiments." *Journal of Economic Literature* 42, no. 4 (December): 1009–55.

Hastings, Justine S., Brigitte C. Madrian, and William L. Skimmyhorn. 2013. "Financial Literacy, Financial Education, and Economic Outcomes." *Annual Review of Economics* 5, no. 1 (May): 347–73.

Heller, Sara B. 2014. "Summer Jobs Reduce Violence among Disadvantaged Youth." *Science* 346, no. 6214: 1219–23.

Heller, Sara B., Anuj K. Shah, Jonathan Guryan, Jens Ludwig, Sendhil Mullainathan, and Harold A. Pollack. 2017. "Thinking, Fast and Slow? Some Field Experiments to Reduce Crime and Dropout in Chicago." *Quarterly Journal of Economics* 132, no. 1 (February): 1–54.

Hendren, Nathaniel, and Ben Sprung-Keyser. 2020. "A Unified Welfare Analysis of Government Policies." *Quarterly Journal of Economics* 135, no. 3 (August): 1209–318.

Hombert, Johan, Antoinette Schoar, David Sraer, and David Thesmar. 2020. "Can Unemployment Insurance Spur Entrepreneurial Activity? Evidence from France." *Journal of Finance* 75, no. 3 (June): 1247–85.

Hoynes, Hilary, Diane Whitmore Schanzenbach, and Douglas Almond. 2016. "Long-Run Impacts of Childhood Access to the Safety Net." *American Economic Review* 106, no. 4 (April): 903–34.

Hurst, Erik, and Benjamin Wild Pugsley. 2011. "What Do Small Businesses Do?" *Brookings Papers on Economic Activity* (Fall): 73–143. https://doi.org/10.1353/eca .2011.0017.

Jackson, C. Kirabo, Rucker C. Johnson, and Claudia Persico. 2016. "The Effects of School Spending on Educational and Economic Outcomes: Evidence from School Finance Reforms." *Quarterly Journal of Economics* 131, no. 1 (February): 157–218.

Kline, Patrick, and Enrico Moretti. 2014a. "Local Economic Development, Agglomeration Economies, and the Big Push: 100 Years of Evidence from the Tennessee Valley Authority." *Quarterly Journal of Economics* 129, no. 1 (February): 275–331.

Kline, Patrick, and Enrico Moretti. 2014b. "People, Places, and Public Policy: Some Simple Welfare Economics of Local Economic Development Programs." *Annual Review of Economics* 6, no. 1 (August): 629–62.

Laibson, David. 1997. "Golden Eggs and Hyperbolic Discounting." *Quarterly Journal of Economics* 112, no. 2 (May): 443–78.

Ludwig, Jens, Greg J. Duncan, Lisa A. Gennetian, Lawrence F. Katz, Ronald C. Kessler, Jeffrey R. Kling, and Lisa Sanbonmatsu. 2013. "Long-Term Neighborhood Effects on Low-Income Families: Evidence from Moving to Opportunity." *American Economic Review* 103, no. 3 (May): 226–31.

Ludwig, Jens, and Douglas L. Miller. 2007. "Does Head Start Improve Children's Life Chances? Evidence from a Regression Discontinuity Design." *Quarterly Journal of Economics* 122, no. 1 (February): 159–208.

Lusardi, Annamaria, and Olivia S. Mitchell. 2014. "The Economic Importance of Financial Literacy: Theory and Evidence." *Journal of Economic Literature* 52, no. 1 (March): 5–44.

Madrian, Brigitte C., and Dennis F. Shea. 2001. "The Power of Suggestion: Inertia in 401(k) Participation and Savings Behavior." *Quarterly Journal of Economics* 116, no. 4 (November): 1149–87.

Mani, Anandi, Sendhil Mullainathan, Eldar Shafir, and Jiaying Zhao. 2013. "Poverty Impedes Cognitive Function." *Science* 341, no. 6149: 976–80.

Mian, Atif, and Amir Sufi. 2015. *House of Debt: How They (and You) Caused the Great Recession, and How We Can Prevent It from Happening Again.* Chicago: University of Chicago Press.

Miller, Cynthia, Lawrence F. Katz, Gilda Azurdia, Adam Isen, Caroline B. Schultz, and Kali Aloisi. 2018. *Boosting the Earned Income Tax Credit for Singles: Final Impact Findings from the Paycheck Plus Demonstration in New York City.* New York: MDRC.

Miller, Sarah, and Laura R. Wherry. 2019. "The Long-Term Effects of Early Life Medicaid Coverage." *Journal of Human Resources* 54, no. 3: 785–824.

Mullainathan, Sendhil, and Eldar Shafir. 2013. *Scarcity: Why Having Too Little Means So Much.* New York: Macmillan.

Oliner, Stephen D., Tobias J. Peter, and Edward J. Pinto. 2020. "The Wealth Building Home Loan." *Regional Science and Urban Economics* 80 (January): 103389.

Parolin, Zachary, Megan Curran, Jordan Matsudaira, Jane Waldfogel, and Christopher Wimer. 2020. "Monthly Poverty Rates in the United States during the COVID-19 Pandemic." Poverty and Social Policy Discussion Paper, Center on Poverty and Social Policy, New York. https://www.povertycenter.columbia.edu/s/COVID-Projecting -Poverty-Monthly-CPSP-2020.pdf.

Royer, Heather. 2009. "Separated at Girth: US Twin Estimates of the Effects of Birth Weight." *American Economic Journal: Applied Economics* 1, no. 1 (January): 49–85.

Ryan, Rebecca, Ariel Kalil, Susan Mayer, and Rohen Shah. 2020. "COVID-19 Could Erase Parenting Gains of the Last 30 Years." Brookings. October 26. https://www.brookings .edu/blog/up-front/2020/10/26/covid-19-could-erase-parenting-gains-of-the-last-30 -years/.

Thaler, Richard H., and Shlomo Benartzi. 2004. "Save More Tomorrow: Using Behavioral Economics to Increase Employee Saving." *Journal of Political Economy* 112, no. S1: S164–S187.

Wainer, Allison, and Jeffrey Zabel. 2020. "Homeownership and Wealth Accumulation for Low-Income Households." *Journal of Housing Economics* 47 (March): 101624.

COVID-19 and Educational Disparities

9. Latinx Immigrant Parents and Their Children in Times of COVID-19: Facing Inequities Together in the "Mexican Room" of the New Latino South

MARTA SÁNCHEZ, MELANIA DIPIETRO, LESLIE BABINSKI, STEVEN J. AMENDUM, AND STEVEN KNOTEK

The Mexican Room was a segregated space for the instruction of Mexican immigrant and Mexican American school-aged children attending school during the first half of the twentieth century in Arizona, Texas, and Southern California (Ruiz 2001; Valencia 2005). The Mexican Room was sometimes located within a school and at times was built as a separate structure and referred to as the Mexican School. There were no laws that allowed for segregation; nonetheless, school districts unlawfully established these spaces, often to uphold notions of white racial superiority even as Mexicans were considered white under the law (Powers and Patton 2008). The Mexican Room was a site of racial subordination and a place of great isolation, where children of Mexican descent languished academically under the guise of receiving specialized instruction delivered by poorly prepared teachers. These segregated spaces were prevalent in part to appease the demands of white parents (Gándara and Orfield 2010) but mostly as part of a larger web of discriminatory practices against Mexicans and Mexican Americans, practices that were also enacted in California and Texas (Powers 2008). The 1951 *Gonzales v. Sheely* court decision ended the Mexican Rooms in Arizona. Noting the deleterious effects segregation had on students' learning of English as well as on their sense of self, the justices wrote: "The methods of segregation prevalent in the respondent school district foster antagonisms in the children and suggest inferiority among them where none exists" (Gándara and Orfield 2010, 3).

We evoke this construct of the Mexican Room (Gándara and Orfield 2010) to capture Latino[1] English Learners' and their parents' experiences as they navigate children's remote learning at the intersection of English-language learning, the use of virtual technologies, and COVID-19. From the onset of shelter-in-place orders in the early stages of the COVID-19 pandemic in March 2020 and extending beyond that, and even as educators quickly adapted and continue to adapt, Latinx English Learners (ELs)[2] have, nonetheless, been in a de facto virtual Mexican Room.

Marta Sánchez and Melania DiPietro are two educators of Mexican descent, each with a long history of working in educational settings with Latinx immigrant families. The first author has thirty years of experience in early childhood education, bilingual education, reading instruction within bilingual education, Latinx immigrant family literacy, and Latinx family support in urban and rural areas. She is also a professor at a comprehensive regional university and conducts research in local and transnational spaces with Latinx families and teachers. The second author has thirty years of experience as an English as a Second Language resource staff. Throughout the years, we have engaged in conversations about the education of Latinx children, the relationship schools establish with their parents, the work conditions that Latinx parents experience, how these impact family life, and the general precarity Latinx parents face as brown, laboring bodies in the geographies of the New Latino South, whether they are undocumented immigrants, documented immigrants, or citizens.

Leslie Babinski, Steven J. Amendum, Steven Knotek, and Marta Sánchez have collaborated on two studies funded by the Institute of Education Sciences, the first of which was a pilot study called Developing Consultation and Collaboration Skills (DCCS): English as a Second Language (ESL) and Classroom Teachers Working Together with Students and Families (Babinski et al. 2018). They are now conducting an efficacy trial to test the DCCS teacher professional development program for impacts on teachers and students. Babinski, Amendum, Knotek, and Sánchez have a long trajectory of conducting research individually, together, and as part of other research teams. All teach at the university level.

We come together to outline the state of affairs for Latinx families in the southeastern United States in times of COVID-19, and to situate what is happening within the broader experiences of the Latinx community in the United States, using a sociohistorical approach to understand the struggle and current inequities in the education of Latinx children and how these are further exacerbated by COVID-19. We make no claim that the impacts are unique to Latinx children and their families; it would be impossible to ascertain this without studying all the children and families of the world. We do seek to highlight the ways in which Latinx children, their families, and teachers are navigating the COVID-19 pandemic, what lessons their experiences teach us, and what the policy implications are moving forward.

We draw from multiple texts that include COVID-19-related literature on Latinx immigrants and Latinx school-aged ELS, brief histories of Latinx education in US public schools, the first and second author's experiences with families of K-5 Latinx students in the southeastern United States, lessons learned by other programs that have publicly reported on these, studies conducted by the authors, and preliminary DCCS survey data with Latinx parents of kindergarten and first grade ELS. These diverse texts begin to define the context and offer distinct perspectives that should be considered when seeking to draft policy. We discuss the intersections of aspiration and precarity to understand the unique positioning of Latinx ELS in schools; we examine how a global pandemic emerges as an actor in the resegregation of Latinx ELS through the establishment of a virtual Mexican Room; and we point to possible ways out.

The Broader Context

LATINX ELS AND THEIR PARENTS

COVID-19 has had a disparate impact on immigrant communities, and especially on Latinx immigrants (Cano et al. 2020), who tend to be essential workers without essential protections. Latinx immigrants disproportionately work in retail and service industries where they have greater exposure to the public. These jobs cannot be carried out from home, the consequences of which are that only 16.2 percent of Hispanics can work from home (Gould and Shierholz 2020). Not speaking English is associated with a higher risk of COVID-19 infection (Rodriguez-Diaz et al. 2020; Rozenfeld et al. 2020). Latinos report lacking health insurance, having mistrust of the medical profession, and having no access to paid leave (Cano, Snow, and Anderson 2020). Moore and colleagues (2021) found that individuals who live in multigenerational homes and in communities with high concentrations of foreign-born noncitizens and food-service workers are at increased risk of contracting COVID-19. Perhaps, consequently, their COVID-19-related deaths are 2.3 times higher than that of whites (CDC 2021), and while Latinos may represent 18.5 percent of the US population (US Census Bureau 2020), they have a higher rate of infection than Asians, blacks, and whites, similar to that of the indigenous community (CDC 2021). In the early stages of the pandemic, Latinos had more confirmed cases in proportion to the percentage they represent of the total US population. In North Carolina, for example, Cano, Snow, and Anderson (2020) report that while Latinos represent 10 percent of the state's population, they accounted for 45 percent of coronavirus cases in that state. This pattern held in forty-two states and Washington, DC. In the other eight states, the number of confirmed cases among Latinos was "more than four times greater than any other group" (Godoy and Wood 2020, para. 9). Latinos continue to have higher infection and mortality rates than most of the population (Wood 2020). Risk of exposure to the virus is also present because of household occupancy density (Rodriguez-Diaz et al. 2020). Finally, many Latinx immigrants experience a higher incidence of preexisting health conditions, like diabetes (Cano et al. 2020), which can make having COVID-19 worse.

Many Latinx adults work in jobs designated as essential. Essential workers who are undocumented are vulnerable not only to becoming infected because of the frontline jobs they have, but because they are unlikely to have health insurance and also may not seek to be vaccinated or receive medical attention for fear of being detained or deported (Cano et al. 2020; Goodman 2020). According to the Institute of Taxation and Economic Policy, undocumented immigrants contributed $11.7 billion in local and state taxes (Goodman 2020), and they fuel two economies: the US economy with the purchases they make, the taxes they pay, and the cheap labor they supply; and their homeland's economy with the remittances they send. Mexico, for instance, received 34 billion dollars in remittances in 2018 (World Bank 2019, April 8). However, their contribution does not translate into individual or group access to basic healthcare. These families toil and see only modest gains in their quality of life and a limited ability to provide their children with twenty-first-century learning tools, such as computers and household internet access.

In 2005, the Pew Research Center issued a report on changing demographics in the southeastern United States, highlighting the exponential growth of the Latinx population in the 1990–2000 decade in six southern states: Arkansas, Alabama, Georgia, North Carolina, South Carolina, and Tennessee. The report dubbed these "the New Latino South," recognizing that the six states had become new settlement sites for internal migration of Latinos from other states and for immigrants from Mexico and Central America. Ethnographer Enrique Murillo was among the early chroniclers of these migrations (1996–1998) and was able to isolate Siler City, North Carolina, as one of the first southeastern settlement sites for immigrants from Mexico. Drawn to the area's poultry farms, this migration was quickly followed by Mexican migration to the southeastern hog, turkey, and chicken processing farms. The fast-paced linework at these farms requires that one stand almost shoulder to shoulder with fellow workers as hogs and chickens are butchered to prepare them for the family-size packaging available at the grocery store. While declared essential workers during COVID-19, animal processing line workers were hardly cherished by their employers. Many workers spoke about the fear of being fired if they took a sick day, and those who filled in for absent coworkers were not adequately compensated for the extra work. The work has long-term sequelae, such as joint pain and pain resulting from repetitive movements and working in rooms where the temperature must be kept low. A 2018 Guardian investigative report found that there are two amputations a week among workers in US meat processing plants. Risk of injury rises as plants increase speed time on the line without increasing the number of line employees (Wasley, Cook, and Jones 2018). The Latinx immigrant parents with whom Melania DiPietro has had extensive contact for three decades work in these plants and worry about working in such close proximity with others in a COVID-19 context but fear speaking to their supervisors about it. They also fear becoming sick, as this would mean missing workdays and possibly losing their job as a result.

Moreover, for many Latinx immigrant parents in the New Latino South, their skin color and language make them hypervisible in rural geographies, and for some, their immigration status is a daily worry. In a 2017 study that the first two authors undertook, a mother narrated how the local sheriff would park outside the trailer park where she lived and stop her on her way to the grocery store. He would ask for her driver's license, which she could not furnish. The state she lived in did not issue driver's licenses to undocumented immigrants. The sheriff would ticket her regularly, and she would then pay the fine. Through these encounters, she accumulated approximately $700 worth of fines that she was paying monthly. The mother said, "Sé que jamás me van a deportar porque le ganan dinero cada vez que me multan y me dan el ticket" (I know that they will never deport me, because they make money every time they fine me and give me a ticket).

Further defining the immigrant experience in the southeastern United States is immigration code 287g. Code 287g allows for Immigration and Customs Enforcement, or ICE, to enter into a memorandum of agreement (MOA) with local sheriff's offices so that sheriffs can act as de facto ICE agents and have the ability to detect, detain, and deport undocumented immigrants. Many counties within the states that constitute the New Latino South received funding to implement 287g. This allowed sheriffs to set up checkpoints on highway exit ramps and on any road in their jurisdiction. Latino parents in a study in the same southeastern region of the country (Knotek and Sánchez 2017) reported that sheriffs would station themselves on roads commonly used by parents to get to their children's school. In many counties, 287g was defunded, but because of MOAS that are still in force with local sheriffs, the possibility of being detained and deported continues to concern Latinx immigrants in the southeast.

LABORING ALONE TOGETHER

It is in these contexts that Latinx immigrant parents and their children navigate toward their aspirations. COVID-19's arrival introduced greater vulnerability to Latinx immigrant parents and their emergent bilingual children. A public panel presentation with Latina immigrant mothers convened by a regional nonprofit revealed that amid the uncertainty of the COVID-19 pandemic, Latina mothers remained focused on supporting their children's education at home even as they faced challenges with technology and their inability to help their children with the unfamiliar content of the assignments. The mothers made two observations not yet brought up by any of the literature or survey research: (1) their children missed their peers; and (2) the pandemic will go on, which has consequences for their children when all of the adults in the household reassume a regular work schedule and return to their worksites. DiPietro, in her work with Latinx ELS, provides evidence to support the mothers' claims about children missing their peers. It is not only within a social dimension that children look for the company of their peers; for Latinx ELS, their peers help unlock meaning during the school day. Peers can be asked in a quick sidebar what the teacher said or be asked to translate a key word. Peers can help ELS complete an assignment successfully. For Latinx ELS, their bilingual peers are an indispensable resource that facilitates their learning and emerging sense of belonging. In a separate public discussion facilitated by school and government leaders about COVID-19 and bilingual children from distinct ethnic backgrounds, a call was made to fulfill the federal mandate to provide translation at all parent meetings and establish internet access as a universal right for all, "like water" (Center for Applied Linguistics 2021). These conversations with the Latinx and other immigrant communities and educators signaled the importance of having policies and practices that prioritize the needs of the most vulnerable.

LATINX ELS, THEIR TEACHERS, AND SCHOOLING

As Latinx immigrant parents labor in precarious situations, their children labor in virtual spaces where the communication is not circular but unidirectional, bereft of native language support, either from the teaching staff or from peers, and they are unable to navigate or access necessary technologies because of lack of hardware and internet access. In this virtual Mexican Room, Latinx ELS are unable to ask a bilingual peer for help to orient them to the learning task, an action they would be able to take in a face-to-face context.

Of the 50.2 million students enrolled in public schools, 13.6 million (27 percent) are Hispanic[3] (National Center for Education Statistics 2021). Hispanic students comprise over 75 percent of the EL population (National Center for Education Statistics 2018). As Latinx emergent bilinguals or emergent multilinguals—as is the case with indigenous children from Latin American countries, who arrive to US schools speaking Spanish and an indigenous language—the students are academically vulnerable. These students are vulnerable not because of their linguistic abilities, but because of a lack of teacher preparation and support to teach students with this more complex student profile. The instructional mismatch can have significant consequences: Latinx students can experience loss of the home language, thus severing their connection to family, culture, and knowledge (Hinton 2015; Valenzuela 1999; Fillmore 1991).

Despite the continuous growth of the Latinx emergent bilingual student population and other ELs in public schools, US educators are not receiving adequate training, professional development, or support to teach this population. Teacher preparation programs often do not require future teachers to have any formal preparation in teaching linguistically diverse students, and while federal law explicitly states that school districts must provide professional development to all school personnel working with ELs (ECS 2014, para. 5), thirty-two states have zero certification requirements for general classroom teachers in the teaching of emergent bilinguals, or ELs. The result is that teachers may be entering classrooms with little to no formal education on how to teach and support ELs while ELs continue to grow as a student group. Because the majority of US ELs are Hispanic, policy decisions in preservice teacher education programs and in-service teacher professional development disproportionately impact Latinx ELs. COVID-19 exacerbates an already problematic reality for Latinx families and their school-aged children, a reality that can reverberate into the future. It is not uncommon to hear teachers and researchers refer to the "lost cohort" when speaking about students who may simply not be able to catch up after schooling became virtual to comply with COVID-19 protocols.

Latinx Education in the United States: A History of Struggle and Triumph and Struggle and Loss

COVID-19 has revealed the long-standing marginalization of Latinx families and the sustained effort to subordinate Latinx immigrants through immigration, labor, and education policies and practices, and to disenfranchise them from our healthcare system because of their immigration status, dynamics that have characterized the US-Latin American relationship. Schooling has been a primary site of Latinx struggle, a place where Latinx education in the United States has been a process of substantive gains and equally substantive losses. This phenomenon represents one of the urgent social and educational equity issues in the country, and this moment of living and learning through a global pandemic is exposing many of the historical vulnerabilities that remain to be addressed. The impact of systemic and structural inequalities for Latinx families and their children contributes to creating the conditions that generate the Mexican Room.

All actors—administrators, teachers, parents, and students—are ensnared by the Mexican Room's arrival to the New Latino South and face the challenge of dismantling it. These inequities are not new; for example, a 2019 report indicated that the Latino family faced a digital divide because of either not having access to the internet or having limited access to the internet (Cano, Garcia, and Thompson 2020). In a nationally representative survey conducted with Latinx families (Latino Decisions 2020), families reported not having access or the necessary supports to access the internet for their children's remote instruction and learning. Disruptions in communication with teachers and having to navigate diverse web applications and learning management systems, as well as encountering broken links, were noted by survey respondents as barriers to their children's participation in remote learning. Indeed, DiPietro has found that Latinx immigrant parents mostly have access to the internet on their cell phones, and their children have to wait until their parents come home in the evening from work in order to connect to the school-based applications and assignments.

The long struggle for education and language rights among Latinx families is characterized by three cross-cutting themes: (1) Latinx parents were key actors in agitating for transformation; (2) a "rights" discourse was advanced through Latinx parents' struggle; and (3) their actions achieved the pathbreaking changes they sought. The following court cases are a series of negotiations of educational rights at the intersection of race, language, ethnicity, aspirations, and precarity.

In these court cases, Latinx parents resisted efforts to segregate their children on the basis of color; argued against schools' claims that they wanted to alleviate overcrowded schools by constructing new schools to which only children of Mexican descent would be assigned; and rejected schools' claims that they sought to address the special needs of children of Mexican descent, such as learning English. In all instances, Latinx parents found the support of the courts and secured a better model of education for their children. These lessons matter when schools have not yet reliably transitioned to successful virtual course delivery to Latinx ELS.

Struggle and Triumph

From 1931 to 1951 three desegregation court cases resulted in improved education for children of Mexican descent and Mexican American children and progressively challenged the "separate but equal" doctrine. In all three cases, parents were the impetus for change. The Lemon Grove Incident of 1931, *Mendez v. Westminster* (1946), and *Gonzales v. Sheely* (1951) involved the school district seeking to require Mexican immigrant and Mexican American children to enroll in Mexican Schools: schools within the United States in the same general locale of the schools the children were already attending. In other cases, students were relegated to the Mexican Room. Phenotype (*Mendez v. Westminster*), ethnicity (all three cases), deficit discourses, and racism (all three cases) played roles in the segregation of Mexican immigrant and Mexican American children.

The Lemon Grove Incident of 1931 in San Diego, California, resulted in the country's first school desegregation case: *Roberto Alvarez v. The Board of Trustees of the Lemon Grove School District*. The parents' legal action was galvanized by the school principal's action of barring Mexican and Mexican American students from entering Lemon Grove Elementary School in January 1931. The students were redirected to the Mexican School that supposedly had been built for them. The children and the parents refused, sought legal recourse, and won (Madrid 2008).

Mendez v. Westminster (1946) is about Silvia Mendez, a Mexican American student who, upon the start of the school year in Westminster County, was told she had to attend the Mexican School. Her parents refused to comply. The Mendez case is important for several reasons. First, unlike the Lemon Grove incident, the Mendez plaintiffs did not argue that the Mexican School was inferior; instead they argued against the practice of segregation, thus challenging the doctrine of "separate but equal" (Blanco 2010, 2; Wallace 2013). The triumph of Mendez was a triumph over historical segregation, first legislated to segregate blacks in 1854 (Wallace 2013, 125), followed by *Ward v. Flood* (1874), which established the right for all Californians to receive a public education but maintained separate facilities for groups by race, which was considered legal to do (Wallace 2013, 126). Finally, Mendez was viewed as a "dry run" for *Brown v. Board of Education* (Wallace 2013, 128). Jared Wallace warns not to overstate the role of *Mendez* in the success of *Brown*. *Brown* is the result of unprecedented massive civil uprising in search of racial justice; however, the case does symbolize ethnic and racial unity. Maria Blanco (2010) highlights "the important crossover between different ethnic and racial groups who came together to argue in favor of desegregation" (2).

Porfirio Gonzales and the Latinx parents of three hundred children who attended schools in Tolleson Elementary School District in Arizona sued the board of trustees and the principal, arguing that the school district broke the law when segregating children of Mexican descent, because there was no law requiring Latinx children to be segregated (Valencia 2005). That is, *Gonzales v. Sheely* (1951) did not challenge the doctrine of separate but equal; the parents simply cited unlawfulness. This is in contrast to the 1925 case in Arizona of Adolfo "Babe" Romo, who sued two school districts on behalf of his children. Romo cited racism and the misclassification of his children as being "colored," a racial designation referring to black children and which, he argued, should not be applicable to children of Mexican descent (Valencia 2008). Jeanne Powers and Lirio Patton (2008) point out how segregation invariably meant an inferior education for children. For example, there were no reliable assessments of children's English language development or for reassignment out of the Mexican Schools, when at the same time, the rationale for segregating children of Mexican descent through placement in the Mexican Schools was so that they might be taught English more intensively. The courts ruled in favor of the parents, declaring that the segregation of children of Mexican descent was unconstitutional.

Advancing a Rights Discourse through Latinx Parent Struggle for Educational Equity

The Bilingual Education Act of 1968 was an outcome of the broader civil rights movement that recruited not only Latinx parents to its vision but also other groups who sought to have their children's language rights guaranteed through school-based bilingual education programs (Cervantes-Soon et al. 2017). The Bilingual Education Act was not about becoming competitive global polyglot citizens or enhancing cognitive functioning through bilingualism. Rather, it was about basic civil rights—rights won through peaceful resistance and collective mobilization.

In subsequent years, the No Child Left Behind Act of 2001 (NCLB) represented a loss of gains made in previous decades, specifically because it ushered in nativist language policies emphasizing English language learning only rather than continuing the civil rights ethos inscribed in the Bilingual Act of 1968. The commitment of honoring children's right to both the language of the home and English was replaced by English immersion—also known as the "sink or swim" model—and English as a second language models of English language instruction, both considered to be among the weakest forms of second language learning. As English established itself as a global language and the world's lingua franca, achieving a hegemonic status, monolingual English speakers were established as the new desirable citizens. The Bilingual Education Act came to an end and was replaced by the No Child Left Behind Act, which officially sought to improve teacher quality and student outcomes through curricular reforms and standardized testing (Mangual Figueroa 2013). Also, officially, Title III of NCLB establishes English as the language of instruction. In practice, for ELS, NCLB accelerated leaving the home language behind and relying on standardized curricula to teach and standardized tests to assess student and school progress, including ELs. Standardization of curricula and testing in schooling has long been studied, and we have learned that standardized tests are inscribed with gender, racial, socioeconomic, and linguistic bias. In an NCLB context, school districts can opt to omit children with special needs and ELs—not to avoid subjecting these students to biased tests, but to keep the school's overall achievement scores high.

Under NCLB, school districts use student testing data in problematic ways. Some states grade schools based on these data, using an A-F system. The outcomes can be punitive, as schools face state intervention if they do not make progress, as measured by these test scores. At the same time, there is no consideration for underfunded schools and schools with disproportionate numbers of early career or uncertified teachers, as is the case in schools with high African American and Latino student populations (Au 2004).

NCLB has also been criticized for ranking teachers as "highly qualified" simply for passing "a computer exam to receive their professional teaching credentials" (Au 2004, para. 3), even as the federal definition is that teachers must have a bachelor's degree, be certified, and demonstrate content knowledge through coursework and testing (Au 2004). NCLB also violates basic principles of social justice in requiring ELs who have just entered ESL or other English language instruction programs to be tested (Gándara and Baca 2008). NCLB's implicit English-only mandate; its lack of strong, additive models of language instruction; and its use of standardized curricula and standardized testing with nonwhite, bilingual and multilingual children create an acute academic disadvantage for Latinx ELs and an academic advantage for monolingual whites, thus perpetuating historical US racial and ethnic hierarchies. It is with this understanding that NCLB is seen as a threat and is detrimental to Latinx academic and social advancement.

It is important to remember that language is a vast epistemological, ontological, and social resource that connects us to family, culture, history, and ways of thinking and being. To willfully create the conditions that facilitate and expedite the loss of language constitutes deculturalization (Fillmore 1991; Spring 2016) and creates precarity for children and adults in a country that historically has engaged in both their exploitation as cheap labor and their expulsion as undocumented workers. The unique positioning of Latinx immigrant children is that their bilingualism will keep them connected to their heritage but also connect their family linguistically to English-dominant spaces. In a crisis like COVID-19, language disarticulations can feel disorienting, threatening, and violent. To deny a child any of their languages is epistemological violence and can render them unable to be that vital link for their family. This understanding of the Latinx immigrant child is that they can intervene in cultural and social processes through linguistic and cultural knowledge and help the family and others navigate new languages, cultures, societies, practices, and expectations (Faulstich Orellana 2009). Latinx parents and their children now enter another era of struggle for educational equity.

How Are Parents of Latino English Learners Faring in the COVID-19 Pandemic?

As part of a larger survey, Latinx immigrant parents of K-1 English learners responded to a series of questions about remote learning in times of COVID-19. The questions asked were designed to require a narrative response. Fifty-one of ninety-one parents from seventeen elementary schools within one school district responded. Although not all parents answered the questions about remote learning and COVID-19, those who did provide a snapshot of how Latinx parents of young ELs were faring as they navigated remote learning with their children.

The fifty-one respondents were thirty Mexican parents, eight Honduran parents, four Guatemalan parents, four El Salvadoran parents, two parents from the Dominican Republic, one Colombian parent, one parent from Spain, and one parent from Venezuela. The questions examined three areas: access to hardware and apps, ease of use and access (e.g., reliable connectivity), and teacher presence and support. Parents emphasized an appreciation for the school's efforts to provide each child with a computer. They expressed frustration with the hardware—four parents noted that they did not receive their child's computer until two weeks after remote learning sessions had started—with the malfunctioning passcodes, and with the lack of teacher presence (via videos or written posts) to help students and parents navigate the assignments.

Three more themes emerged from parents' responses: a sense of gratitude toward the school or the teacher; a disposition of thoughtful involvement in their children's education as evidenced by requests for more scaffolds or services to support their children; and the role of siblings in teaching, learning, and serving as a bridge between the parents' Spanish-language dominance and the siblings' English-language dominance.

One parent expressed frustration with the process and loss of essential and valuable educational supports for her child with special needs, but she nevertheless was maintaining a positive attitude about the challenge she was facing together with her son. Appealing to collective, collaborative action, she said that "in talking with other parents, this was frustrating for everybody. They [school personnel] should do a video to help. He needs help with speech therapy. There has not been support for children who have a speech problem as is my son's case. He used to receive services before. It has been a new challenge for all of us, but if all collaborate, together, we will achieve it."

Other responses indicated that remote learning could be disrupted by a number of factors: illness in the family, a parent not understanding how to help the child because of language differences, lack of connectivity, an access code not working that then prevented the child from accessing academic content, unreliable internet service, a complicated login process, and having to be at work when the child needed help with academic content. While many parents thanked teachers for their efforts, they also noted that more teacher support was needed to ensure their children's successful completion of assignments. Five parents experienced problems with internet connectivity, with the connection failing or being slow. Accessing the platforms was also a challenge, as one parent said in a comment that was representative of five more comments that described problems with the access codes: "There was a problem with my girl's codes. At the beginning, she could enter but after a week, the code was bad, and she couldn't enter it anymore."

PARENT FRUSTRATIONS AND RECOMMENDATIONS

Parents said they felt disappointed that they could not help their children because they had to work, and others made recommendations, such as providing children with downloadable, printable forms so that children could have something "tangible" that would allow the parent "to be able to see what their day will be like." Other parents advocated for themselves and their child(ren). They wrote how difficult it was, as someone who does not read English, to navigate the online learning system including logging into the system, and then navigating other areas. One parent pointed out that no interpreters were available, which is required by law. She asked, "So how is this being resolved in an online forum?" Additionally, one parent gave a strong critique of the delivery mode, calling out a low-quality approach, she wrote, "This new way of learning is very limited, of very little use if they only send homework to children." Finally, one parent offered this cogent observation: "Parents are not teachers. It was difficult to help with homework in the afternoon. Hard after my work to help with remote learning. For him, he didn't understand what was being explained to him and there were too many children connected. For me, the connection, they should have sent text."

The comments merit serious consideration. The parent above is highlighting the significant difference between being a teacher and being a parent. In recognizing this, she is also recognizing the professionalism of teachers. She made comments about the order of things—perhaps parents should not be asked to engage in a cognitively demanding task immediately after work. She also discussed how class size matters online in the same way it would matter in face-to-face instruction. She advocates for her son. She implies that he needed another explanation, another scaffold in order to understand what was expected of him, revealing a formal understanding of how learning happens. Finally, she recommends the use of text messages to connect. This comment requires follow-up questioning of the parent to determine whether she was referring to WhatsApp, for example, an extraordinarily popular text messaging service among Latinx parents, but her comment is clear about her preference for the use of texts for communication.

In spite of frustrations, many parents thanked the school for the computers and for the teachers' efforts to motivate their children to be interested in learning, as well as for the teachers' broader help and support. Other respondents thanked teachers for their kindness and patience.

Survey Summary

The parents who responded to the survey point the way toward the improvement of remote learning. In their feedback, they offered specific examples of the ways in which the current approaches to education remain challenging and how some of these could be improved. The parents explained how malfunctioning codes shut them out of being able to use the computer, and they reminded teachers and the school that the staff who support parent involvement and student learning in a face-to-face context are also needed in a remote learning context (e.g., interpreter, speech therapist). At least three parents introduced the idea of how important siblings are as English language brokers, helping younger siblings with assignment instructions and helping them read the texts. Parents asked teachers not to leave them or their children behind as they navigated the technology to access the academic content. Finally, in sharing how they felt sadness, guilt, or a sense of failure for not being able to help their child either because they were tired from a long day of work, did not have an interpreter to support their participation, or were at work, these parents could help schools reconceptualize the distribution of personnel and how to support Latinx parents so that they are successful supporting their children's online learning.

Accompanying Latinx Families as They Navigate COVID-19: A View from the Field

ESTABLISHING LINES OF COMMUNICATION

The arrival of COVID-19 has made virtual communication essential to facilitating the delivery of education to students around the world. Virtual tools allow educators to be in direct contact with their students for the purposes of instruction; however, for this approach to teaching and learning to be effective, or at least for it to be possible to some degree, all actors (e.g., teachers, parents, caregivers, students, principals) in the processes of schooling must be involved, trained, and have access to all tools. We focus this discussion on the experiences of Latinx K-5 students for whom English is a new or developing language and who are enrolled in schools in the southeastern United States. We draw from the lived experience of the second author, who has affiliations as English as second language support staff in area schools (where the first and second author conducted research from 2017–2019). We highlight the differential impacts that the Latinx community is experiencing in times of COVID-19 and acknowledge that these occur within school districts that have made and continue to make extraordinary efforts to equip families with the needed tools so that the students can continue their education in virtual spaces.

In the aftermath of COVID-19's emergence in North Carolina, schools surveyed parents and personnel about the curriculum delivery options that were under consideration. Each county offered various possibilities similar to those that were proposed around the country: face-to-face classes only (option A), online synchronous classes only (option B), and a hybrid option with 50 percent face-to-face classes and 50 percent remote classes (option C). In many cases, schools polled families and teachers and they elected to start classes remotely (option B). An orientation to the "new normal" proceeded, followed by the distribution of materials and digital devices (e.g., iPads, Chromebooks, laptops, and MacBooks). These were assigned to students according to grade level and in consideration of each school's preferred technologies. The schools assessed the students' ability to access and use the applications within the digital devices. The array included StateEdCloud, Google Mail, Google Meet, Class Dojo, IStation, and other applications. The setup involved the tedious process of having schools create student accounts so that through these applications students could be in remote contact with their teachers in a multitude of ways. These efforts were undergirded by a sincere commitment to fulfill the state's obligation to its youngest citizens of providing a free K-12 education. In the context of the pandemic, as with other state efforts related to public goods such as the delivery of healthcare, the process was fraught with challenges that included technical glitches and logistical difficulties gathering and distributing the apparatuses.

Under option B (online synchronous classes only), policymakers overlooked what this choice entailed and for whom this option might not work at all. That is, the degree to which option B could serve as an adequate substitute for face-to-face instruction was contingent upon a family's access to the internet; a students' fluency in English; the family's broader English-language resources; the students', parents', and/or caregivers' ability to navigate the hardware and various applications; the presence and knowledge of an adult or more competent peer to help the student; the teacher's fluency with these applications; the teacher's ability to differentiate instruction according to student need in a virtual format where they might or might not be able to structure peer interactions or intervene directly to support a student and groups of students; and the ability of the child to complete tasks with little adult support. For Latinx ELs and for those whose immigrant parents may also not be fluent in English, the challenges felt insurmountable. In many cases, parents had to work during the day and had to leave their children with caregivers. Suddenly caregivers, many of whom were Latinx immigrants with diverse levels of English-language knowledge, were now responsible for overseeing connectivity, guaranteeing students logged in to their remote classes, and responding to children's questions. In many cases, caregivers had multiple children in their care, each from different families, and each at different grade levels, levels of English-language acquisition, and levels of digital literacy. Many Latinx ELs were and continue to be in the care of people who have not had experience with or exposure to the specific technologies of schooling, such as Google Classroom and the StateEdCloud site, nor have the caregivers received any instruction or support from anyone on how these sites work. Unlike teachers who receive ongoing professional development and students who would have received instruction on how to use virtual technologies (as time allowed for it), parents and caregivers are not prepared for this role. Yet parenting and caregiving now included ensuring that the student was connected during the hours that each teacher offered instruction. Caregivers had to understand how to guide the student to check assignments and homework that had been sent to the teacher in order to receive a grade.

Many caregivers simply lacked the means to provide this support. For instance, caregivers (and families of students) may not have internet access at home or the possibility of providing transportation to take students to a site that offered a free WiFi connection to students. The connectivity and use of applications for virtual teaching and learning revealed a formidable challenge: Latinx students were not receiving assistance with their assignments and homework at home, because their parents worked in essential businesses. The parents in the school districts under discussion lived in a harsh reality. They worked in such business, places like the hog, chicken, and turkey factories, and they continued to go to work because of economic reasons. As members of the lower echelons of the socioeconomic class, they could not simply stop working or work from home. Their family economy was then further affected, under option B, by having to pay someone to care for one or more students in the same family.

A small percentage of students (the more fortunate ones) may have had access to digital devices at home—devices purchased, often with great sacrifice, by parents so that the children had the hardware to access the internet. The less fortunate, however, who in many cases were Latino EL students, were overlooked. To some degree these schools provided digital devices that were integrated with the programs and applications necessary to begin to open the portals of communication with the teachers in the different classes to which the students had to connect, so that they could receive the education that by law they needed to receive—an education that is, hopefully, of quality. But not each and every student could truly access a digital device. In some cases, especially when families had more than one child receiving some type of virtual education, the school lacked sufficient digital devices to provide one to each student at home. Such a scenario led to another situation in which schools provided only a certain number of digital devices per family to be shared among siblings. This situation had consequences: students had to connect at different times with teachers, and teachers had to plan live classes at times that did not conflict with siblings' schedules, a titanic task for teachers in terms of creating schedules and planning.

THE PERFECT TRIANGLE OF EDUCATION

It is important to consider that education has three parts that make up the "education triangle": students, teachers, and parents. Quality of education cannot be possible if the triangle is unequally balanced, or if one leg of the triangle is unable to properly support the others. Recently, teachers have had to be trained even more to provide the education that our students need. They must continue to train, through online courses, to make remote classes accessible and understandable and to meet the standards required by the state and board of education. They train and, through remote classes, in turn train the students.

Forgotten in this picture are the parents. Remote classes are taken at home, and it is at home where, instead, the support of the teacher has to be provided by the parents. Here, the parents' roles will go beyond those of providers and guardians to those of active participants in the classes that their children receive through remote teaching. Parents then face the situation that they are the only ones who have not received previous training on how to use the tools and digital devices that they have received from the school. In this way, giving digital devices to a parent who does not have an internet connection is like giving them a car without gasoline in it. Also, teachers and students are trained to understand how to use the different applications, devices, programs, and so on, but parents are not. To continue the metaphor, the situation results in parents having cars without gasoline that they, moreover, cannot use because they do not know how to drive.

A QUALITY EDUCATION?

The arrival of COVID-19 was the impulse for initiating a new way of providing elementary education or remote education that many educators were also not accustomed to implementing. Remote education emerges as a challenge for all, and it can, in some cases, be experienced by Latinx ELs as a "silent and passive" and isolating process—like being in the historical Mexican Room.

The difference between face-to-face teaching and remote learning is vast. On the one hand we have the scenario in which an EL student arrives for the first time at a school in the United States without knowing English or is at a beginning level of English language learning. This student has the opportunity to integrate into a classroom and can receive the support of the teacher, new classmates, and direct English as a second language services through its different modalities. These opportunities differ from remote or digital classes, where the student is seated in front of a monitor or screen where all the information, either synchronous or asynchronous, is provided by the educator completely in English; the student and parents find themselves in total silence unable to understand or know what to respond to in front of a screen where a group of students and their teachers speak completely in English. An education is being offered, but Latinx ELs sit in total silence with a lack of understanding.

THE BRIDGES TOWARD UNITY

There is a new form of communication between Spanish-speaking teachers, students, and parents that COVID-19 has brought about. COVID-19 highlighted the importance of ESL personnel, the school receptionist, and translators in serving as bilingual support. These key members of the school community have become the bridges toward unity that make the triangle of education possible by providing a network of support. ESL educators, for example, have gone above and beyond the line of duty in one way or another, all with the purpose of offering students and parents the support they deserve, opening the lines of connection between each and every one of the members that make up the school staff to make it possible to approximate a quality education. In schools with a high percentage of Latinx students, the active participation of these staff is "overloaded" by having to support teachers in contacting Latinx students and to communicate with parents. Latinx staff are taxed with giving families training in the use of digital devices as well as instruction on how to use the different applications. In the midst of the shift to digital technologies, the ESL teacher must continue planning and creating lessons for ELs *and* provide the necessary content and scaffolds for English language learning and development. The bilingual personnel go beyond the established schedule by having to contact parents after they arrive home from their jobs; receive calls from students and parents who do not understand how to connect with the teacher because the digital device presents a problem; explain assignments and homework from different classes; and make occasional home visits—taking all necessary measures to avoid direct contact with families—to help parents who need guidance and support in the use of digital devices and applications.

Although the scenarios created by the COVID-19 pandemic could not have been imagined, the events of this era have revealed the lack of preparation to provide and receive education; the lack of training with and understanding of the use of digital devices and their various applications; and the reality that language knowledge makes education go through a "test" in which great inequality in learning regionally and nationally is being revealed. It is only as a community that we can dismantle the Mexican Room.

Conclusion and Implications

We examined histories of Latinx education evoking the Mexican Room to heed a warning about how remote learning can be detrimental to emergent bilingual students who rely heavily on bilingual peers for information about the social practices of language use and for translation and clarification of learning tasks. We sounded a similar alarm for their parents, who have a disproportionate classification as essential workers and who, in the geographies of the New Latino South, may face working conditions that put them in daily peril, creating precarity and risk in the era of COVID-19. We pointed to emerging studies on COVID-19 that consider the impacts on Latinx populations and to a chronology of how COVID-19 unfolded in a public school of the southeastern United States in which the transition from a pre-COVID-19 set of agreements about schooling had to be set aside as the world shifted into a COVID-19 reality. Finally, we examined emerging survey data of Latinx parent respondents. These narratives all suggest that, again, Latinx parents are leading transformations in their children's schooling through their assertions about the shortcomings in remote learning, and they signal that their children's learning profiles are more complex and thus require appropriate supports—making suggestions about pedagogy and how to meet special needs. They offer ideas on how to support Latinx parent involvement, reminding schools to include interpreters in the remote learning environment. As they have done throughout history, Latinx parents assume their role in transforming their children's formal learning environments, rejecting the segregation and isolation of the Mexican Room.

Latina/o/x parents, educators, and public servants have made insightful observations that begin to set policy recommendations for providing a higher quality education to Latina/o/x ELS. Latino parents have pointed out the complex learning profile that bilingual children bring to the classroom and the implication this has for sustaining language supports (e.g., interpretation and translation) in virtual learning environments; structuring peer interactions so that Latinx ELS can interact with bilingual peers for academic support; providing school support to Latinx EL students and parents around the use of hardware, software, and access to the internet; and not interrupting the specialized services that children with special needs receive. Public servants have called for universal access to technology for all students (Valade et al. 2021). David Valade, a language acquisition specialist at the Massachusetts Department of Elementary and Secondary Education, has also amplified parent voices by calling for on-demand interpreters, as federal law mandates but rarely guarantees. Valade and colleagues (2021) notes that providing language interpretation must be a priority in schools in recognition of the need to support families: "We need to reach out to our families, be able to speak their languages, have cultural brokers. We cannot rely on the kindness of staff; we need to do this professionally. We need to bridge that gap; it is a community—we are all together. We are not isolated from others."

Fordham University professor Diana Rodríguez, participating in that same forum, put forth a framework for schools and communities to ensure that lessons learned from the COVID-19 pandemic are not lost. She notes that coordination, collaboration, communication, and continuity are critical to improving services for ELs and their families. Coordination must include understanding family needs and availability with regard to family members' work schedules; moreover, it implies having effective communication, of which interpretation services and providing continuous support to parents of ELs are essential components. Continuity of services should include a one-on-one support line as well as a bilingual homework hotline. Effective models have emerged. For example, Hannah Gill at the University of North Carolina at Chapel Hill prepared undergraduate students with some knowledge of Spanish to tutor Latinx elementary school–aged students by phone and on online platforms. An instant waiting list emerged as information on this program reached the Latino community.

Extrapolating from what teachers and parents have observed during remote teaching and learning is that students may need mental-health support as they return to the physical classroom. Latinx ELs, as well as other students, may have experienced the loss of family members, prolonged food insecurity, and isolation. The loss of structure and social life that school can offer may have had a profound impact on K-5 students, and teachers, social workers, parents, and the entire school community will want to be vigilant and proactive. Federal law on school-based interpretation services must be followed and school leaders (e.g., superintendents, parents, and principals) must agitate for adequate funding and aggressively hire bilingual staff and interpreters. Schools must offer parent workshops on the use of technology, potentially partnering with universities that offer degrees in instructional technology, and they must use these resources to develop e-learning modules in multiple languages for parents and caregivers. Schools must agitate for lush federal funding to develop or improve disaster-preparedness plans that include partnerships with healthcare providers, foodbanks and local/corporate grocers, mental-health specialists, and bilingual volunteers to formulate community responses to local problems. Schools must consider the distinct student profiles among their student populations and include in their disaster-response plans specific contingencies and interventions to support student groups according to their unique needs and strengths.

The COVID-19 pandemic has resulted in the critical interaction with EL teaching and learning and a renewal of commitments made long ago with ELS and their families and teachers. Any sufficient response will (at least) require proposing equity-focused policy and practices, such as universal access to technology, equitable education for children with complex learning profiles, support for parents through on-demand interpretation, similar supports for their children with online homework hotlines, and one-to-one academic support. The message has been that education, like health, cannot be a by-product of privilege. To make such an education a reality will require a reimagining of the community we constitute, and through that, an emphatic rejection of the re-emergence and permanence of the Mexican Room.

NOTES

The parent survey reported here was supported by the Institute of Education Sciences, US Department of Education, through Grant R305A180336 to Duke University. The opinions expressed are those of the authors and do not represent views of the Institute or the US Department of Education.

1. It is now common to use Latinx as a nonbinary designation of the Latino community. Following the decision of the Latina/o/x Research Special Interest Group of the American Educational Research Association, we use Latina, Latino, Latinx and Latina/o/x interchangeably to recognize both binary and nonbinary gender identification and the distinct areas of research that Latina/o/x researchers and others undertake (e.g., Chicana feminist research, Latino masculinities research, Latinx Trans research, etc.).

2. English Learners (ELS) is the federal designation for students whose home language is not English and, therefore, must learn English while they learn academic content in English (Education Commission of the States [ECS] 2014). English as a Second Language (ESL) is the English-language instructional program most bilingual school children are enrolled in; some may be enrolled in dual language programs, which require a balanced population of monolingual English speakers and emergent bilingual students, and all students learn both English and the dominant second language simultaneously. Finally, some ELS may be enrolled in bilingual programs, in which children academically develop their home language as they are introduced to and develop English. Dual language and some bilingual programs are considered additive programs because they add a second language through the academic instruction of literacy and academic content in both languages, while ESL programs are considered subtractive because they do not engage or develop students' home language academically, resulting in language loss of that language.

3. Hispanic is a federal designation; Latina/o/x are designations used by the community, media and in academic writing. Latina/o/x is inclusive of individuals and nations in which Spanish is not spoken (e.g., Brazil, Haiti) but that are geopolitically linked to Latin America. We use Hispanic when the source cited uses this term.

REFERENCES

Au, Wayne. 2004. "No Child Left Untested: The NCLB Zone—Where 'Highly Qualified' Can Mean Low-Quality Teaching." *Rethinking Schools* 19, no. 1 (Fall). https://rethinkingschools.org/articles/the-nclb-zone/.

Babinski, Leslie M., Steven Amendum, Steven Knotek, Marta Sánchez, and Patrick Malone. 2018. "Improving Young English Learners' Language and Literacy Skills through Teacher Professional Development: A Randomized Controlled Trial." *American Educational Research Journal* 55, no. 1 (February): 117–43.

Blanco, Maria. 2010. "Before Brown, There Was Mendez: The Lasting Impact of *Mendez v. Westminster* in the Struggle for Desegregation." *Perspectives.* March, 1–6. https://socialequity.duke.edu/wp-content/uploads/2022/01/BEFORE-BROWN-THERE-WAS-MENDEZ-PERSPECTIVES-MARCH-2010-THE-LASTING-IMPACT-OF-MENDEZ-V.-WESTMINSTER-IN-THE-STRUGGLE-FOR-DESEGREGATION.pdf.

Cano, Regina Garcia, Bryan Anderson, Meghan Hoyer, Adrian Sainz, and David Collins. 2020. "COVID-19 Is Ravaging Latino Communities." *Hispanic Outlook in Higher Education.* July. https://www.hispanicoutlook.com/articles/covid-19-ravaging-latino-communities.

Cano, Regina Garcia, Anita Snow, and Bryan Anderson. 2020. "COVID-19 Is Ravaging America's Vulnerable Latino Communities." *AP News.* June 19.

Cano, Regina Garcia, and Carolyn Thompson. 2020. "ELLs Face Unique Challenges during Pandemic." *Hispanic Outlook in Higher Education.* April. https://www.hispanicoutlook.com/articles/ells-face-unique-challenges-during-pandemic.

CDC (Centers for Disease Control and Prevention). 2021. "Risk for COVID-19 Infection, Hospitalization, and Death by Race/Ethnicity." February 18. https://www.cdc.gov/coronavirus/2019-ncov/covid-data/investigations-discovery/hospitalization-death-by-race-ethnicity.html.

Cervantes-Soon, Claudia G., Lisa Dorner, Deborah Palmer, Dan Heiman, Rebecca Schwerdtfeger, and Jinmyung Choi. 2017. "Combating Inequalities in Two-Way Language Immersion Programs: Toward Critical Consciousness in Bilingual Education Spaces." *Review of Research in Education* 41, no. 1 (March): 403–27.

ECS (Education Commission of the States). 2014. "50-State Comparison: What ELL Training, if Any, Is Required of General Classroom Teachers?" November. http://ecs.force.com/mbdata/mbquestNB2?rep=ELL1415.

Faulstich Orellana, Marjorie. 2009. *Translating Childhoods: Immigrant Youth, Language, and Culture.* New Brunswick, NJ: Rutgers University Press.

Fillmore, Lily Wong. 1991. "When Learning a Second Language Means Losing the First." *Early Childhood Research Quarterly* 6, no. 3 (September): 323–46.

Gándara, Patricia, and Gabriel Baca. 2008. "NCLB and California's English Learners: The Perfect Storm." *Language Policy* 7, no. 3 (September): 201–16.

Gándara, Patricia, and Gary Orfield. 2010. *A Return to the Mexican Room: The Segregation of Arizona's English Learners.* The Civil Rights Project/Proyecto Derechos Civiles, University of California, Los Angeles. https://files.eric.ed.gov/fulltext/ED511322.pdf.

Godoy, Maria, and Daniel Wood. 2020. "What Do Coronavirus Racial Disparities Look Like State by State?" *NPR.* May 30. https://www.npr.org/sections/health-shots/2020/05/30/865413079/what-do-coronavirus-racial-disparities-look-like-state-by-state.

Goodman, James. 2020. "The Essential, the Undocumented: COVID-19 Exposes the Fallacy and Danger of Donald Trump's Anti-immigrant Crusade." *Progressive* 84, no. 3 (June): 38–41.

Gould, Elise, and Heidi Shierholz. 2020. "Not Everybody Can Work from Home: Black and Hispanic Workers Are Much Less Likely to be Able to Telework." *Working Economics Blog,* Economic Policy Institute. March 19. https://www.epi.org/blog/black-and-hispanic-workers-are-much-less-likely-to-be-able-to-work-from-home/.

Hinton, Kip Austin. 2015. "We Only Teach in English": An Examination of Bilingual-in-Name-Only Classrooms. In *Research on Preparing In-Service Teachers to Work Effectively with Emergent Bilinguals,* edited by Yvonne S. Freeman and David E. Freeman, 265–89. Bingley, UK: Emerald Group.

Knotek, Steven E., and Marta Sánchez. 2017. "Madres Para Niños: Engaging Latina Mothers as Consultees to Promote Their Children's Early Elementary School Achievement." *Journal of Educational and Psychological Consultation* 27, no. 1: 96–125.

Latino Decisions. 2020. "Momento Latino—COVID-19 y Nuestros Niños: School Re-Opening Survey." https://latinodecisions.com/polls-and-research/momento-latino-covid19-y-nuestros-ninos-school-re-opening-survey/.

Madrid, E. Michael. 2008. "The Unheralded History of the Lemon Grove Desegregation Case." *Multicultural Education* 15, no. 3 (Spring): 15–19.

Mangual Figueroa, Ariana. 2013. "Citizenship Status and Language Education Policy in an Emerging Latino Community in the United States." *Language Policy* 12, no. 4 (November): 333–54.

Moore, Jazmyn T., Jessica N. Ricaldi, Charles E. Rose, Jennifer Fuld, Monica Parise, Gloria J. Kang, Anne K. Driscoll et al. 2020. "Disparities in Incidence of COVID-19 among Underrepresented Racial/Ethnic Groups in Counties Identified as Hotspots during June 5–18, 2020—22 States, February–June 2020." *Morbidity and Mortality Weekly Report* 69, no. 33: 1122–26.

National Center for Education Statistics. 2018. "Number and Percentage Distribution of English Language Learner (ELL) Students in Public Schools and Number of ELL Students as a Percentage of Total Public School Enrollment, by the 10 Most Commonly Reported Home Languages of ELL Students: Fall 2018." https://nces.ed.gov/programs/coe/indicator/cgf.

National Center for Education Statistics. 2021. "Racial/Ethnic Enrollment in Public Schools." https://nces.ed.gov/programs/coe/pdf/2021/cge_508c.pdf.

Powers, Jeanne M. 2008. "Forgotten History: Mexican American School Segregation in Arizona from 1900–1951." *Equity and Excellence in Education* 41, no. 4: 467–81.

Powers, Jeanne M., and Lirio Patton. 2008. "Between *Mendez* and *Brown: Gonzales v. Sheely* (1951) and the Legal Campaign against Segregation." *Law and Social Inquiry* 33, no. 1: 127–71.

Rodriguez-Diaz, Carlos E., Vincent Guilamo-Ramos, Leandro Mena, Eric Hall, Brian Honermann, Jeffrey S. Crowley, Stefan Baral et al. 2020. "Risk for COVID-19 Infection and Death among Latinos in the United States: Examining Heterogeneity in Transmission Dynamics." *Annals of Epidemiology* 52 (December): 46–53.e2. https://doi.org/10.1016/j.annepidem.2020.07.007.

Rozenfeld, Yelena, Jennifer Beam, Haley Maier, Whitney Haggerson, Karen Boudreau, Jamie Carlson, and Rhonda Medows. 2020. "A Model of Disparities: Risk Factors Associated with COVID-19 Infection." *International Journal for Equity in Health* 19, article 126 (July): 1–10.

Ruiz, Vicki L. 2001. "South by Southwest: Mexican Americans and Segregated Schooling, 1900–1950." *OAH Magazine of History* 15, no. 2 (Winter): 23–27. https://doi.org/10.1093/maghis/15.2.23.

Spring, Joel. 2016. *Deculturalization and the Struggle for Equality: A Brief History of the Education of Dominated Cultures in the United States.* 8th ed. New York: Routledge.

US Census Bureau. 2020. Quick Facts: United States. https://www.census.gov/quickfacts/fact/table/US/RHI725219.

Valade, David, Diane Rodriguez, Francesca Di Silvio, and Shondel Nero. 2021. "Family Engagement and Digital Equity: Strategies for Staying Connected with Families of Multilingual Students." Webinar, Center for Applied Linguistics, Washington, DC. June 24. https://www.cal.org/resource-center/research-to-policy-series/family-engagement-and-digital-equity.

Valencia, Richard R. 2005. "The Mexican American Struggle for Equal Educational Opportunity in *Mendez v. Westminster*: Helping to Pave the Way for *Brown v. Board of Education*." *Teachers College Record* 107, no. 3 (March): 389–423.

Valencia, Richard. 2008. *Chicano Students and the Courts: The Mexican American Legal Struggle for Educational Equality.* New York: NYU Press.

Valenzuela, Angela. 1999. *Subtractive Schooling: US-Mexican Youth and the Politics of Caring.* Albany: State University of New York Press.

Wallace, Jared. 2013. "*Mendez et al. v. Westminster et al.*'s Impact on Social Policy and Mexican American Community Organization in Mid-century Orange County." *Voces Novae* 5, article 8: 124–47.

Wasley, Andrew, Christopher D. Cook, and Natalie Jones. 2018. "Two Amputations a Week: The Cost of Working in a US Meat Plant." *Guardian.* July 5. https://www.theguardian.com/environment/2018/jul/05/amputations-serious-injuries-us-meat-industry-plant.

Wood, Daniel. 2020. "As Pandemic Deaths Add Up, Racial Disparities Persist—and in Some Cases Worsen." *NPR.* September 23. https://www.npr.org/sections/health-shots/2020/09/23/914427907/as-pandemic-deaths-add-up-racial-disparities-persist-and-in-some-cases-worsen.

World Bank. 2019. "Record High Remittances Sent Globally in 2018." Press release. April 8. https://www.worldbank.org/en/news/press-release/2019/04/08/record-high-remittances-sent-globally-in-2018.

10. COVID-19, Higher Education, and Social Inequality

ADAM HOLLOWELL AND N. JOYCE PAYNE

More than four thousand institutions of higher education enroll nearly twenty million students in the United States across a mixture of public and private nonprofit colleges and universities and for-profit entities. Among those four thousand institutions are 101 Historically Black Colleges and Universities (HBCUS); 32 Tribal Colleges and Universities (TCUS); and 539 Hispanic-Serving Institutions (HSIS); community colleges, research universities, women's colleges, cosmetology colleges; and Christian, Jewish, and Islamic universities. Higher education is at once sprawling and stretched thin.

This chapter considers what impact social and economic changes stemming from the COVID-19 pandemic will have on existing racial and class inequalities in higher education in the years ahead. From the economic forces of global recession to the installation of plexiglass barriers in college classrooms, the pandemic has wrought havoc across all sectors of higher education. Colleges and universities now must face long-term questions that cut to the very core of their mission: Are campuses safe? Can institutions remain financially solvent? How will online education transform the on- and off-campus experience? Can college be an engine of social mobility?

We consider these questions, and others, through the lenses of economic trends in higher education, campus closures and online learning, student and faculty experiences, and student debt and for-profit education. We also consider the future of pedagogy in higher education and conclude with reflections on the state of the sector in the years and decades to come.

Economic Trends and Impacts on Higher Education

Higher education is big business, but its financial foundations are increasingly unstable. The sector employs about three million people and contributed $600 billion of spending to the US gross domestic product in 2017–2018 (Paxson 2020). State aid to public colleges and universities plummeted during the Great Recession, and in most states spending per student, adjusted for inflation, remains well below prerecession spending (Altschuler and Wippman 2020).[1] In fact, inflation-adjusted state funding for public two- and four-year colleges in the 2017–2018 school year was $6.6 billion below what it was in 2007–2008 (Mitchell, Leachman, and Saenz 2019). In November 2019, months before the pandemic hit the United States, *Forbes* examined the financial health of nine hundred private colleges and universities, giving more than six hundred schools a rating of C or D (Schifrin and Coudriet 2019).

Economic losses associated with COVID-19 will drive drastic financial changes in higher education in the years ahead. First, the repercussions of federal austerity will be vast. The CARES Act, signed into federal law on March 27, 2020, included $14 billion for higher education; it also suspended federal loan payments for six months for some holders and offered protections from collectors garnishing wages for loan payments (Snyder 2020). These federal dollars were woefully insufficient and inequitably distributed. The ten largest for-profit universities in the United States received more than $32 million in direct cash assistance (Wakamo 2020). Meanwhile, community colleges received just 27 percent of funds while enrolling 39 percent of all college students (Whistle 2020).

By August 2020 over five hundred colleges and universities showed signs of financial distress (Dennis 2020). Robert Zemsky, professor at the Graduate School of Education at the University of Pennsylvania, predicted that two hundred schools will close permanently in the coming five years (Korn, Belkin, and Chung 2020). This is in part due to the paucity of the federal response—while the CARES Act supplied $14 billion to higher education, the American Council on Education estimated that colleges and universities would need more than $120 billion to cover health-related preparations, expected losses in revenue, and emergency financial aid in the 2020–2021 academic year alone (Lomax et al. 2020).

Second, endowments and philanthropic contributions will remain down, as evidenced by recent economic downturns. During the Great Recession, from 2007 to 2008, philanthropic giving dropped nearly 12 percent from 2007 to 2008, and university endowments dropped on average by 23 percent (Friga 2020). HBCUS will face particularly acute challenges in the wake of the COVID-19 pandemic.

HBCU endowments are, on average, one-eighth the size of endowments at historically white colleges and universities (Thurgood Marshall 2020). Gregory N. Price, professor of economics at the University of New Orleans, noted that in 2019 the top seven historically white universities received $2.94 billion in donations. During that same year the 101 HBCUs received $43 million total (Toldson, Price, and Gasman 2020).

Smaller endowments mean a greater reliance on tuition, which entails greater financial volatility in unstable economic times. In other words, relative to wealthier historically white institutions, HBCUs operate on thinner margins and with a disproportionately higher risk of financial trouble as a result of the pandemic (Lomax et al. 2020). Since financial stability is one aspect of accreditation renewal, colleges and universities—and especially HBCUs and TCUs—may risk losing their accreditation (Toldson, Price, and Gasman 2020). If schools lose accreditation, it will be nearly impossible for them to retain students and survive.

Third, enrollments may not return to prepandemic levels. Even before the pandemic, college enrollments were down 11 percent since 2011 across every sector of higher education—spanning public state schools, community colleges, for-profits, and private liberal arts schools (Nadworny 2019, 2020). COVID-19's arrival drove even sharper declines. The National Student Clearinghouse Research Center found that undergraduate enrollment dropped 2.5 percent in fall 2020 and 5.9 percent in spring 2021 (St. Amour 2020c; Weissman 2021). Community colleges faced particularly sharp declines—down 9.5 percent in fall 2020 and 11.3 percent in spring 2021 (Weissman 2021).

Enrollments typically rise during economic recessions, but widespread unemployment and wealth depreciation because of the COVID-19 pandemic will force institutions to provide higher levels of support to students with financial need in the years ahead, and concerns about campus health and safety are expected to depress enrollment numbers independent of economic factors (Friga 2020). The challenges will be even greater at HBCUs, which serve a disproportionate number of first-generation students (52 percent) and Pell Grant eligible students (74 percent), those whose family income is less than $20,000 per year. Ninety-four percent of students at public HBCUs receive some form of financial aid (Thurgood Marshall 2020).

Friga (2020) provides a concrete example of how drastically these three factors can impact a state university's budget. In 2009, in the wake of the Great Recession, the University of North Carolina at Chapel Hill lost $25 million in state support, $30 million in philanthropic giving, and $297 million in endowment returns—a total loss of revenue of $352 million, or 25 percent of the previous year's operating revenue (Friga 2020). A gap of that size cannot be closed with a mere increase of tuition rates, a development push for additional gifts, or spending from the "rainy day" portion of an endowment base. In late July 2020 UNC Board of Governors Chairman Randall Ramsey asked each chancellor of the seventeen universities in the UNC system to prepare a proposal that would reflect a budget cut of up to 50 percent (Brown and Rao 2020).

The UNC system includes five HBCUs that serve around 27,000 students and have produced nearly a half million graduates. A system-wide budget cut of 50 percent would drastically curtail the economic and social benefits that thriving HBCUs, as well as their students and alumni, provide to the state, in addition to the vast benefits of the entire UNC system. To give just two examples, in 2018–2019, students at North Carolina Central University contributed nearly 200,000 hours in public service, adding the equivalent of $5.1 million to the state's economy. A report by the United Negro College Fund (UNCF) estimates that HBCUs in North Carolina added more than $7 billion to the state economy in 2014 and $14 billion annually to the US economy (UNCF 2020).

Robert Kelchen (2020) has noted that previous financial shocks "have generally hit colleges on either the revenue or the expenditure sides of the ledger, but the coronavirus pandemic has hit both, simultaneously." The changes wrought by COVID-19 were swift, devastating, and tumultuous. From month to month, week to week, and even day to day in 2020, higher education was confronted with new and daunting challenges. These began with campus closures and the abrupt transition to entirely online learning.

Campus Closures and Online Learning

By the end of March 2020, over one thousand colleges and universities had closed their campuses because of COVID-19, immediately thrusting fourteen million students into remote online learning (Hess 2020). By the end of May, the California State University system announced that each of its twenty-three campuses would be closed to in-person instruction in the fall 2020 semester, even after the system lost $460 million in nonmedical campus operations through the end of the spring 2020 semester (Burke 2020; APLU 2020). In early August, Harvard announced that 20 percent of its incoming class had deferred enrollment (Krantz and Fernandes 2020). On August 17 the University of North Carolina at Chapel Hill—which had tried to remain open for the fall semester—had 177 positive coronavirus cases among students and a 14 percent positivity rate for student tests. The school closed the campus and sent students packing after less than two weeks of in-person instruction (Fausset 2020).

The impact of campus closures and remote learning on higher educational attainment may not be clear for several years, but early indications are deeply troubling, especially for students from disadvantaged populations. In general, students in online classes withdraw more often and earn lower grades than students in traditional classrooms (Glazier 2016). According to Bettinger et al. (2017), enrolling in an online course reduces student grades in future courses by one-eighth of a standard deviation. It also lowers the probability of the student remaining enrolled in college one year later by more than 10 percent (2017). Online students are more likely to drop out of college altogether, as compared to students enrolled in in-person or hybrid courses (Dynarski 2018). These trends might be explained by a weaker commitment to education among remote students, but the evidence points instead to more traditional vectors of disparity and disadvantage. Bettinger and Loeb observe that online courses are especially challenging for "the least well-prepared students," a notably strange euphemism (2017, 2). Additional research found that for the most academically disadvantaged students, college retention in online courses was 28 percent lower than for students in face-to-face classes (Patel 2020).

Students may also have faced a host of challenges in their quarantine homes, including food insecurity, financial stress, housing concerns, and a lack of resources to complete their academic work (Wood 2020; Cohen 2019; Fry and Barroso 2020). Moreover, campus closures likely exacerbated economic and racial disparities in online education and broadband access, particularly at schools that already serve disproportionately higher numbers of economically vulnerable students. Thirty-four percent of black Americans did not have high-speed internet access at home in 2019, compared to 21 percent of white Americans (Pew Research Center 2021). Lower-income students may not have had reliable internet access or private spaces for studying during the pandemic (Paxon 2020). An open letter published on August 3, 2020, from the presidents of six organizations that represent over six million students at minority serving institutions (MSIS) named federal funding for broadband access as an essential component of educational equality amid COVID-19 and in the years ahead (Lomax et al. 2020).

Opening campuses threatened even worse outcomes in the form of racialized health vulnerabilities. From the start of the pandemic, members of black, American Indian, and Hispanic groups were at greater risk for severe illness and death from COVID-19 as a result of long-standing health inequities in the United States (Braithwaite and Warren 2020, 2). Risk of death from COVID-19 among young adults was five to nine times higher among black, Hispanic, and indigenous young adults (Bansal, Carlson, and Kraemer 2020). The same health disparities visible throughout the population were present on college and university campuses among both students and staff when campuses pushed to reopen in 2020–2021. A survey of more than five thousand students across seventeen HBCUs in June 2020 found that many were dealing with difficulties such as sick family members, worsening mental health, financial trouble, and stress from the pandemic and visible anti-black police violence (St. Amour 2020b).[2]

Student, Staff, and Faculty Experiences in Higher Ed during the COVID-19 Pandemic

It has long been argued that race and class influence educational content and delivery in ways that perpetuate inequality (e.g., Watkins, Ayers, and Quinn 2001). In recent years, colleges and universities have frequently touted progress in admitting and graduating greater numbers of students facing social, racial, and economic inequalities. Schools that are successful in closing attainment gaps often point to the efficacy of "high touch" wraparound services for vulnerable students, including social, physical, and mental-health services; financial aid, professional development, and career preparation; and early interventions for academic support. Perhaps no school has been more highly praised and profiled in this area than Georgia State University, an urban research university that has nearly doubled its graduation rate in the past twenty years through a combination of predictive analytics, targeted micro-grants, and other student support programs (Goral 2016; Stern 2017; McMurtrie 2018).

Campus-based services shuttered overnight in the wake of widespread campus closures and the abrupt transition to entirely remote learning due to COVID-19. As Vimal Patel (2020) notes, "How do you do high touch in what has suddenly become a 'no touch' world? . . . For students who already struggle to stay enrolled, and for the institutions who say they are committed to keeping them, the COVID-19 crisis may be a make-or-break moment." Many students were enrolled in "no-touch" higher education well before COVID-19's arrival, and many will continue to do so long after the rollout of vaccines. Forty percent of high school graduates who enroll in college enroll in community colleges, which are less likely to have on-campus student health offices (Zimmerman 2020).[3]

Colleges and universities are now facing intensified scrutiny about worker safety, fair compensation, and stratified benefits in a post-COVID labor market. Nearly three-fourths of all teaching jobs in higher education today are not tenure eligible, and nontenure-track positions offer lower wages, fewer benefits, and little job security (Al-Gharbi 2020, 21; Nzinga 2020, 56).[4] Financial and institutional benefits accrue along lines of race and gender—tenure-track faculty are disproportionately white and male, while adjuncts are disproportionately women and nonwhite (Al-Gharbi 2020, 22; Afinogenov 2020, 44). The pandemic highlighted this increasing precarity: in one instance, the State University of New York denied an instructor's request to teach remotely in 2020 given that K-12 schools and day cares were closed, saying that caring for a child did not qualify as a reason to stay home under the federal Americans with Disabilities Act (Hartocollis 2020).[5]

College students are also college workers more now than ever before. In 1960, 25 percent of full-time college students between the ages of sixteen and twenty-four worked while enrolled. Five decades later, national statistics show that, on average, more than 70 percent of all undergraduates are working. Twenty percent of all undergraduate students are employed full time, year-round. Among the 52 percent of all students who work part time, half work more than twenty hours per week (Goldrick-Rab 2016). Forty-three percent of HBCU students rely on jobs to cover their basic living expenses (Williams 2020a).

And then there are staff—who often have even fewer protections than students and faculty. Roopika Risam has noted that "while research shows that administrators, tenure-line faculty and librarians at universities are overwhelmingly white, black, brown, and indigenous people are relatively better represented in staff positions and among service employees," positions like student services, dining services, maintenance, groundskeeping, and custodians (2020). The same reasons that explain disproportionate incidence of COVID-19 and mortality among black Americans in the general labor force apply to black Americans working in higher education: an overrepresentation in "essential" jobs where social distancing is impossible, an underrepresentation in access to healthcare, and a higher probability of being poor (Graham et al. 2020). These workers faced even greater vulnerability at smaller rural colleges, which were more likely to be farther from hospitals with sufficient capacity during times of peak COVID-19 hospitalizations (Dynarski 2020).

Illustratively, when Florida State University announced a policy that staff could lose their right to work from home if they were discovered to be simultaneously caring for children or other dependents, the policy applied to university staff but not faculty (Mangan 2020). While the public discourse around universities reopening has largely focused on faculty teaching remotely or students missing out on the campus experience, the workers most likely to face penalties for school closures, dependent care, and health risks were, and continue to be, staff in lower-paid, less-protected positions.

COVID-19, Student Debt, and "Lower Ed"

Many Americans imagine higher education as a space of social mobility. As Jonathan Zimmerman notes, "We like to imagine college as an egalitarian force, which reduces the gap between rich and poor. But over the past four decades it has mostly served to reinforce or even to widen that gap" (Zimmerman 2020; Nzinga 2020).[6] According to Jeffrey Aaron Snyder, "Nine in ten children with family incomes above $100,000 access postsecondary education, compared to six in ten of children with family incomes below $50,000" (2020). Stratification is particularly drastic at top-tier private research universities. A 2017 *New York Times* report found that thirty-eight colleges in America, including five in the Ivy League, enroll more students from the top 1 percent of household income than from the bottom 60 percent (Aisch et al. 2017).

Education debt reinforces inequalities in enrollment and rising costs, with Americans holding, in total, more than $1.5 trillion in student debt (Zimmerman 2020). Even with access to federal Pell Grants and institutional financial aid, low-income students have a higher likelihood of borrowing money to pay for college than their peers (Mitchell, Leachman, and Saenz, et al. 2019). Debt is particularly prevalent among black students: in 2016, 85 percent of black graduates across all higher education institution types graduated with debt, compared to just under 70 percent of their white peers (Mitchell et al. 2019).

Debt becomes particularly burdensome for students enrolled in for-profit colleges, where "the new economy's job crisis produced the behemoth for-profit college crisis of debt, constrained choices, and poor labor market returns, not the other way around" (Cottom 2018, 14). In *Lower Ed*, Tressie McMillan Cottom describes how for-profit colleges and universities "organized to commodify social inequalities," noting that prospective for-profit college and university students "are considered a valuable asset only insofar as our social conditions keep producing them" (2018, 11, 21). For example, enrollment at for-profit colleges climbed 24 percent at the height of the Great Recession (Butrymowicz and Kolodner 2020), demonstrating the link between economic crisis for students and economic boon for lower ed. The COVID-19 pandemic compounded and exacerbated this pattern, suggesting that the current moment will generate the asset value of potential students and present an economic opportunity to for-profit colleges.

Unlike many smaller private schools with little to no endowment and public schools that are subject to state budgets, the parent companies of for-profit colleges often have considerable cash reserves to bolster marketing and student retention services (Butrymowicz and Kolodner 2020). The *New York Times* reported that the for-profit Ashford University hired two hundred new "enrollment advisers" in summer 2020 to handle the uptick in inquiries from potential students during the pandemic (Butrymowicz and Kolodner 2020). It was reported that the University of Arizona "acquired" Ashford University in early August 2020, but the fine print outlined an agreement by the University of Arizona to provide services to Ashford's parent company, Zovio, which also receives 19.5 percent of the revenue from the partnership (Korn, Belkin, and Chung 2020). Tellingly, Zovio's stock price hit its all-time high at closing two days after the partnership was announced (MacroTrends 2020).

As for-profit college becomes an even higher-risk, more expensive proposition for students, it will nonetheless be a risk that students will likely feel compelled to take. As Cottom (2017) notes, "The more insecure people feel, the more they are willing to spend money for an insurance policy against low wages, unemployment, and downward mobility. Those least likely to have an insurance policy that our labor market values are people for whom higher education has always been a long shot: poor people, single parents, the socially isolated, African Americans, the working class." Higher education must create additional and more accessible avenues to debt-free public college, and federal regulations must keep the predatory operations of for-profit colleges in check.

Higher Education after COVID-19: Bold Ideas for Reform

The COVID-19 pandemic made it clear that the status quo of higher education will have to change in the decades to come. In the final section, we outline bold ideas for higher education reform that can increase access, equalize outcomes, and facilitate social mobility.

State and federal leaders should prioritize equitable and debt-free access to higher education as well as the widespread alleviation of crippling student-loan debt. The widespread temporary suspension during the COVID-19 pandemic of SAT and ACT test requirements for undergraduate college admissions should become permanent. Nikole Hannah-Jones has recommended special legacy admissions programs for native-born black descendants of American slavery (2020). An immediate step would be to double the maximum Pell Grant award for students (Lomax et al. 2020).

Expanding access is a necessary but insufficient first step.[7] As Patel (2020) notes, "The promise of higher education as an engine of social mobility rests on whether it can deliver on the commitment to get [students] to the finish line." The most vulnerable students will face the greatest obstacles in the years after this pandemic—from a lack of internet access and other technologies at home, to unsafe homes or lack of money for travel, to a loss of access to campus jobs, healthcare, and other support services. Higher education must establish and develop the resources and networks to enable its students to thrive in classrooms of all formats.

For example, John Warner has called for universities to conduct expansive research on effective methods to provide student support through distance learning programs (2020). William A. Darity Jr., an editor of this book, has called for targeted research on admissions practices for racial inclusion (2019). Sara Goldrick-Rab has called for higher education to implement robust antipoverty programs, including cash transfers directly to students in times of crisis and modernization of emergency aid programs. Colleges should also increase administrative aid to students who are eligible for federal unemployment insurance and Supplemental Nutrition Assistance Program (SNAP) benefits, just as they help students fill out their Free Application for Federal Student Aid (FAFSA) (Godrick-Rab 2020). All student services, including health, psychological, and financial services, should be made accessible remotely for students who will not return to a traditional campus environment (Mintz 2020; Hollowell, Swartz, and Proudman 2021).

The shift to online learning provides new opportunities to assess the racial equity and disability accessibility of higher education for students and faculty (St. Amour 2020a; Hamraie 2020). Immediately, colleges and universities should require that all online course materials contain image descriptions and alt-text for all images and videos, captions and/or transcripts for all videos, and OCR (optical character recognition) for all PDF documents (Hamraie 2020). Attendance should no longer be a part of course grades, and the system of requiring doctor's notes for excused absences should end, permanently.

Pedagogy will also have to stretch beyond the classroom in ways that advance equity and access.[8] As Zimmerman (2020) has observed, there is a sad irony in the increasingly common suggestion that higher education needs a "student success movement." How did higher education come to be about anything else? In reality, just 20 percent of two- and four-year college professors cite institutional reasons for student failure. Most professors blame lack of student effort or skill, even as research demonstrates the crucial role played by active instruction, student support, and institutional equity as drivers of success (Zimmerman 2020).

One tangible step would be to expand the formats and requirements for student work across levels and promotion in graduate programs toward greater equity and public service in academic research outputs (Foley 2020, 19). Another would be to set new course design expectations for faculty to ensure equitable education access for disabled students and others who may face periodic interruptions to health, internet access, and/or on-campus resources. Regardless of *why* a student may not operate according to prepandemic faculty standards, universities must require faculty to provide nondiscriminatory avenues to participation and completion of course requirements (Hamraie 2020).

The Social Sciences Feminist Network (SSFN) has called for colleges and universities to elevate the visibility of "invisible" labor. For example, women perform a disproportionate amount of "care work" within the academy, including teaching, mentoring, and service, which leaves them less time for the things that really "count" for tenure and promotion at research institutions (2017, 231).[9] Deborah Harley uses the phrase "Maids of Academe" to describe the disproportionate institutional assignment of service labor to black women in predominantly white institutions (2008). The SSFN suggests linking this work to the economic value of student retention, which can validate nonresearch faculty work and offers "an effective strategy for encouraging institutions to see, count, and reward these labors" (2017, 241). This same strategy would serve to increase the visibility of nonwhite faculty, who face unequal service burdens within the academy (Joseph and Hirshfield 2011).

Marybeth Gasman, executive director of the Rutgers Center for Minority Serving Institutions, has noted the essential function of wraparound services to student success and retention at HBCUs, whose budgets rely heavily on enrollment and tuition. She told Safiya Charles and Byron Dobson (2020) that "one of the things we've noticed is they are working really, really hard to foster a sense of community. . . . That's a big deal. Some might argue that this is touchy-feely, but touchy-feely equals retaining students, which equals enrolling students, which equals alumni donations, which equals an overwhelming positive impression of the institution." Similar to SSFN's call to recognize care work, this call to name and claim the economic value of wraparound services to overall institutional financial sustainability is of the utmost importance.

Targeted support for black students is crucial, not just in the aftermath of the COVID-19 pandemic but in preparation for future global public-health events. Ronald Braithwaite and Rueben Warren have called for comprehensive access to early, sustained, and affordable access to healthcare for vulnerable students, including coverage of hospitalization (2020, 2). Representatives of over six million students at MSIs called for the creation of a National Institute on Minority Health and Health Disparities (Lomax et al. 2020).

The federal government should pass legislation to support economically vulnerable higher education institutions, especially HBCUs and TCUs. For example, Gregory Price recommended a federal coronavirus stimulus package that would provide $1,000 for every enrolled student at an HBCU per academic year (Toldson, Price, and Gassman 2020).[10] Other MSI leaders have called for federal investment of $10 billion in HBCUS, TCUS, HSIS, PBIS, and other institutions (Lomax et al. 2020). These funds are as necessary now as they were in 2020, even as we have passed the worst of the pandemic's threats to public health.

Research must be a central focus of federal funding to MSIS. Of $5.558 billion expenditures in fiscal year 2017 for federal research funding from the National Science Foundation (NSF), less than one-fourth of 1 percent ($13.8 million) went to TCUS. And of all federal spending on research and development in FY 2018, HBCUS received $400.349 million—a mere 0.67 percent of total federal spending. If the federal government set aside 15 percent of all spending on research and development for MSIS, the net investment would be $6.5 billion in funding (Lomax et al. 2020). Moreover, colleges and universities must increase access to STEM fields for students from traditionally underrepresented populations, given projected employment sector growth in engineering, life and physical sciences, and computer and information systems (Tippett and Stanford 2019; Mammen and Guerdan 2019).

Research is essential to the mission of higher education in the United States and around the world. The coming decades must include new avenues of international exchange and a rejection of regressive nationalist policies that overshadow the myriad benefits of conducting research with scholars around the world on global health, energy, and the environment. There is an urgent need to recognize that higher education can serve as a "pathway to the empowerment of people" only inasmuch as it promotes and expands social mobility (Altbach and Salmi 2011, xiii).

Conclusion

The measure of a country's greatness is its ability to retain compassion in times of crisis. —US Supreme Court Justice Thurgood Marshall

Historically Black Colleges and Universities have served as a counterforce to exclusionary politics since the founding of Cheyney University of Pennsylvania in 1837. They have educated students to be powerful agents in the work of social transformation, as evidenced sixty years ago when four black students from

North Carolina A&T State University walked into a Woolworth's for lunch and helped ignite the civil rights movement. Against these daunting and tumultuous times, HBCUs have continued to offer what Thurgood Marshall called the greatness of retaining compassion in a time of crisis.

The years after the COVID-19 pandemic will be no time for business as usual, and HBCUs can provide the model for resilient institutions that build resilient students. "HBCUs have an important tradition and history of helping black students to be successful to weather any storm," Bennett College President Suzanne Walsh told the *Washington Post*. "We help our students while they're on campus learn how to be successful, how to navigate a volatile, uncertain, complex, and ambiguous world in a safe place" (Ferguson 2020). Harry Williams, president of the Thurgood Marshall College Fund, echoes Walsh: "The presidents and chancellors at HBCUs are steeped in the knowledge and experience of leading under pressure. In spite of limited resources, they have demonstrated the kind of dogged determination they've always shown during times of crisis" (Williams 2020b). As we build the postpandemic academy, we must look for new ways of teaching and learning as well as for new ways of using this opportunity to create and assiduously defend a new social order that reaffirms rising expectations for HBCUs and the students they serve.

Hua Hsu (2020) issued the prophet's call to higher education in the heat of 2020: "If we survive this pandemic, we must wean ourselves off the hierarchies and inequalities of our profession. They hinder our ability to engage with the broader public, whose support and patronage we need to survive." This call will ring true until we heed it. Labor and justice movements outside of the academy have offered a vision of the way forward: rent strikes amid economic devastation; walkouts by Amazon fulfillment workers and service employees throughout the gig economy; and growing demands for loan and debt forgiveness, prison abolition, and the defunding of police forces across the country (Kanuga and Dhillon 2020). Racial justice protests during the spring and summer of 2020 also brought issues of social equity to the center of the conversation about higher education.

Whatever colleges and universities will look like in the years and decades to come, the moral demand for racial justice is clear: Center on the health and safety of black students, staff, and faculty. Prioritize social mobility through equitable and debt-free access to higher education. Abandon the commitment to hierarchy and inequality that has characterized so much of higher education's past. Teach and learn in ways that build lasting communities of social, racial, and political equity.

NOTES

Thank you to Rachel Proudman for research assistance in the preparation of this chapter.

1. During the Great Recession, for example, between 2008–2009 and 2009–2010, the average financial-aid grant per undergraduate increased by 22 percent. Colleges, universities, and the federal government picked up about 70 percent of the increase, with loans from the federal government also increasing substantially (Altschuler and Wippman 2020).

2. For this reason, on July 20, Spelman College, Morehouse College, and Clark Atlanta University announced that they would move to virtual instruction for the fall 2020 semester, well before wealthier southern historically white institutions such as the University of North Carolina at Chapel Hill (Guzman 2020). Morehouse College led the way in cancelling fall sports in late June (Risam 2020), while Clemson University had an outbreak with thirty-seven football players testing positive for COVID-19 in June and July (Kreidler 2020).

3. Even students in "high touch" campus environments will face obstacles to health and other wraparound services as schools face budget shortfalls in the years ahead. One in six traditional four-year colleges and universities does not provide on-campus, school-run student health services (Lemly et al. 2014).

4. Disparities are most pronounced at the level of full professor (Social Sciences Feminist Network 2017, 228). Among the lower ranks, more than 40 percent of faculty at four-year and two-year colleges don't have full-time positions, which decreases access to health insurance coverage (Pettit 2020, 34).

5. Malav Kanuga and Jaskiran Dhillon have noted that during COVID-19, college instructors—60 percent of them adjuncts and nontenure track—"have been asked to do the impossible: to maintain the university's status quo as the world breaks apart" (2020).

6. Sekile Nzinga's recent book observes that "neoliberalism's economic and social stronghold on higher education is not evenly distributed but is racialized and gendered, which disproportionately impacts underrepresented women of color" (2020, 12).

7. As Cottom has noted, "Access is a useful frame for some questions but is anemic in the face of globalization, growing inequality, and privatization" (2019, xv).

8. As Aimi Hamraie (2020) has noted, many of the "hacks" that higher education is promoting to increase accessibility to remote students were first developed as survival strategies by disabled and immunocompromised students who wanted equal access to classroom learning.

9. According to the Social Sciences Feminist Network, women make up 51 percent of nontenured instructors and lecturers, 46 percent of assistant professors, 36 percent of associate professors, and only 21 percent of full professors" (2017, 229–230). Similar trends operate along lines of race, with white faculty occupying almost 90 percent of positions at the ranks of associate and full professors (2017, 230).

10. Price notes that for a private HBCU like Bennett College in Greensboro, North Carolina, "this would translate into approximately $500,000 to offset declines in housing revenue" and other losses due to the pandemic (Toldson, Price, and Gassman 2020).

REFERENCES

Afinogenov, Greg. 2020. "Tenure Is Not Worth Fighting For." *Chronicle of Higher Education*. January 24. https://www.chronicle.com/article/tenure-is-not-worth-fighting-for/.

Aisch, Gregor, Larry Buchanan, Amanda Cox, and Kevin Quealy. 2017. "Some Colleges Have More Students from the Top 1 Percent Than the Bottom 60. Find Yours." *New York Times*. January 18. https://www.nytimes.com/interactive/2017/01/18/upshot/some-colleges-have-more-students-from-the-top-1-percent-than-the-bottom-60.html.

Al-Gharbi, Musa. 2020. "Universities Run on Disposable Scholars." *Chronicle of Higher Education*. May 1. https://www.chronicle.com/article/universities-run-on-disposable-scholars/.

Altbach, Philip G., and Jamil Salmi, eds. 2011. *The Road to Academic Excellence: The Making of World-Class Research Universities*. Washington, DC: World Bank Publications.

Altschuler, Glenn C., and David Wippman. 2020. "Higher Education's 'To-Do' List—The Consequences of Coronavirus." *The Hill*. July 20. https://thehill.com/opinion/education/494687-higher-educations-coronavirus-to-do.list.

APLU (Association of Public and Land Grant Universities). 2020. "Public Higher Ed Groups Urge Congress to Extend Coronavirus Response Tax Relief to Public Institutions." July 20. https://www.aplu.org/news-and-media/News/public-higher-ed-groups-urge-congress-to-extend-coronavirus-response-tax-relief-to-public-institutions.

Bansal, Shweta, Colin Carlson, and John Kraemer. 2020. "There Is No Safe Way to Reopen Colleges This Fall." *Washington Post*. June 30. https://www.washingtonpost.com/outlook/2020/06/30/there-is-no-safe-way-reopen-colleges-this-fall/.

Bettinger, Eric, and Susanna Loeb. 2017. "Promises and Pitfalls of Online Education." *Evidence Speaks Reports* (Economic Studies at Brookings) 2, no. 15 (June): 1–4.

Bettinger, Eric P., Lindsay Fox, Susanna Loeb, and Eric S. Taylor. 2017. "Virtual Classrooms: How Online College Courses Affect Student Success." *American Economic Review* 107, no. 9 (September): 2855–75. https://doi.org/10.1257/aer.20151193.

Braithwaite, Ronald, and Rueben Warren. 2020. "The African American Petri Dish." *Journal of Health Care for the Poor and Underserved* 31, no. 2 (May): 491–502. https://doi.org/10.1353/hpu.0.0026.

Brown, Stacia, and Anita Rao. 2020. "Budget Cuts, Health Risks Loom for UNC System Campuses and Workers." WUNC.org. July 22. https://www.wunc.org/post/budget-cuts-health-risks-loom-unc-system-campuses-and-workers.

Burke, Michael. 2020. "First in Nation, California State University to Close Campuses for In-Person Instruction This Fall." EdSource. May 12. https://edsource.org/2020/california-state-university-classes-to-continue-mostly-online-in-fall/631381.

Butrymowicz, Sarah, and Meredith Kolodner. 2020. "For-Profit Colleges, Long Troubled, See Surge amid Pandemic." *New York Times*. June 17. https://www.nytimes.com/2020/06/17/business/coronavirus-for-profit-colleges.html.

Charles, Safiya, and Byron Dobson. 2020. "Historically Black Colleges Fight for Survival, Reopening amid Coronavirus Pandemic." *USA Today*. June 9. https://www.usatoday.com/story/news/education/2020/06/09/coronavirus-hbcu-colleges-fall-semester-2020/5286165002/.

Cohen, Diedre. 2019. "Homelessness on Campus." CBS News. January 20. https://www
.cbsnews.com/news/homelessness-on-campus-the-toughest-test-faced-by-tens-of
-thousands-of-college-students-in-america/.

Cottom, Tressie McMillan. 2017. "For-Profit Colleges Thrive Off of Inequality." Atlantic.
February 22. https://www.theatlantic.com/education/archive/2017/02/the-coded
-language-of-for-profit-colleges/516810/.

Cottom, Tressie McMillan. 2018. Lower Ed: The Troubling Rise of For-Profit Colleges in the
New Economy. New York: New Press.

Cottom, Tressie McMillan. 2019. "Foreword." In The Credential Society: An Historical
Sociology of Education and Stratification, by Randall Collins. New York: Columbia University Press. First published 1979.

Darity, William A., Jr. 2019. A New Agenda for Eliminating Racial Inequality in the United
States: The Research We Need. New York: William T. Grant Foundation.

Dennis, Marguerite J. 2020. "Evaluate Post-COVID-19 Threats to Higher Education."
Student Affairs Today 23, no. 9 (December): 6. https://doi.org/10.1002/say.30822.

Dynarski, Susan. 2018. "Online Courses Are Harming the Students Who Need the
Most Help." New York Times. January 19. https://www.nytimes.com/2018/01/19
/business/online-courses-are-harming-the-students-who-need-the-most-help.html.

Dynarski, Susan. 2020. "College Is Worth It, but Campus Isn't." New York Times. June 29.
https://www.nytimes.com/2020/06/29/business/college-campus-coronavirus-danger
.html.

Fausset, Richard. 2020. "Outbreaks Drive UNC Chapel Hill Online after a Week of
Classes." New York Times. August 17. https://www.nytimes.com/2020/08/17/us/unc
-chapel-hill-covid.html.

Ferguson, Amber. 2020. "How the Protest Movement Could Help HBCUs through
Higher Education's Financial Crisis." Washington Post. July 2. https://www
.washingtonpost.com/education/2020/07/02/how-protest-movement-could-help
-hbcus-through-school-year-upended-by-covid-19/.

Foley, Nadirah Farah. 2020. "Don't Forget about Graduate Students." Chronicle of Higher Education. March 31. https://www.chronicle.com/article/dont-forget-about-graduate-students/.

Friga, Paul N. 2020. "Under COVID-19, University Budgets Like We've Never Seen Before." Chronicle of Higher Education. Accessed May 4, 2020. https://www.chronicle.com
/article/Under-Covid-19-University/248574.

Fry, Richard, and Amanda Barroso. 2020. "Amid Coronavirus Outbreak, Nearly Three-
in-Ten Young People Are Neither Working nor in School." Pew Research Center (blog).
July 29. https://www.pewresearch.org/fact-tank/2020/07/29/amid-coronavirus
-outbreak-nearly-three-in-ten-young-people-are-neither-working-nor-in-school/.

Glazier, Rebecca A. 2016. "Building Rapport to Improve Retention and Success in Online Classes." Journal of Political Science Education 12, no. 4: 437–56. https://doi.org/10
.1080/15512169.2016.1155994.

Goldrick-Rab, Sara. 2016. Paying the Price: College Costs, Financial Aid, and the Betrayal of
the American Dream. Chicago: University of Chicago Press.

Goldrick-Rab, Sara. 2020. "Real College for Real Students." Chronicle of Higher Education.
April 10. https://www.chronicle.com/article/How-Will-the-Pandemic-Change/248474.

Goral, Tim. 2016. "Creating the Modern Urban Research University: Behind Georgia State University's Data-Driven Success." *University Business* 19, no. 3: 10.

Graham, Carol, Yung Chun, Michal Grinstein-Weiss, and Stephen Roll. 2020. "Well-Being and Mental Health amid COVID-19: Differences in Resilience across Minorities and Whites." *Brookings Institute* (blog). June 24. https://www.brookings.edu/research /well-being-and-mental-health-amid-covid-19-differences-in-resilience-across -minorities-and-whites/.

Guzman, Joseph. 2020. "As Coronavirus Surges in Georgia, HBCUs Move to Online Classes for Fall Semester." *The Hill*. July 20. https://thehill.com/changing-america/well-being /prevention-cures/508203-atlanta-hbcus-move-to-online-classes-for-fall.

Hamraie, Aimi. 2020. "Accessible Teaching in the Time of COVID-19." Mapping Access. March 10. https://www.mapping-access.com/blog-1/2020/3/10/accessible-teaching-in -the-time-of-covid-19.

Hannah-Jones, Nikole. 2020. Twitter, August 14, 9:23 a.m. https://twitter.com /nhannahjones/status/1294263294178594816.

Harley, Debra A. 2008. "Maids of Academe: African American Women Faculty at Pre-dominately White Institutions." *Journal of African American Studies* 12, no. 1 (March): 19–36. https://doi.org/10.1007/s12111-007-9030-5.

Hartocollis, Anemona. 2020. "A Problem for College in the Fall: Reluctant Professors." *New York Times*. July 3. https://www.nytimes.com/2020/07/03/us/coronavirus-college -professors.html.

Hess, Abigail. 2020. "How Coronavirus Dramatically Changed College for over 14 Million Students." CNBC. March 26. https://www.cnbc.com/2020/03/26/how-coronavirus -changed-college-for-over-14-million-students.html.

Hollowell, Adam, Jonas J. Swartz, and Rachel Proudman. 2021. "Telemedicine Access and Higher Educational Attainment." *Journal of American College Health*, March 24. https://doi.org/10.1080/07448481.2021.1891085.

Hsu, Hua. 2020. "The Purpose of Our Profession Is at Risk." *Chronicle of Higher Education*. April 10. https://www.chronicle.com/article/How-Will-the-Pandemic-Change /248474.

Joseph, Tiffany D., and Laura E. Hirshfield. 2011. "'Why Don't You Get Somebody New to Do It?' Race and Cultural Taxation in the Academy." *Ethnic and Racial Studies* 34, no. 1: 121–41. https://doi.org/10.1080/01419870.2010.496489.

Kanuga, Malav, and Jaskiran Dhillon. 2020. "Beyond Survival Strategies." *Chronicle of Higher Education*. April 10. https://www.chronicle.com/article/How-Will-the-Pandemic -Change/248474.

Kelchen, Robert. 2020. "Liquidity, Liquidity, Liquidity." *Chronicle of Higher Education*. April 10. https://www.chronicle.com/article/How-Will-the-Pandemic-Change/248474.

Korn, Melissa, Douglas Belkin, and Juliet Chung. 2020. "Coronavirus Pushes Colleges to the Breaking Point, Forcing 'Hard Choices' about Education." *Wall Street Journal*. April 30, 2020. https://www.wsj.com/articles/coronavirus-pushes-colleges -to-the-breaking-point-forcing-hard-choices-about-education-11588256157.

Krantz, Laura, and Deirdre Fernandes. 2020. "At Harvard, Other Elite Colleges, More Students Deferring Their First Year." *Boston Globe*. August 6. https://www.bostonglobe

.com/2020/08/06/metro/harvard-other-elite-colleges-more-students-deferring-their
-first-year/.

Kreidler, Mark. 2020. "Coronavirus Is Placing College Sports on Hold, Putting Students, University Budgets, and Entire Towns at Risk." *Time*. August 3. https://time.com /5874483/college-football-coronavirus/.

Lemly, D. C., K. Lawlor, E. A. Scherer, S. Kelemen, and E. R. Weitzman. 2014. "College Health Service Capacity to Support Youth with Chronic Medical Conditions." *Pediatrics* 134, no. 5 (November): 885–91. https://doi.org/10.1542/peds.2014-1304.

Lomax, Michael L., Harry L. Williams, Lezli Baskerville, Antonio R. Flores, Carrie L. Billy, and Rita Pin Ahrens. 2020. "Letter to Richard Shelby and Lamar Alexander." August 3. https://www.hacu.net/images/hacu/govrel/08032020ResponseToHEALSAct.pdf.

MacroTrends. 2020. "Zovio Inc—Stock Price History | ZVO." Accessed August 7, 2020. https://www.macrotrends.net/stocks/charts/ZVO/zovio-inc/stock-price-history.

Mammen, Taylor, and Ryan Guerdan. 2019. "2019 STEM Job Growth Index." RCLCO.com. January 31. https://www.rclco.com/publication/2019-stem-job-growth-index/.

Mangan, Katherine. 2020. "Working While Parenting Is a Reality of Covid-19. One University Tried to Forbid It." *Chronicle of Higher Education*. July 1. https://www.chronicle .com/article/Working-While-Parenting-Is-a/249107.

McMurtrie, Beth. 2018. "How Georgia State U. Made Its Graduation Rate Jump." *Chronicle of Higher Education*. May 25. https://www.chronicle.com/article/georgia-state-u -made-its-graduation-rate-jump-how/.

Mintz, Steven. 2020. "Reimagining Higher Education Post-coronavirus." *Higher Ed Gamma* (*Inside Higher Ed* blog). April 14. https://www.insidehighered.com/blogs /higher-ed-gamma/reimagining-higher-education-post-coronavirus.

Mitchell, Michael, Michael Leachman, and Matt Saenz. 2019. "State Higher Education Funding Cuts Have Pushed Costs to Students, Worsened Inequality." Center on Budget and Policy Priorities. October 24. https://www.cbpp.org/research/state-budget -and-tax/state-higher-education-funding-cuts-have-pushed-costs-to-students.

Nadworny, Elissa. 2019. "Fewer Students Are Going to College. Here's Why That Matters." NPR.org. December 16. https://www.npr.org/2019/12/16/787909495/fewer -students-are-going-to-college-heres-why-that-matters.

Nadworny, Elissa. 2020. "Can Colleges Survive Coronavirus? 'The Math Is Not Pretty.'" NPR.org. April 20. https://www.npr.org/2020/04/20/833254570/college-brace-for -financial-trouble-and-a-big-question-will-they-reopen-in-fall.

Nzinga, Sekile M. 2020. *Lean Semesters: How Higher Education Reproduces Inequity*. Baltimore, MD: Johns Hopkins University Press.

Patel, Vimal. 2020. "COVID-19 Is a Pivotal Moment for Struggling Students. Can Colleges Step Up?" *Chronicle of Higher Education*. April 14. https://www.chronicle.com /article/Covid-19-Is-a-Pivotal-Moment/248501.

Paxson, Christina. 2020. "College Campuses Must Reopen in the Fall. Here's How We Do It." *New York Times*. April 26. https://www.nytimes.com/2020/04/26/opinion /coronavirus-colleges-universities.html.

Pettit, Emma. 2020. "The New Tenured Radicals." *Chronicle of Higher Education*. April 23. https://www.chronicle.com/article/the-new-tenured-radicals/.

Pew Research Center. 2021. "Demographics of Internet and Home Broadband Usage in the United States." *Pew Research Center: Internet, Science and Tech* (blog). https://www.pewresearch.org/internet/fact-sheet/internet-broadband/.

Risam, Roopika. 2020. "Reopening Schools Safely Can't Happen without Racial Equity." CNN. July 2. https://www.cnn.com/2020/07/02/opinions/covid-19-colleges-racial-equality-risam/index.html.

Schifrin, Matt, and Carter Coudriet. 2019. "Dawn of the Dead: For Hundreds of the Nation's Private Colleges, It's Merge or Perish." *Forbes*. November 27. https://www.forbes.com/sites/schifrin/2019/11/27/dawn-of-the-dead-for-hundreds-of-the-nations-private-colleges-its-merge-or-perish/.

Snyder, Jeffrey Aaron. 2020. "Higher Education in the Age of Coronavirus." *Boston Review*. April 30. http://bostonreview.net/forum/jeffrey-aaron-snyder-higher-education-age-coronavirus.

Social Sciences Feminist Network Research Interest Group. 2017. "The Burden of Invisible Work in Academia: Social Inequalities and Time Use in Five University Departments." *Humboldt Journal of Social Relations* 39: 228–45.

St. Amour, Madeline. 2020a. "Financial Disparities among HBCUs, and between the Sector and Majority-White Institutions." *Inside Higher Ed*. July 27. https://www.insidehighered.com/news/2020/07/27/financial-disparities-among-hbcus-and-between-sector-and-majority-white-institutions.

St. Amour, Madeline. 2020b. "Survey: HBCU Students Struggling during Pandemic." *Inside Higher Ed*. July 31. https://www.insidehighered.com/quicktakes/2020/07/31/survey-hbcu-students-struggling-during-pandemic.

St. Amour, Madeline. 2020c. "Final Fall Enrollment Numbers Show Pandemic's Full Impact." *Inside Higher Ed*. December 17. https://www.insidehighered.com/news/2020/12/17/final-fall-enrollment-numbers-show-pandemics-full-impact.

Stern, Gary M. 2017. "How Georgia State University's Micro-grants Are Keeping Students Enrolled and Raising Graduation Rates." *Hispanic Outlook in Higher Education* 28, no. 2: 9–10.

Thurgood Marshall College Fund. 2020. "About HBCUs." *Thurgood Marshall College Fund* (blog). Accessed August 12, 2020. https://www.tmcf.org/about-us/member-schools/about-hbcus/.

Tippett, Rebecca, and Jessica Stanford. 2019. *North Carolina's Leaky Educational Pipeline and Pathways to 60 Percent Postsecondary Attainment*. Report for the John M. Belk Endowment, Carolina Population Center, University of North Carolina at Chapel Hill. https://NCedpipeline.org.

Toldson, Ivory A., Gregory N. Price, and Marybeth Gasman. 2020. "COVID-19 Closures Could Hit Historically Black Colleges Particularly Hard." *Conversation*. March 24. http://theconversation.com/covid-19-closures-could-hit-historically-black-colleges-particularly-hard-134116.

UNCF. 2020. "HBCU Economic Impact Report." Accessed August 8, 2020. https://uncf.org/programs/hbcu-impact.

Wakamo, Brian. 2020. "Instead of Bailing Out For-Profit Colleges, Congress Should Cancel Student Debt." Inequality.org. June 15. https://inequality.org/great-divide/private-colleges-student-debt/.

Warner, John. 2020. "Lurching toward Fall, Disaster on the Horizon." *Just Visiting (Inside Higher Ed* blog). June 28. https://www.insidehighered.com/blogs/just-visiting/lurching-toward-fall-disaster-horizon.

Watkins, William H., William Ayers, and Therese Quinn. 2001. *The White Architects of Black Education: Ideology and Power in America, 1865–1954*. New York: Teachers College Press.

Weissman, Sara. 2021. "Spring Brings Even Steeper Enrollment Declines." *Inside Higher Ed*. April 29. https://www.insidehighered.com/news/2021/04/29/spring-brings-even-steeper-enrollment-declines.

Whistle, Wesley. 2020. "Next Stimulus Should Help Community Colleges." *Forbes*. August 4. https://www.forbes.com/sites/wesleywhistle/2020/08/04/next-stimulus-should-help-community-colleges/.

Williams, Harry L. 2020a. "How TMCF Is Responding to COVID-19." *Thurgood Marshall College Fund* (blog). Accessed August 8, 2020. https://www.tmcf.org/events-media/tmcf-in-the-media/how-tmcf-is-responding-to-covid-19/.

Williams, Harry L. 2020b. Personal communication to N. Joyce Payne, August 20, 2020.

Wood, Sarah. 2020. "Coronavirus Pandemic Has Impacted College Students' Mental Health." *Diverse Issues in Higher Education*. April 14. https://diverseeducation.com/article/173412/.

Zimmerman, Jonathan. 2020. "What Is College Worth?" *New York Review of Books*. July 2. https://www.nybooks.com/articles/2020/07/02/what-is-college-worth/.

11. The Rebirth of K-12 Public Education: Postpandemic Opportunities

KRISTEN R. STEPHENS, KISHA N. DANIELS, AND ERICA R. PHILLIPS

Given the challenges we face, education doesn't need to be reformed—it needs to be transformed. —Sir Ken Robinson

What can the future of education be for every student? The opportunity to urgently respond to and act upon this question is perhaps the silver lining of the COVID-19 pandemic. Over the last several decades in education, there has been "so much reform and so little change" (Payne 2008), almost as if equity-based reform efforts have been on a treadmill with advocates working tirelessly while gaining limited traction. This lack of progress in ameliorating inequities in K-12 education is due to many factors, including (1) the inability to sustain reforms—even those that show promise—due to lack of adequate resources, a desire for a "quick fix," and/or the inability to scale-up the reform effort; (2) other education reform initiatives (i.e., school choice, standardized testing) that serve to counter or cancel the impact of equity-based education reform initiatives (Selig 2020); and (3) structural fragmentation and a lack of coherence that has prevented widespread institutionalization of equity-based reforms (Fullan 2000).

While the literature base is replete with examinations of the issues surrounding equity and access issues in education, the aim of this chapter is to present a path forward by detailing a systematic process (in phases) by which a new education model can be born with equity at its heart. It is important to note that the proposed "rebirth" process is not meant to merely "tweak" the current education paradigm but is presented to support efforts to completely reconceptualize how an equity-focused, K-12 education should look moving forward. The goal is to leave the past system behind and begin anew, to vigorously challenge existing education paradigms, and to audaciously think and plan for the future of K-12 education in the United States.

The COVID-19 Pandemic's Impact on Students and Learning

In mid-March 2020, when COVID-19 spread across the United States, school districts, concerned about the health and well-being of students and staff, shifted to remote learning. This decision impacted almost fifty-one million public school students, all of whom had no other option but to learn from home (Decker, Peele, and Riser-Kositsky 2020). Teachers immediately began modifying their lesson plans and teaching methodology to begin teaching remotely, often using technology they had never used before. However, despite these efforts, many educators were dismayed by technology glitches, poor attendance in virtual classes, and the lack of student participation—especially from nonwhite students and those with low-income backgrounds.

Teachers grew frustrated when they were unable to get into contact with their most vulnerable students. Some students were absent because they did not have access to the technology or WiFi to participate in virtual classes. Others were unable to complete their school work because they had to take on additional familial responsibilities, such as becoming the primary caregivers for younger siblings stuck at home while their parents worked. Students also expressed to their counselors that their parents or family members had fallen ill and that they were just trying to survive and, as a result, could not focus on school (Strauss 2020). Richard Rothstein (2020) highlighted the experiences of families as follows:

> Many white-collar professionals with college degrees [were operating] home schools, sometimes with superior curricular enhancements. . . . Meanwhile, many parents with less education have jobs that even during the coronavirus crisis cannot be performed at home—supermarket clerks, warehouse workers, delivery truck drivers. Even with distance learning being established by schools and teachers—many of whom are now busy with their own children at home—too many students in low-income and rural communities don't have internet access: 35 percent of low-income households with school-aged children don't have high-speed

internet (Anderson and Perrin 2018); for moderate-income families it is 17 percent, and only 6 percent for middle-class and affluent families. When measured by race and ethnicity, the gap is greater for African American and Hispanic families.

The catastrophe of the COVID-19 pandemic exposed the inequities of schooling, not just to those who participated in K-12 schooling efforts but also to the entire nation.

LEARNING LOSS AND THE ACHIEVEMENT GAP

In the midst of the pandemic, research projected that students nationwide would return to school in the fall of 2020 with roughly 70 percent of learning gains in reading relative to a typical school year and less than 50 percent gains in math (Kuhfeld et al. 2020). However, most students did not return to traditional, face-to-face instruction in fall 2020 as anticipated. Educators, parents, and others feared that learning losses would continue to expand the longer schools remained closed. Both the lack of assessment data and wide variances in learning loss projections among researchers have complicated the process of quantifying the pandemic's effect on student learning progress.

There is no precedent for the extended absences from school that the COVID-19 pandemic has created. The largest span of time that has been studied previously is the traditional summer break. Harris Cooper and his team were among the first to prove that extended periods away from school and learning can produce an average of one-tenth of a standard deviation reduction in test scores—and that around two months away from school can equal one month of learning regression (Cooper et al. 1996). This phenomenon is commonly referred to as "summer slide." As mentioned previously, the effects of summer slide are more detrimental for low-income students, as they may not have access to academic enrichment over the summer months. Conversely, students from middle- and upper-class backgrounds gain approximately one month of reading skills because of their participation in summer enrichment opportunities (Cooper et al. 1996). The data regarding summer learning loss have been reproduced time and time again, proving that when students experience extended periods of absence from school, it can be detrimental—especially for students from lower socioeconomic backgrounds, because of their lack of access to resources and opportunities to practice school skills over the summer break.

As more data are collected, academics are convinced that the impact of remote learning during the COVID-19 pandemic will be much more significant than a traditional summer slide. Using the framework from Cooper and colleagues

(1996), if students have a learning loss accounting for approximately half of the time they are away from school, this would mean that students may have potentially lost nearly an entire academic year of learning during the pandemic. However, educational researchers from Brookings reported that COVID-19-related learning loss (coined "the COVID slump") may be even more detrimental than previous estimates because of the psychological tolls accompanying the pandemic (Golinkoff et al. 2020). Neuroscientists have long studied the impact of toxic stress on certain areas of the brain, specifically the amygdala, which assists in retaining long-term memories. The Brookings team projected that the toxic stress associated with living in a pandemic will exacerbate the usual rate in which the summer slide is typically calculated. As can be assumed, these extra stressors will have an even greater effect on low-income students who, being disproportionately nonwhite students, have an even higher stress level because of uncertain financial status and unpredictable housing, and whose family members may have higher exposure to COVID-19 through their duties as essential workers (Golinkoff et al. 2020). The impacts of the COVID slump can only be tabulated once schooling resumes in a stable, traditional sense, but it can be reasonably inferred that the results will be concerning and detrimental for these students in the long term.

Even in instances where learning resumed remotely, learning loss is expected. McKinsey and Company created a statistical modeling estimate to analyze three different scenarios of remote learning: (a) students with an average-quality remote instruction; (b) students with lower-quality remote instruction; and (c) students with inconsistent or no remote instruction. The estimate shows that in any of the epidemiological scenarios, whether in person, remote for one semester, or remaining remote for the entire school year, all three types of student learning environments led to students experiencing "significant" learning loss, with students with inconsistent or low engagement losing over one year of learning (Dorn et al. 2020, 4).

Low-income students and students of color are projected to feel the effects of the learning loss the most, stemming from poorly funded schools and inadequate teacher preparation paired with a lack of resources at home. An average student with remote learning for approximately one year will experience an average of seven months of learning loss, but a black student will have 10.3 months of loss; a Hispanic student 9.2 months of loss; and low-income students (a category overly represented by black and Hispanic students) will lose 12.4 months of academic learning. With these contrasting remote-learning environments, the achievement gap between white students and nonwhite students is projected to widen (Dorn et al. 2020, 4).

Although the United States spends more than almost every other country on public education—over seven hundred billion dollars per year—disparities of opportunities and outcomes remain, especially between white students and students of color (Hussar et al. 2020). The achievement gap—"the statistically significant difference between the average test scores of white students compared to other groups, such as black or Latino students"—varies by state and subject but exists in essentially every academic area across all regions of the United States (Phillips 2019). Student performance on assessments reveals that only 18 percent of black fourth graders scored proficient or above in reading, compared to 45 percent of their white peers who scored at this level, with similar gaps in reading proficiency existing between eighth-grade black and white students (McFarland et al. 2019).

McKinsey and Company estimate that learning loss resulting from remote learning will "exacerbate existing achievement gaps by 15 to 20 percent" (Dorn et al. 2020, 6). The gaps have expanded because remote learning requires many assumed physical and environmental materials such as personal computer devices, hotspots, and dedicated work spaces, as well as assistance from others in the home. Furthermore, a blaring digital divide exists.

THE DIGITAL DIVIDE

Perhaps the most visible access challenges that were magnified during the pandemic were those dealing with technology. Regardless of how a student was performing prior to the COVID-19 pandemic, projections indicate a greater learning loss for "minority and low-income children who have less access to technology" (Hobbs and Hawkins 2020). The disparity in access to technology is often referred to in education as "the digital divide."

The sudden shift from face-to-face to virtual learning revealed the real consequences of the digital divide. Suddenly, many students lacked access to education because of the absence of devices and internet access. New York City and Philadelphia were two cities already aware of the large number of students with no computers or internet access. New York City cited approximately 300,000 students without computers (Rothstein 2020), and the Philadelphia School District stated that "many" of its 200,000 students "lack computers or high-speed internet at home" (Dale 2020). Both cities were hesitant to provide any online instruction when the pandemic shifted learning because of these technological inequities. Philadelphia's school superintendent stated, "If it's [online instruction] not available to all children, we cannot make it available to some" (Dale 2020).

In order to accommodate students and proceed with learning, Philadelphia and New York City schools decided to provide weekly work packets for students to pick up until relief could be provided to families in the form of free devices and internet access. However, the majority of school districts across the country did not pursue such an approach. Most decided to try to continue with as much normalcy as possible, with teachers teaching lessons online via Zoom, Google Meet, and similar software, and assigning work via Google Classroom or Canvas. As Tawnell Hobbs and Lee Hawkins succinctly summarize, "problems began piling up almost immediately. In many places, lots of students simply didn't show up online, and administrators had no good way to find out why not. Soon, many districts weren't requiring students to do any work at all, increasing the risk that millions of students would have big gaps in their learning" (2020). Without even measuring academic progress, but in just tracking attendance and work completion, disparities could be seen between students with adequate digital access and those without such access—exposing the potential for learning gaps to widen. Essentially, the digital divide "show[ed] the cracks in the system between the 'have-nots' and the 'haves.'" (Dale 2020).

The digital divide existed long before the pandemic, but COVID-19's arrival merely amplified these disparities in access. Data from the 2013 census, and further investigation from the Pew Research Center, revealed that, on average, one in five teens do not have reliable access to the internet when at home, a share that increases for low-income students. One out of three students whose parents earn $30,000 or less annually do not have internet or technology access at home, compared to less than one in ten students who live in households that earn incomes of $75,000; as Monica Anderson and Andrew Perrin (2018) state, "these broadband disparities are particularly pronounced for black and Hispanic households with school-age children—especially those with low household incomes." Black students are overrepresented in the low-income category, as one in four black students have reported not being able to complete their homework because of a lack of technological resources.

The pandemic not only provided an opportunity to proactively address the digital divide, but it also served to adjust the role technology plays in schools moving forward. Some school districts found ways to provide resources to students and families to ensure that every student had access to the needed technology to maximize their education (i.e., supplying every child with a laptop, tablet, hotspot, etc.). Such initiatives to remedy existing technological disparities, though born out of necessity, now provide opportunities for how schools and learning might be structured in the future. Lifting the barrier of access to technology can encourage the exploration of innovative instructional practices that may never have been fully realized without the pandemic.

ADDITIONAL CHALLENGES

Along with technical challenges, students and families face many practical challenges that have been exacerbated by COVID-19. The loss of family income, food instability, disrupted schedules, changes in household responsibilities, separation from peers, and the sharing of work spaces within the home can all impact a child's learning. As students engage in virtual learning from home, the role of the parent/caregiver in their child's education has intensified.

Parents/caregivers must balance their own work responsibilities while also supporting their child's academic and social-emotional needs. Parental engagement has long been a goal of educators and should be even more of a priority during a pandemic. If parents are to support their child's education at home, they must be equipped with the knowledge and resources to do so effectively; otherwise, educational inequalities will deepen. The COVID-19 pandemic has provided a critical opportunity to reset the relationship between teachers and parents to reveal the true power of parental engagement in helping students learn (Seale 2020).

The pandemic has also given rise to emotional challenges that impact student learning. Stress, anxiety, and trauma-induced depression are expected during times of unprecedented change in a student's life; a pandemic, then, provides an ideal ecosystem for an emotional tsunami to hit. Adverse experiences also negatively impact cognitive functioning, and the more trauma that is experienced, the greater the deficit in learning (Blodgett and Lanigan 2018). The adverse conditions created by COVID-19's arrival have presented an opportune time to strategically develop partnerships between schools and mental-health providers within the community. This is particularly critical given that prior to the pandemic, the average student-to-counselor ratio (430:1) was nearly double the American School Counselor Association's (ASCA) recommended ratio (ASCA 2020).

From Catastrophe to Opportunity

One of the few benefits of the COVID-19 pandemic was the opportunity it facilitated for many to get a glimpse into institutional inequities. More than just the oft-suggested "band-aids" of additional summer school or increased early childhood education will be needed to solve the problems exacerbated by COVID-19.

The challenges that have arisen and/or intensified as a result of COVID-19's arrival are difficult to navigate, but they also present a unique opportunity to reimagine what the US educational system could be if racial, ethnic, and economic disparities were eradicated. Of course, educational policies alone cannot remedy these inequities; massive, systemic social reform must occur in tandem. As the general public comes to recognize the K-12 education system as essential to the success of the country's economic recovery, perhaps it will finally become a national issue of high priority.

Change will not be easy, as current educational paradigms are deeply rooted and the status quo is a strong inertial foe. Nonetheless, reforms must be bold, as the current educational system was based on supporting an industrial model and was born out of segregation. Creating a new education system designed to align with the needs of the future is daunting, especially since we can only make predictions about what lies ahead for the next generation. However, it no longer makes sense to keep renovating an increasingly inequitable system—especially since the overall infrastructure has weakened considerably under the strain of competing ideologies. The system must be rebuilt upon a foundation with a sturdy frame designed to shepherd all students equitably into the twenty-second century.

Toward a K-12 Education Rebirth: A Plan Forward in Phases

Following is a plan for moving substantive education change forward in phases. Each phase toward a K-12 education rebirth must be thoroughly and thoughtfully considered to ensure every student has an equitable and accessible education.

PHASE 1: RECLAIMING

In recent years, education reform has become of great interest to a variety of political actors. From businesses to think tanks to entrepreneurs, many new voices have entered the K-12 education landscape to promote their ideas for transforming education. Noticeably absent from many of these conversations are teachers. While teachers have been marginalized within the education policy dialogue, their critical role as change agents in school reform efforts is beginning to receive some traction (Imants and Van der Wal 2020; Robinson 2012). This renewed focus on the value of teachers is most likely due to increased insight into the valuable role teachers play in the change capacity of schools, and their role as advocates for students who have frequently been abandoned by the system. The professional judgment of teachers must be restored, as they are best positioned to respond to localized needs by "strategically embracing, reframing, and resisting educational policy as necessary" on behalf of their students (Dover, Henning, and Agarwal-Rangnath 2016, 466)

Albert Bandura (2001) acknowledges that beliefs about one's own efficacy are foundational to agency; however, the efficacy of teachers has been consistently challenged in recent years by politicians, parents, and other education stakeholders. As a result, teachers, to some degree, have lost their agency within their own profession. Their voices must be reclaimed as schools need social justice warriors who stand in direct opposition to those policies and practices that have marginalized children of color. If teachers are not heard or choose not to engage in this important dialogue, then they simply become props in a system that continues to perpetuate inequities (Khan 2016).

Educators must reclaim their voices and agency within the education policy arena. According to social cognitive theory (Bandura 2001), there are three forms of agency:

1. personal, or one's own efforts to influence;
2. proxy, or enlisting others with expertise to influence; and
3. collective, or acting with others on a shared belief to prompt change.

While it seems that educators have been most successful in using collective forms of agency (i.e., unions), in order for substantive equity-based reform to take place, they must employ all three forms of agency. Teachers must find their points of personal power and not underestimate their individual value to education reform efforts. In addition, teachers should seek formidable and influential community, state, and national allies to promote an equity-based education agenda.

In order to reclaim the voices of teachers in education decision making, it is important to consider the structure of the educational system that has contributed to the silencing of teachers. From a sociological perspective, the design of schools has greatly contributed. The lack of classroom autonomy, isolation during the workday, and the use of silence to protect against insubordination have all been cited as reasons for why the voices of teachers have been suppressed (McDonald 1986). In addition, teachers have been recipients of education policy rather than active participants in the policy-making process (McDonald 1986). Often there is the illusion that those in power are sympathetic to teachers, but these sympathies are often disingenuous and result in perceived tokenism. For example, policy makers may speak and write about the important role that teachers have in educating K-12 students but, in practice, fail to obtain testimony and/or insight from teachers when crafting and enacting education policy. In turn, teachers resent and become wary of those who consistently patronize and undercut and exclude them (see Boyer 1983).

Moving forward, it is important to eliminate those factors that constrain teacher agency and support those designed to enable and empower educators (Robinson 2012). Educators are vital benefactors to students who have been neglected by the system. The following recommendations will support teacher agency and assist teachers in reclaiming their critical voice in the education policy arena.

1. *Break the silence.* Build a culture of collegiality and collaboration in schools. The structural design of schools physically separates and isolates educators from one another (McDonald 1986). Schools must be transformed—both in physical space and climate (i.e., interpersonal relationships)—to support and encourage conversation and collaboration among educators around equity and access issues.

2. *Listen.* As internal actors, teachers are intimately connected with the day-to-day functions of the school. As such, they must be repositioned as a central voice in policy making to ensure continuity of policy implementation and the realization of desired results (Ellison et al. 2018; Priestley, Edwards, and Priestley 2012). Teachers must have a "seat at the table," and policy makers, as external actors, should listen and proactively engage with teachers in developing education policy as "externally initiated educational change . . . is highly problematic" (Priestley et al. 2012, 210).

3. *Prepare.* It is essential that preservice and in-service teachers are prepared for "active and constructive roles in education policy" (Heincke, Ryan, and Tocci 2015, 392). Teachers must learn about education policy and understand how policies have historically perpetuated equity and access issues in education. Teachers must engage with policy makers and advocate for those policies designed to counteract deeply rooted practices that have contributed to these persistent inequities. In other words, teachers must be equipped to be active and ardent contributors rather than "passive targets" as schools are revisioned toward equity.

PHASE 2: REFOCUSING

"What is the purpose of education for *all* children?" This purpose has evolved and will continue to fluctuate based on societal needs, but as the world continues to change—more rapidly than ever—the revisiting of this purpose must occur with greater frequency, and the education system must be able to pivot and adapt nimbly as the needs of our country, our communities, and broader humanity shift.

The new purpose of K-12 education should be considered within the context of equity. The purpose should not only consider civic knowledge but also address the dispositions and skills needed to effectively contribute to the well-being of the populace. The purpose should also go beyond meeting workforce needs and seek to improve the human condition (see Strauss 2015).

The public isn't in agreement as to the purpose of education. Roughly 45 percent of citizens indicate that academic achievement is the primary purpose of education followed by citizenship and workforce preparation (both cited at approximately 25 percent; Walker 2016). When Magdalena Slapik (2017) asked students their thoughts on the purpose of education, more profound responses emerged. Students stated the role of education is to broaden one's mind and learn about other cultures, empower students, assist students in finding their passion, and help advance the human race. These student perspectives are more in alignment with what a refocused purpose of education should be moving forward. An equity-focused purpose must extend beyond consideration of the "mind" and also encompass the desired outcomes for the "heart" and "soul" of K-12 students—capturing our hope for the future of humanity.

A collective purpose of education must be grounded in equity. For decades, schools have been working to remedy equity and access issues in education. When the killing of George Floyd in May 2020 spurred national protests and broader actions to address racism and racial inequalities, schools were already hard at work to overcome legacies of inequality. However, the pandemic certainly set schools even further behind on these equity goals. Our current educational system exists within our country's unjust realities; therefore, our education system continues to reflect the broader injustices of society. Inattention to inequities in schools only serves to exacerbate inequities within our broader social systems. Any postpandemic plan for the rebirth of schools that lacks a resounding purpose to eradicate existing inequities will be inherently flawed.

In her 2019 book, *We Want to Do More Than Survive: Abolitionist Teaching and the Pursuit of Educational Freedom*, renowned education professor Bettina Love offers the opinion that our schools today are "spaces of whiteness, white rage, and white supremacy, all of which function to terrorize students of color" (13). Perhaps in response to this view, and in recognition of ongoing events and persistent student achievement gaps, the American Association of School Administrators (AASA) announced that "the work on equity must go further to become actively antiracist. . . . Leading a system-wide effort requires that we ensure that cultural responsiveness permeates all levels of a district" (Brown, Lenares-Solomon, and Deaner 2019, 88). For some, this might sound like a tenable response in the wake of a tragic injustice; however, for most, it comes with the task of accepting the fact that we've all been raised in a society that elevates white culture over others. Thus, a new purpose of education must exude antiracism. It's not enough to eliminate racist practices; we must also champion antiracist policies (see Kendi 2019).

Antiracism means more than "equal treatment and respect." It is an all-encompassing ideology that should enact the constant questioning of one's own actions, motives, and implicit biases along with the actions, motives, and implicit biases of others (Nielsen 2020). Therapist Resmaa Menakem suggests that the process is similar to going through the stages of grief (Farber 2019). Likely, education will go through the same pains of denial, anger, bargaining, depression, and finally acceptance, as a paradigm shift is made to reimagine schools that work for the most marginalized populations.

The following considerations will support the articulation of a new, equity-focused purpose for education.

1. *Focus on mind, heart, and soul.* If the purpose of education is to improve the human condition, a new purpose for education must harmoniously coalesce all aspects of the human experience, as knowledge alone cannot solve equity issues. Compassion; perspective taking; hope; understanding of how privilege, oppression, and power operate; and an awareness of one's own identity, assumptions, and biases should all be foundational components to a refocused purpose of education.

2. *Champion antiracism.* As protests unfolded around police violence against African Americans in Ferguson, Minneapolis, Louisville, and other communities, many education organizations released statements from their leadership calling for solidarity and critical conversations around racism, power, privilege, and oppression (Barnum and Belsha 2020). These support statements often call for the deployment of antiracist and trauma-informed education practices. The attention to such practices needs to expand beyond a reaction to "a moment" and become a proactive and consistent focus of our education system.

3. *Revisit.* As the world continues to change at unprecedented speeds, the purpose of education needs to be revisited with greater frequency to ensure it accurately reflects our aspirations. As systems, policies, and demographics shift, the purpose of education should be assessed and recalibrated as needed to ensure a constant vision toward equity.

How do we imagine our ideal K-12 education system with equity at the heart rather than on the periphery? First, we must both ensure alignment between K-12 education's stated purpose and the overall structure and design of the education system and clarify its relationship between and among other societal systems. By all accounts, the structure of K-12 education has largely been created in a vacuum reflective of a deterministic system; as a result, we have primarily relied on one way of thinking about educational challenges. While the pandemic has further exposed the importance of essential workers and the pernicious flaws within our social, civic, and economic systems, it has also given birth to new debates and insights regarding just how much schools do to support these other public systems.

Schools have served as a staunch safeguard, delivering students warm meals, mental-health support, and instruction while also supervising children as parents and caregivers work (Jesso 2020). The absence of a robust social welfare system in the United States means that schools have become the de facto primary alternative. Listening to political education debates, one would conclude that there is nothing more important to this country than educating our children. However, bureaucrats continue to shoulder K-12 schools with the responsibility of eradicating systemic inequities, often at the expense of the primary task of educating students. While resources wane from year to year, the education system is still expected to do it all. Furthermore, as societal inequities persist, the education system is the convenient scapegoat for deeper, systemic problems that perpetuate inequities.

As schools are newly envisioned, it is imperative that we audit all of the responsibilities that schools have been tasked with and make decisions about which ones are sustainable within the new structure and which ones might be transferred to the responsibility of other community organizations and entities. Presently, educational systems are overtasked with additional roles and responsibilities; in serving those roles, they allow those who should be responsible for tackling systemic racism to remain both blameless and unaccountable.

Revisioning a system of education can level the playing field for all students if we can agree that remedying inequities is nonnegotiable and will require sustained will and resources. The COVID-19 pandemic has highlighted several realities regarding face-to-face versus remote learning, and, moving forward, reconsidering the role of technology in education will be central to any discussion pertaining to educational transformation. As we plan for the future of K-12 education, we must acknowledge these realities: that digital platforms are here to stay, but they are incapable of functioning equitably without large investments in teachers and instructional development; that teachers are irreplaceable and that a highly trained teacher can make a big difference in the lives of students; and that a hybrid delivery approach to schooling isn't just about the reliance on dependable technology and highly qualified personnel but also about a constant desire for innovation and a steadfast appreciation for flexibility.

The teaching and learning process has completely been transformed as a result of COVID-19's presence. Hybrid learning models should become part of the modern education vernacular as well as a component of systematic design for transformation. In a future scenario, schools should be designed to provide a variety of learning options that support unique, individual learning plans—whether instruction is delivered within brick-and-mortar settings or virtually, as well as synchronously or asynchronously.

During the COVID-19 pandemic, many schools made unprecedented pivots in policy and eschewed traditional practices that, for years, had been foundational to our educational system (most notably, grading practices and testing). As we move out of this phase, some of these amended policies should be continued and become the new standard (Pandey 2020). Consequently, as tough as the pandemic has been for families and schools, for many disenfranchised students of color, it has provided an opportunity to shift focus away from targeted compliance and toward equity-driven initiatives.

With the broadening of the conceptualization of the teaching-learning process, the inflexibility of past education paradigms can be challenged. For example, any or all of the following might be considered:

1. Restructuring (or deconstructing) the school day, week, and/or calendar year.
2. Shifting from reliance on high-stakes tests where students solve contrived problems toward performance-based assessments, where students solve relevant, authentic problems.
3. Eliminating grading systems that are purely quantitative and summative (provided at the end of a learning experience) toward use of qualitative, formative measures that provide students with constructive feedback throughout the duration of the learning experience and encourage continued progress and growth toward expertise.
4. Integrating a combination of innovation and flexibility that allows for multiple instructional designs to accommodate diverse learners (face-to-face/synchronous remote; asynchronous virtual/synchronous remote; face-to-face/asynchronous virtual; work site/synchronous remote;

asynchronous virtual/face-to-face and project-based learning [PBL]; work site/face-to-face/asynchronous virtual and PBL, etc.).

5. Reallocating local education agency (LEA) funds to increase or support the reconstitution of school personnel to ensure that every child has a dedicated instructional team (teachers, counselors, instructional coaches, and other support staff). This cluster focus would provide a sustainable model for individualized support that includes both academic instruction and prevention and intervention of student emotional learning (SEL).

6. Allocating federal funding to public and private teacher preparation (undergraduate and graduate) programs that specifically target innovative recruitment and retention efforts to increase black and Latino teachers in classrooms.

Rejuvenation: What We All Gain from Eliminating Racial, Ethnic, and Economic Inequities in Our Pre-K-12 School System

A rejuvenated education system with equity at its heart would greatly improve all our lives. First, a new era of education would ensure that every student's individual learning path is acknowledged, by providing an appropriate range of learning options, methods, and resources. There should be no linear "one size fits most" approach, a dynamic that has held education hostage for decades (Reimers 2020). A true, individualized design could foster a culture of mastery that also increases intellectual, social, and emotional competencies without impending barriers.

Another benefit of an equity-focused education system is that students and families will have increased options within the structure of the public education system. Additionally, school environments will become spaces of expression and pleasure rather than control and regulation (Kirkland 2018), thereby ensuring that every student's individual learning path is acknowledged via options for learning that are as diverse as the students that the system is tasked to serve.

The rebirth of the pre-K-12 education system will mean a different role for government: one that restores public confidence by deeming education as an essential component to a community's infrastructure. Of the sixteen infrastructure sectors identified by the Department of Homeland Security (i.e., agriculture, communications, electricity, financial services, healthcare, transportation systems, water, etc.), education is notably neglected. The aforementioned sectors are defined as those that are "so vital to the United States that their incapacitation or destruction would have a debilitating effect on security, national economic security, national public health, or safety" (Kayyem 2020). Based on this definition, the COVID-19 pandemic has caused education to be considered as essential infrastructure by Americans, elected officials, and communities. This renewed commitment to education could result in a designation of resources, financial and complementary, necessary to reinvent education. Fundamentally, doing what is right for education will require substantial civic mobilization.

We are currently at a crossroads that has provided America with an opportunity to make an ambitious choice. We cannot be deterred by either the existence of deepened tribalism or the push to silence and discredit progressives and social-justice education warriors (see Freedberg 2020; Mac Donald 2018). A true reinvention of how this country educates students goes far beyond the scope of distributing Chromebooks and issuing Zoom links. Public schools deserve a plan that requires a critical and systematic deep dive into its fissures. It is only through this effort that we can design a system that is not only resilient but equitable for all.

REFERENCES

ASCA (American School Counselor Association). 2020. "Student-to-School-Counselor Ratio 2018–2019." https://www.schoolcounselor.org/getmedia/c0351f10-45d1-4812 -9c88-85b071628bb4/Ratios18-19.pdf.

Anderson, Monica, and Andrew Perrin. 2018. "Nearly One-in-Five Teens Can't Always Finish Their Homework Because of the Digital Divide." Pew Research Center. October 26. https://www.pewresearch.org/fact-tank/2018/10/26/nearly-one-in-five-teens -cant-always-finish-their-homework-because-of-the-digital-divide/.

Bandura, Albert. 2001. "Social Cognitive Theory: An Agentic Perspective." *Annual Review of Psychology* 52, no. 1 (February): 1–26. https://doi.org/10.1146/annurev.psych.52.1.1.

Barnum, Matt, and Kalyn Belsha. 2020. "How the Education World Is Responding to George Floyd's Killing." *Chalkbeat*. June 2. https://www.chalkbeat.org/2020/6/2 /21278591/education-schools-george-floyd-racism.

Blodgett, Christopher, and Jane D. Lanigan. 2018. "The Association between Adverse Childhood Experience (ACE) and School Success in Elementary School Children." *School Psychology Quarterly* 33, no. 1: 137–46. https://doi.org/10.1037/spq0000256.

Boyer, E. L. 1983. *High School: A Report on Secondary Education in America*. New York: Harper and Row.

Brown, Margaux H., Denise Lenares-Solomon, and Richard G. Deaner. 2019. "Every Student Succeeds Act: A Call to Action for School Counselors." *Journal of Counselor Leadership and Advocacy* 6, no. 1: 86–96. https://doi.org/10.1080/2326716X.2018.1557574.

Cooper, Harris, Barbara Nye, Kelly Charlton, James Lindsay, and Scott Greathouse. 1996. "The Effects of Summer Vacation on Achievement Test Scores: A Narrative and Meta-Analytic Review." *Review of Educational Research* 66, no. 3 (Fall): 227–68. https://doi .org/10.3102%2F00346543066003227.

Dale, Maryclaire. 2020. "Philadelphia Schools, Citing Inequity, Won't Teach Online." *US News and World Report*. March 18. https://apnews.com/article/00bc1279d8f94a37c071 39ebdfa78fef.

Decker, Stacey, Holly Peele, and Maya Riser-Kositsky. 2020. "The Coronavirus Spring: The Historic Closing of US Schools (a Timeline)." *Education Week*. February 1. https://www.edweek.org/leadership/the-coronavirus-spring-the-historic-closing-of-u-s -schools-a-timeline/2020/07.

Dorn, Emma, Bryan Hancock, Jimmy Sarakatsannis, and Ellen Viruleg. 2020. "COVID-19 and Student Learning in the United States: The Hurt Could Last a Lifetime." McKinsey and Company. https://www.mckinsey.com/industries/public-and-social-sector /our-insights/covid-19-and-student-learning-in-the-united-states-the-hurt-could-last-a -lifetime.

Dover, Alison G., Nick Henning, and Ruchi Agarwal-Rangnath. 2016. "Reclaiming Agency: Justice-Oriented Social Studies Teachers Respond to Changing Curricular Standards." *Teaching and Teacher Education* 59 (October): 457–67. https://doi.org/10 .1016/j.tate.2016.07.016.

Ellison, Scott, Ashlee B. Anderson, Brittany Aronson, and Courtney Clausen. 2018. "From Objects to Subjects: Repositioning Teachers as Policy Actors Doing Policy Work." *Teaching and Teacher Education* 74 (August): 157–69. https://doi.org/10.1016/j .tate.2018.05.001.

Farber, Brianna. 2019. "Dismantling White Supremacy Starts Inside." *Anthropology News* 60, no. 3 (May/June): e166–e170. https://doi.org/10.1111/AN.1192.

Freedberg, Louis. 2020. "President Trump Accuses Schools of 'Extreme Indoctrination' of Children." EdSource. July 6. https://edsource.org/2020/president-trump-accuses -schools-of-extreme-indoctrination-of-children/635299.

Fullan, Michael. 2000. "The Three Stories of Education Reform." *Phi Delta Kappan* 81, no. 8 (April): 581–84.

Golinkoff, Roberta Michnick, Helen Shwe Hadani, and Kathy Hirsh-Pasek. 2020. "Avoiding the COVID-19 Slump: Making Up for Lost School Time." Brookings. April 30. https://www.brookings.edu/blog/education-plus-development/2020/04/30 /avoiding-the-covid-19-slump-making-up-for-lost-school-time/.

Heineke, Amy J., Ann Marie Ryan, and Charles Tocci. 2015. "Teaching, Learning, and Leading." *Journal of Teacher Education* 66, no. 4: 382–94. https://doi.org/10 .1177%2F0022487115592031.

Hobbs, Tawnell D., and Lee Hawkins. 2020. "The Results Are In for Remote Learning: It Didn't Work." *Wall Street Journal*. June 5. https://www.wsj.com/articles/schools -coronavirus-remote-learning-lockdown-tech-11591375078.

Hussar, Bill, Jijun Zhang, Sarah Hein, Ke Wang, Ashley Roberts, Jiashan Cui, Mary Smith, Farrah Bullock Mann, Amy Barmer, and Rita Dilig. 2020. *The Condition of Education 2020*. Washington, DC: US Department of Education, NCES (National Center for Education Statistics). https://nces.ed.gov/pubs2020/2020144.pdf.

Imants, Jeroen, and Merel M. Van der Wal. 2019. "A Model of Teacher Agency in Professional Development and School Reform." *Journal of Curriculum Studies* 52, no. 1: 1–14. https://doi.org/10.1080/00220272.2019.1604809.

Jesso, Tanner. 2020. "Public Education System Isn't about Kids Anymore: Commentary." *Orlando Sentinel*. August 19. https://www.orlandosentinel.com/opinion/guest-commentary/os-op-education-isnt-about-kids-anymore-20200819-rn5bzhm6cnb3zjuicvma44tygi-story.html.

Kayyem, Juliette. 2020. "Trump Leaves States to Fend for Themselves." *Atlantic*. April 9. https://www.theatlantic.com/ideas/archive/2020/03/america-has-never-had-50-state-disaster-before/608155/.

Kendi, Ibram X. 2019. *How to Be an Antiracist*. New York: One World.

Khan, LeeAndra. 2016. "Our Schools Need Social Justice Warriors, Not Status-Quo Embracers." *Education Post*. October 24. https://educationpost.org/our-schools-need-social-justice-warriors-not-status-quo-embracers/.

Kirkland, David E. 2018. "Learning to Teach Reading across Racial Contexts: A Focus on Transforming Teacher Mindsets." *Michigan Reading Journal* 50, no. 2. https://scholarworks.gvsu.edu/mrj/vol50/iss2/10.

Kuhfeld, Megan, James Soland, Beth Tarasawa, Angela Johnson, Erik Ruzek, and Jing Liu. 2020. "Projecting the Potential Impacts of COVID-19 School Closures on Academic Achievement." EdWorkingPaper 20-226, Annenberg Institute for School Reform, Brown University, Providence, RI. https://doi.org/10.26300/cdrv-ywo5.

Love, Bettina L. 2019. *We Want to Do More Than Survive: Abolitionist Teaching and the Pursuit of Educational Freedom*. Boston: Beacon Press.

Mac Donald, Heather. 2018. *The Diversity Delusion: How Race and Gender Pandering Corrupt the University and Undermine Our Culture*. New York: St. Martin's Press.

McDonald, Joseph P. 1986. "Raising the Teacher's Voice and the Ironic Role of Theory." *Harvard Educational Review* 56, no. 4 (Winter): 355–79.

Nielsen, Carolyn. 2020. *Reporting on Race in a Digital Era*. Switzerland: Springer.

Pandey, Erica. 2020. "The Silver Linings of Online School." *Axios*. August 8. https://www.axios.com/online-school-what-works-85668c44-c31b-4b06-b1e6-4a55cb7d4730.html.

Payne, Charles M. 2008. *So Much Reform, So Little Change: The Persistence of Failure in Urban Schools*. Cambridge, MA: Harvard Education Press.

Phillips, Erica Roberson. 2019. "Yes, 'All Students Can Be Taught How to Be Smart': How Anti-Bias Teacher Preparation Paired with Scaffolding of Rigorous Curriculum Can Eradicate the Achievement Gap." Capstone project, Duke University. https://hdl.handle.net/10161/18951.

Priestley, Mark, Richard Edwards, Andrea Priestley, and Kate Miller. 2012. "Teacher Agency in Curriculum Making: Agents of Change and Spaces for Manoeuvre." *Curriculum Inquiry* 42, no. 2: 191–214. https://doi.org/10.1111/j.1467-873X.2012.00588.x.

Reimers, Fernando. 2020. *Educating Students to Improve the World*. Singapore: Springer Open.

Robinson, Sarah. 2012. "Constructing Teacher Agency in Response to the Constraints of Education Policy: Adoption and Adaptation." *Curriculum Journal* 23, no. 2 (June): 231–45. https://doi.org/10.1080/09585176.2012.678702.

Rothstein, Richard. 2020. "The Coronavirus Will Explode Achievement Gaps in Education." *Working Economics Blog* (Economic Policy Institute). April 14. https://www.epi.org/blog/the-coronavirus-will-explode-achievement-gaps-in-education/.

Seale, Colin. 2020. "Parent Involvement Has Always Mattered. Will The COVID-19 Pandemic Finally Make This the New Normal In K-12 Education?" *Forbes*. May 19. https://www.forbes.com/sites/colinseale/2020/05/19/parent-involvement-has-always-mattered-will-the-covid-19-pandemic-finally-make-this-the-new-normal-in-k-12-education/?sh=c2d22c05e465.

Slapik, Magdalena. 2017. "What Students Think Public Education Is For." *Atlantic*. October 1. https://www.theatlantic.com/education/archive/2017/10/the-purpose-of-education-according-to-students/541602/.

Strauss, Valerie. 2015. "What's the Purpose of Education in the 21st Century?" *Washington Post*. February 12. https://www.washingtonpost.com/news/answer-sheet/wp/2015/02/12/whats-the-purpose-of-education-in-the-21st-century/.

Strauss, Valerie. 2020. "How Relationships between Teachers and Students Are Being Tested in COVID-19 Crisis." *Washington Post*. April 22. https://www.washingtonpost.com/education/2020/04/22/how-relationships-between-teachers-students-are-being-tested-covid-19-crisis/.

Walker, Tim. 2016. "What's the Purpose of Education? Public Doesn't Agree on the Answer." *NEAToday*. August 29. https://www.nea.org/advocating-for-change/new-from-nea/whats-purpose-education-public-doesnt-agree-answer.

EUGENE T. RICHARDSON

From legacies of enslavement to legal segregation; white terrorism; hyperincarceration; lethal policing; and ongoing discrimination in housing, employment, education, credit markets, and healthcare, this collection of essays has traced the major structural determinants of disproportionate COVID-19 incidence and mortality among people of color in the United States. It has also highlighted a number of reparative and redistributive policies to ameliorate such disparities in future pandemics.

Many of these calls for social justice are not novel. As such, how is it that our ability to imagine social alternatives to the racist status quo in this country has been so stunted over centuries of struggle? In a word: ideology.

Ideology can be thought of as "the distortion of knowledge to conform with an inequitable social structure" (Hamilton 1974). Since time immemorial—from the caste system in India to the evolution of racial capitalism across the Atlantic (Yengde 2019; Robinson 2000)—groups of people have been effectively dominated by the control, through knowledge production, of how they perceive themselves and their relationship to the world (wa Thiong'o 1986).

If we understand the enslavement of black people as foundational to American capitalism, the country's subsequent development can be depicted as an extension of this oppressive social order (Lemman 2020; Johnson 2020)—and as Charles Mills teaches, "If exploitative socioeconomic relations are indeed foundational to the social order, then this is likely to have a fundamental shaping effect on social ideation" (Mills 2017).

White supremacy has been the effective ideology of the United States since prior to its founding (Fields 1990), and it has dominated dialectically the ideation of politicians, jurists, religious leaders, philosophers, academics, artists, and other intellectuals whose work involves interpreting social phenomena (Rehmann 2014). Economists have been key in this epistemic effort; as Rubinstein explains, "Economics [is] an academic field that tends toward conservatism and helps the strong in society maintain their dominance. . . . Economic models generally ignore the aspiration of individuals to gain power and control over other people . . . [and] economic questions that ought to be decided democratically via the political system are treated there as if they were professional matters and are deferred to experts to decide. . . . [This] is a ploy that serves the stronger members of society (including, just by chance, the community of experts)" (Rubinstein 2012).

The $10–12 trillion racial wealth gap in the United States is in no small part a result of the efforts of economists (Darity and Mullen 2020). When analyzed globally, the $152 trillion net appropriation by high-income countries from the Global South can also be tied to the work of this cadre of so-called experts, who are essentially the organic intellectuals—or status-quo propagandists—of racial capitalism (Gramsci 1971; Richardson 2020; Hickel, Sullivan, and Zoomkawala 2021; Marglin 2008; Amin 1973; Rodney 1972; Wilson Gilmore 2003).

With respect to COVID-19 and other diseases that disproportionately affect the marginalized, epidemiologists have taken on these reins by translating pandemic data into thought forms that actively delimit—through their exaggerated precision and acceptance of government interventions as status quo—the public's ability to imagine social alternatives (Graeber 2007). As we move from the superstructure of social science to the base of racial capitalism, we begin to see how the former colludes in the material deprivation and physical oppression of people of color.

Take, for example, the COVID-19 forecasts developed by the Institute for Health Metrics and Evaluation (IHME) at the University of Washington.[1] The models it developed in the spring of 2020 varied wildly over a matter of weeks, and the true number of next-day deaths from COVID-19 in the United States fell outside their prediction intervals as much as 70 percent of the time (Jewell, Lewnard, and Jewell 2020; Marchant et al. 2020). In addition, their plunging estimates were used to endorse the Trump administration's COVID-19 response as competent and effective (Richardson 2020).

But of greater consequence, they made no recommendations about risk structure—that is, the way people are enabled or constrained in their associations with others (Richardson et al. 2021). As such, they could also be deemed racist (Kendi 2017), since their analyses endorse a future where COVID-19 disparities continue to exist, institutionalized racism is rampant, hyperincarceration is ongoing, and universal health coverage is denied. In other words, their supposedly value-free epidemiology espouses valuations peculiar to racial capitalism (Marcuse 2009), preventing the measures and interventions outlined in this volume from being considered in the social imaginary. Indeed, such work filters out information vital to demonstrating the ways white supremacy generates health inequities in the United States.

The IHME aims to improve the health of the world's populations by providing the best information on population health, which is somewhat like saying they could have improved the health of people enslaved in the United States in the seventeenth to nineteenth centuries by counting and reporting how many died from strokes, heart attacks, and malnutrition. There is, in short, no analysis of power (Richardson 2020; Honneth 1991; Farmer 2005; Fanon 1967).

For the most part, public-health data and forecasting are curated in a manner that occults "administered dehumanization and dispossession" (Kabel and Phillipson 2020), thus furthering status-quo relations of inequality (Richardson 2021). The hegemonic status achieved by such knowledge production disciplines us. It shields structural determinants from political contestation (Fraser 1989) and helps ensure—under a pragmatist notion of truth (Rorty 1999; Denzin 1996)—that we do not come to compromise on reparative action when presented with the evidence of disparities by race. In doing so, it coproduces white supremacy (Jasanoff 2004).

The ideological work done by such forecasting is strengthened by its designation as "outbreak science" (Rivers et al. 2019). This coding imparts epistemological currency to a variety of racist discourses so as to invest them with authority and legitimacy (Foucault 1979).

To interpret COVID-19 in an antiracist, relational fashion (Pohlhaus 2012; Emirbayer 1997; Kivinen and Piiroinen 2006; Kendi 2019; Krieger 1999), we could view it not as a *thing*—that is, not a physiological response to viral RNA—but rather as a hub of social distrust, othering, predatory accumulation, and flaunting of evidence (Marx 1976). That a country like Taiwan, with 23.6 million people, can count deaths from COVID-19 in the hundreds—instead of hundreds of thousands as in the United States, Russia, Brazil, and India[2]—demonstrates that the devastating lethality found in these comparatively inegalitarian nations is not a biological inevitability, but rather a socially constructed, reticulate health phenomenon (Berger and Luckmann 1967; Geertz 1973; Mayer 1996; Turshen 1977; Packard 1989; Laster Pirtle 2020).

Consequently, in order to dismantle the inherited ideologies of white supremacy that undergird health disparities in the United States, we must foment a changing of minds—a metapolitics—to enable real cultural reconstruction. The #BlackLivesMatter global movement is showing the way—how struggle in the streets, in the media, in academia, and interpersonally can lead to transformations in how we "capture, orient, determine, intercept, model, control, or secure the gestures, behaviors, opinions, or discourses of [human] beings"

(Agamben 2009). But to reach the ultimate fulfilment of these transformations, we must enact, globally, sweeping material and symbolic reparations programs (Darity Jr. and Mullen 2020; Beckles 2013; Richardson 2020).

NOTES

1. The IHME has been called "the world's premier center for health metrics—the science of measuring and analyzing global health problems" (Butler 2017). It has received more than $600 million from the Gates Foundation alone, which raises the question whether "Gates's billions [are] distorting public health data" (Schwab 2020).

2. As of 2021 (COVID-19 Dashboard by the Center for Systems Science and Engineering at Johns Hopkins University).

REFERENCES

Agamben, Giorgio. 2009. *What Is an Apparatus? And Other Essays*. Translated by David Kishik and Stefan Pedatella. Palo Alto, CA: Stanford University Press.

Amin, Samir. 1973. *Neo-colonialism in West Africa*. Edited by Francis McDonagh. New York: Monthly Review Press.

Beckles, Hilary McD. 2013. *Britain's Black Debt: Reparations for Caribbean Slavery and Native Genocide*. Kingston: University of the West Indies Press.

Berger, Peter L., and Thomas Luckmann. 1967. *The Social Construction of Reality: A Treatise in the Sociology of Knowledge*. New York: Anchor.

Butler, Declan. 2017. "World's Foremost Institute on Death and Disease Metrics Gets Massive Cash Boost." *Nature*. February 2. https://www.nature.com/articles/nature.2017.21373.

Darity, William A., Jr., and A. Kirsten Mullen. 2020. *From Here to Equality: Reparations for Black Americans in the Twenty-First Century*. Chapel Hill: University of North Carolina Press.

Denzin, Norman K. 1996. "Post-pragmatism." *Symbolic Interaction* 19, no. 1 (Spring): 61–75.

Emirbayer, Mustafa. 1997. "Manifesto for a Relational Sociology." *American Journal of Sociology* 103(2): 281–317.

Fanon, Frantz. 1967. *Black Skin, White Masks*. Translated by Charles Lam Markmann. Boston: Grove Press.

Farmer, Paul E. 2005. *Pathologies of Power: Health, Human Rights, and the New War on the Poor*. 2nd ed. Berkeley: University of California Press.

Fields, Barbara Jeanne. 1990. "Slavery, Race and Ideology in the United States of America." *New Left Review* 1, no. 181 (May/June): 95–118.

Foucault, Michel. 1979. *Discipline and Punish: The Birth of the Prison*. Translated by Alan Sheridan. New York: Knopf Doubleday.

Fraser, Nancy. 1989. *Unruly Practices: Power, Discorse, and Gender in Contemporary Social Theory*. Minneapolis: University of Minnesota Press.

Geertz, Clifford. 1973. *The Interpretation of Cultures*. New York: Basic Books.

Graeber, David. 2007. "The Twilight of Vanguardism." In *Possibilities: Essays on Hierarchy, Rebellion, and Desire*, 301–11. Oakland, CA: AK Press.

Gramsci, Antonio. 1971. *Selections from the Prison Notebooks*. Edited and translated by Quintin Hoare and Geoffrey Nowell-Smith. London: Lawrence and Wishart.

Hamilton, Peter. 1974. *Knowledge and Social Structure*. London: Routledge.

Hickel, Jason, Dylan Sullivan, and Huzaifa Zoomkawala. 2021. "Plunder in the Postcolonial Era: Quantifying Drain from the Global South through Unequal Exchange, 1960–2018." *New Political Economy*. March, 1–18. https://doi.org/10.1080/13563467.2021.1899153.

Honneth, Axel. 1991. *The Critique of Power: Reflective Stages in a Critical Social Theory*. Translated by Kenneth Baynes. Cambridge, MA: MIT Press.

Jasanoff, Sheila, ed. 2004. *States of Knowledge: The Co-production of Science and the Social Order*. London: Routledge.

Jewell, Nicholas P., Joseph A. Lewnard, and Britta L. Jewell. 2020. "Caution Warranted: Using the Institute for Health Metrics and Evaluation Model for Predicting the Course of the COVID-19 Pandemic." *Annals of Internal Medicine* 173, no. 3 (August): 226–27. https://doi.org/10.7326/M20-1565.

Johnson, Walter. 2020. *The Broken Heart of America: St. Louis and the Violent History of the United States*. New York: Basic Books

Kabel, Ahmed, and Robert Phillipson. 2020. "Structural Violence and Hope in Catastrophic Times: From Camus' *The Plague* to COVID-19." *Race and Class* 62, no. 4: 3–18. https://doi.org/10.1177/0306396820974180.

Kendi, Ibram X. 2017. *Stamped from the Beginning: The Definitive History of Racist Ideas in America*. New York: Bold Type Books.

Kendi, Ibram X. 2019. *How to Be an Antiracist*. New York: One World.

Kivinen, Osmo, and Tero Piiroinen. 2006. "Toward Pragmatist Methodological Relationalism." *Philosophy of the Social Sciences* 36, no. 3 (September): 303–29.

Krieger, Nancy. 1999. "Questioning Epidemiology: Objectivity, Advocacy, and Socially Responsible Science." *American Journal of Public Health* 89, no. 8 (August): 1151–53.

Laster Pirtle, Whitney N. 2020. "Racial Capitalism: A Fundamental Cause of Novel Coronavirus (COVID-19) Pandemic Inequities in the United States." *Health Education and Behavior* 47, no. 4: 504–8. https://doi.org/10.1177/1090198120922942.

Lemman, Nicholas. 2020. "Is Capitalism Racist?" *New Yorker*. May 25. https://www.newyorker.com/magazine/2020/05/25/is-capitalism-racist.

Marchant, Roman, Noelle I. Samia, Ori Rosen, Martin A. Tanner, and Sally Cripps. 2020. "Learning as We Go: An Examination of the Statistical Accuracy of COVID-19 Daily Death Count Predictions." https://arxiv.org/abs/2004.04734.

Marcuse, Herbert. 2009. *Negations: Essays in Critical Theory*. London: MayFly.

Marglin, Stephen A. 2008. *The Dismal Science: How Thinking Like an Economist Undermines Community*. Cambridge, MA: Harvard University Press.

Marx, Karl. 1976. *Capital: A Critique of Political Economy, Vol. 1*. Translated by Ben Fowkes. London: Penguin Books.

Mayer, J. D. 1996. "The Political Ecology of Disease as One New Focus for Medical Geography." *Progress in Human Geography* 20, no. 4: 441–56.

Mills, Charles W. 2017. *Black Rights/White Wrongs: The Critique of Racial Liberalism.* Oxford: Oxford University Press.

Packard, Randall M. 1989. *White Plague, Black Labor: Tuberculosis and the Political Economy of Health and Disease in South Africa.* Berkeley: University of California Press.

Pohlhaus, Gaile, Jr. 2012. "Relational Knowing and Epistemic Injustice: Toward a Theory of Willful Hermeneutical Ignorance." *Hypatia* 27, no. 4 (Fall): 715–35.

Rehmann, Jan. 2014. *Theories of Ideology: The Powers of Alienation and Subjection.* Chicago: Haymarket Books.

Richardson, Eugene T. 2020. *Epidemic Illusions: On the Coloniality of Global Public Health.* Cambridge, MA: MIT Press.

Richardson, Eugene T. 2021. "The Instruments of Public Health." *Wilson Quarterly.* https://www.wilsonquarterly.com/quarterly/public-health-in-a-time-of-pandemic/the-instruments-of-public-health/.

Richardson, Eugene T., Momin M. Malik, William A. Darity Jr., A. Kirsten Mullen, Michelle E. Morse, Maya Malik, Aletha Maybank, et al. 2021. "Reparations for Black American Descendants of Persons Enslaved in the US and Their Potential Impact on SARS-CoV-2 Transmission." *Social Science and Medicine* 276 (May): 113741. https://doi.org/https://doi.org/10.1016/j.socscimed.2021.113741.

Rivers, Caitlin, Jean-Paul Chretien, Steven Riley, Julie A Pavlin, Alexandra Woodward, David Brett-Major, Irina Maljkovic Berry, et al. 2019. "Using 'Outbreak Science' to Strengthen the Use of Models during Epidemics." *Nature Communications* 10, article no. 3102. https://doi.org/10.1038/s41467-019-11067-2.

Robinson, Cedric J. 2000. *Black Marxism: The Making of the Black Radical Tradition.* Chapel Hill: UNC Press.

Rodney, Walter. 1972. *How Europe Underdeveloped Africa.* London: Bogle-L'Ouverture.

Rorty, Richard. 1999. *Philosophy and Social Hope.* London: Penguin Books.

Rubinstein, Ariel. 2012. *Economic Fables.* Cambridge: Open Book.

Schwab, Tim. 2020. "Are Bill Gates's Billions Distorting Public Health Data?" *Nation,* December 3. https://www.thenation.com/article/society/gates-covid-data-ihme/.

Turshen, Meredith. 1977. "The Political Ecology of Disease." *Review of Radical Political Economics* 9, no. 1: 45–60.

wa Thiong'o, Ngugi. 1986. *Decolonising the Mind: The Politics of Language in African Literature.* London: James Curry.

Wilson Gilmore, Ruth. 2003. "Abolition Geography and the Problem of Innocence." In *Futures of Black Radicalism,* edited by Gaye Theresa Johnson and Alex Lubin. London: Verso.

Yengde, Suraj. 2019. *Caste Matters.* Gurugram: India Viking.

FENABA R. ADDO is an associate professor of public policy at the University of North Carolina at Chapel Hill. Her research program examines the causes and consequences of debt and wealth inequality with a focus on higher education, family, and relationships. Dr. Addo has a PhD in policy analysis and management from Cornell University.

STEVEN J. AMENDUM is a professor in the School of Education in the College of Education and Human Development at the University of Delaware. He studies early reading development, literacy development and instruction for multilingual learners, and evidence-based classroom literacy instruction. He also supports schools and classroom practitioners by providing effective professional learning. He has a PhD in literacy education from the University of North Carolina at Chapel Hill and an MEd in reading education from the University of North Carolina at Charlotte.

LESLIE BABINSKI is an associate research professor and director of the Center for Child and Family Policy in the Sanford School of Public Policy at Duke University. Her areas of expertise are in teacher consultation and collaboration, teacher professional development, and school-based interventions for children and adolescents. Dr. Babinski has an MA and PhD in educational and school psychology from the University of California, Berkeley.

SANDRA L. BARNES is the CV Starr Professor of Sociology and department chairperson at Brown University. She was previously a joint-appointed professor of sociology in the Department of Human and Organizational Development in the Peabody College of Education and Human Development and the Divinity School at Vanderbilt University. Her work focuses on the role of religion and congregations as change agents in society. Her most recent book is *Kings of Mississippi: Race, Religious Education, and the Making of a Middle-Class Black Family in the Segregated South* (2019). Dr. Barnes earned master's degrees from the Georgia Institute of Technology and the Interdenominational Theological Center and a PhD degree in sociology from Georgia State University.

MARY T. BASSETT is health commissioner of the New York State Department of Health. She was previously director of the François-Xavier Bagnoud (FXB) Center for Health and Human Rights and FXB Professor of the Practice of Health and Human Rights in the Department of Social and Behavioral Science at the Harvard T. H. Chan School of Public Health. In her career spent promoting health equity and social justice throughout academia, government, and not-for-profit work, Dr. Bassett has earned numerous awards and accolades, including the Frank A. Calderone Prize in Public Health, a Kenneth A. Forde Lifetime Achievement Award from Columbia University, a Victoria J. Mastrobuono Award for Women's Health, and the National Organization for Women's Champion of Public Health Award. She received her MPH from the University of Washington and her MD from Columbia University's College of Physicians and Surgeons (serving her residency at Harlem Hospital).

KEISHA L. BENTLEY-EDWARDS is an associate professor at Duke University's School of Medicine, General Internal Medicine Division, and the associate director of research and director of the Health Equity Working Group for the Samuel DuBois Cook Center on Social Equity. She is a developmental psychologist who uses a cultural lens to understand the human experience and health outcomes. Her research focuses on how racism, gender, and culture influence social, physical, and emotional health as well as academic outcomes. Dr. Bentley-Edwards has an MA in developmental psychology from the Teachers College at Columbia University and a PhD in interdisciplinary studies in human development from the University of Pennsylvania.

KISHA N. DANIELS is an assistant professor of the practice of education at Duke University. Her lengthy career in the teaching and schooling world has led her to research on teacher quality, collaborative teaching, and community engagement. Her most recent book is *Creating Caring and Supportive Educational Environments for Meaningful Learning* (2018). Dr. Daniels has a doctorate in education leadership, curriculum, and instruction from the University of North Carolina at Chapel Hill.

WILLIAM A. DARITY JR. is the Samuel DuBois Cook Professor of Public Policy, African and African American Studies, and Economics at Duke University and the founding director of the Samuel DuBois Cook Center on Social Equity at Duke University. Darity's research focuses on inequality by race, class, and ethnicity; stratification economics; and schooling and the racial achievement gap. His most recent book is *From Here to Equality: Reparations for Black Americans in the Twenty-First Century* (2020). Dr. Darity holds a PhD in economics from MIT.

MELANIA DIPIETRO is a public elementary school teacher in the southeastern United States. She currently works as an ESL teaching assistant, primarily with students in the middle grades. Previously, DiPietro worked in Mexico as a teacher's assistant in a private Catholic school.

JANE DOKKO is the vice president of the Federal Reserve Bank of Chicago's community development and policy studies division. In this role, she leads research and community engagement to create opportunities and improve economic outcomes for low- and moderate-income people and places. During the Obama Administration, Dokko was the deputy assistant secretary for financial economics at the US Treasury Department and a senior economist at the White House Council of Economic Advisers. Dokko has a master's and PhD in economics from the University of Michigan.

FIONA GREIG is a managing director and the copresident at the JPMorgan Chase Institute and holds adjunct professor appointments at the University of Pennsylvania and Georgetown University. She has published research on topics including household finance, healthcare, labor markets and the online platform economy, gender, and behavioral decision making. Her work has been widely cited in the media, including the *New York Times*, the *Wall Street Journal*, NPR, and CNBC. She has a PhD in public policy from Harvard University.

ADAM HOLLOWELL is a senior research associate at the Samuel DuBois Cook Center on Social Equity and the director of the inequality studies minor at Duke University. He is also the faculty director of the Benjamin N. Duke Scholarship Program. He completed his PhD and MTh in theological ethics at the University of Edinburgh, Scotland.

LUCAS HUBBARD is an associate in research at the Samuel DuBois Cook Center on Social Equity, where he writes articles and press releases to help illuminate and broadcast the Cook Center's research. He also edits reports produced by the Center. His writing has appeared in INDY *Week*, *Duke Magazine*, *Paste*, and *Deadspin*.

DAMON JONES is an associate professor at the University of Chicago Harris School of Public Policy. He conducts research at the intersection of public finance and household finance. His current research topics include inequality, household financial vulnerability, income-tax policy, social security, retirement savings, worker benefits, and labor markets. Dr. Jones has a PhD in economics from the University of California, Berkeley.

STEVEN KNOTEK's research interest focuses on the use of a human-centered design approach to codesign innovations with community stakeholders (i.e., parents and teachers) to promote children's and youths' academic and social-emotional development and thriving. He is also the coordinator of the School Psychology Program at the University of North Carolina at Chapel Hill and is developing an implementation coaching model to bridge the science-to-service gap and allow innovation adopters (e.g., teachers, coaches) to thoughtfully adapt evidence-based programs to be culturally responsive. He has an MA in counseling from the University of San Francisco and a PhD in educational psychology and human development from the University of California, Berkeley.

ARVIND KRISHNAMURTHY is a PhD candidate in political science at Duke University studying the political behavior and race and ethnic politics subfields. He works with the Duke Center for Science and Justice and is a coauthor of *Deadly Justice: A Statistical Portrait of the Death Penalty* (2017). His research also appears in the *Duke Journal of Constitutional Law and Public Policy* and the *Wake Forest Law Review*.

HENRY CLAY MCKOY JR. is the lead entrepreneurship faculty and director of entrepreneurship in the School of Business at North Carolina Central University, as well as professor of practice in strategy and entrepreneurship in the Kenan-Flagler School of Business at the University of North Carolina at Chapel Hill. He is a national speaker and thought leader in the areas of community and economic development, social innovation and entrepreneurship, energy finance and the green economy, sustainability, and sustainable business development. Dr. McKoy has a PhD from the City and Regional Planning Program at the University of North Carolina at Chapel Hill.

N. JOYCE PAYNE is the founder of the Thurgood Marshall College Fund and a long-standing authority on women's issues in relation to higher education and labor force participation. Dr. Payne has published and presented a number of papers on the pursuit of equality for women and African Americans in higher education. She has been inducted into both the District of Columbia's Hall of Fame and the National Black College Alumni Hall of Fame. Dr. Payne earned her master's and doctorate degrees in education from the former Atlanta University.

ERICA R. PHILLIPS is an educational equity and policy specialist at the Samuel DuBois Cook Center on Social Equity. She serves on the Educational Policy working group, focusing on K-12 students, and is a research associate for a federal grant studying the benefits and inequities of gifted programming. She has an MA in educational equity, policy, and reform from Duke University.

EUGENE T. RICHARDSON, MD, PhD, is a physician-anthropologist in the Department of Global Health and Social Medicine at Harvard Medical School, where his overall focus is on biosocial approaches to Ebola and COVID-19 prevention, containment, and treatment in sub-Saharan Africa. He is the author of *Epidemic Illusions: On the Coloniality of Global Public Health* and cochair of the Lancet Commission on Reparations and Redistributive Justice. Dr. Richardson has an MD from Cornell University Medical College and a PhD from Stanford University.

PAUL A. ROBBINS is an assistant professor in the Department of Human Development and Family Studies at Purdue University. He primarily conducts research about the role of families and communities in fostering optimal development and combating academic and health disparities. Dr. Robbins has a PhD in educational psychology from the University of Texas at Austin.

JUNG SAKONG was an economist in the community development and policy studies division of the economic research department at the Federal Reserve Bank of Chicago. His research focuses on household finance and wealth inequality. He has a PhD in economics from the University of Chicago Booth School of Business.

MARTA SÁNCHEZ was an associate professor of social foundations at the University of North Carolina at Wilmington and an educational anthropologist conducting research with students, families, and teachers in the New Latino South. She authored the book *Fathering within and beyond the Failures of the State with Imagination, Work and Love* (2017). She earned a PhD from the School of Education, Culture, Curriculum, and Change at the University of North Carolina at Chapel Hill and an MEd in early childhood education from the Erikson Institute in Chicago.

MELISSA J. SCOTT is a former postdoctoral associate at the Samuel DuBois Cook Center on Social Equity, with interests in environmental health disparities, climate change health impacts, and health equity. She is currently researching the prevalence of heat-related illnesses and deaths in six redlined neighborhoods in Durham, North Carolina, compared to nonredlined neighborhoods to determine whether there are disparities in heat-related illnesses and deaths across races; she is also examining the relationship between religion/spirituality and risk factors for cardiovascular disease, such as depression, in the black community. Dr. Scott has an MA in bioethics from New York University and a PhD in environment and resources at the University of Wisconsin.

KRISTEN R. STEPHENS is the codirector of the Education Policy Working Group at the Samuel DuBois Cook Center on Social Equity and an associate professor of the practice in the program of education at Duke University. Her research explores legal and policy issues with regard to gifted education at the federal, state, and local levels and how teachers assess creative student products to inform future instruction. Dr. Stephens has a PhD from the University of Southern Mississippi.

JOE WILLIAM TROTTER JR. is the Giant Eagle University Professor of History and Social Justice at Carnegie Mellon University in Pittsburgh, Pennsylvania. He is also a member of the American Academy of Arts and Sciences, past chair of the History Department, director and founder of the Center for Africanamerican Urban Studies and the Economy (CAUSE), and president of the Urban History Association. A specialist on African American and US urban, labor, and working-class history, his most recent books include *Pittsburgh and the Urban League Movement: A Century of Social Service and Activism* (2020) and *Workers on Arrival: Black Labor in the Making of America* (2019). Dr. Trotter received his MA and PhD degrees from the University of Minnesota.

CHRIS WHEAT is a managing director and the copresident of the JPMorgan Chase Institute. He worked as an assistant professor at the MIT Sloan School of Management and at the Center for Urban Entrepreneurship and Economic Development at Rutgers Business School. He has a master's degree in sociology and a PhD in organizational behavior, both from Harvard University, as well as a master's degree in computer science from Stanford University.

GWENDOLYN L. WRIGHT is the senior administrator and research scientist for the Samuel DuBois Cook Center on Social Equity at Duke University. Wright's experience spans more than twenty years in organizational administration, research development, and higher education. Her research interests focus on intersectionality and African American women leaders in the academy. Dr. Wright has a doctorate in education from North Carolina State University.

Page numbers in italics indicate maps and figures; those with a *t* indicate tables.

National Partnership for Women and Families, 117

National Student Clearinghouse Research Center, 258

Native Americans. *See* American Indians

New Deal policies, 10, 57–58, 60, 178, 221

Nichols, Christopher, 52

No Child Left Behind Act (2001), 240–42

North Carolina A&T State University, 268

North Carolina Central University, 259

Nzinga, Sekile, 122n3, 269n6

Obama, Barack, 60

obesity, 10, 30, 34, 39

Ogilvie, George, 48

Omicron variant, 20n1, 39

online learning, 2, 15, 277–78; Americans with Disabilities Act and, 262; campus closures and, 259–61; digital divide and, 7, 163, 238, 260, 277–82; Latino children and, 2, 15, 236–37, 242–49; research on, 265

online worship services, 74–76

outbreak curve, 140, *141*

Patel, Vimal, 261, 264

Patton, Lirio, 240

Paul, Mark, 20, 120

Paycheck Plus, 214

Paycheck Protection Program, 6, 130–32, 131t, 138–39, 139t, 147, 158

Payne, Charles M., 276

Pell Grants, 115, 258, 263, 264

Perrin, Andrew, 281

Perry, Tyler, 155

philanthropic giving, 16, 257–58

place-based economic opportunities, 220–21

"poverteering," 151–52

poverty, 5, 10, 137–40, 138t, 170, 265; Du Bois on, 134; housing and, 159–60; wealth gap and, 11, 21n3, 111, 156, 186–96, *191–96*, 210–15, 212

Powers, Jeanne M., 240

PPP. *See* Paycheck Protection Program

preexisting conditions, 12, 234; among prisoners, 88, 89; social determinants of, 30–32; systemic racism and, 29–35

Price, Gregory N., 258, 269n10

prisons, 3, 13, 18, 60, 87–102; COVID infection rates in, 7, 87–88, 96–100, 97–99; jails versus, 89–90; juvenile justice system and, 215–16, 223; Marshall Project study of, 88, 92, 96–97; mortality rates in, 99; overcrowding of, 87, 89; Spanish flu in, 88

public-private partnerships, 166, 174

race, 4, 178; ideologies of, 16, 77, 283, 287, 295–98; social construction of, 3–4, 29

racial capitalism, 70, 101–2, 134–42, 176, 295–97

racism, xii–xiii, 9–10, 40, 69, 176–77, 176–78; Black Lives Matter movement against, 7, 18, 60, 286–87, 297–98; educational reforms versus, 283–91; healthcare and, 37–38; Hispanics and, 239; Jim Crow laws of, 55, 58, 145; preexisting conditions and, 29–35; tuberculosis and, 59; xenophobia and, 17. *See also* segregation

Rajan, Aastha, 204

Reconstruction era, 10, 54, 142

Reich, Steven A., 56

religion, 13, 59, 69–70, 256; civil, 77–78, 81; corporate worship and, 73–77; as pandemic mediator, 78–80

remote learning. *See* online learning

rents, 113, 122, 122n1. *See also* housing

reparations, 9, 20, 60, 298. *See also* slavery

rice plantations, 48–49

Richardson, Eugene T., 20

Risam, Roopika, 262

Robinson, Ken, 276

Rodríguez, Diana, 251

Romo, Adolfo "Babe," 240

Rothstein, Richard, 9

Rubinstein, Ariel, 295–96

Rutgers Center for Minority Serving Institutions, 266

Ryan, Rebecca, 214

Samuel DuBois Cook Center on Social Equity, xi–xii

SAT scores, 264

Savitt, Todd L., 51, 52, 53

Scott, Mackenzie, 156

CPSIA information can be obtained
at www.ICGtesting.com
Printed in the USA
LVHW081147271022
731543LV00013B/464